STROKE

STROKE

A HISTORY OF IDEAS

JAN VAN GIJN

Emeritus of Utrecht University

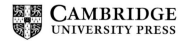

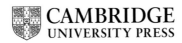

Shaftesbury Road, Cambridge CB2 8EA, United Kingdom

One Liberty Plaza, 20th Floor, New York, NY 10006, USA

477 Williamstown Road, Port Melbourne, VIC 3207, Australia

314–321, 3rd Floor, Plot 3, Splendor Forum, Jasola District Centre, New Delhi – 110025, India

103 Penang Road, #05–06/07, Visioncrest Commercial, Singapore 238467

Cambridge University Press is part of Cambridge University Press & Assessment, a department of the University of Cambridge.

We share the University's mission to contribute to society through the pursuit of education, learning and research at the highest international levels of excellence.

www.cambridge.org
Information on this title: www.cambridge.org/9781108832540

DOI: 10.1017/9781108961134

First published 2023

A catalogue record for this publication is available from the British Library.

Library of Congress Cataloging-in-Publication Data
NAMES: Van Gijn, Jan, 1942- author.
TITLE: Stroke : a history of ideas / Jan van Gijn.
DESCRIPTION: New York, NY : Cambridge University Press, 2023. | Includes bibliographical references and index.
IDENTIFIERS: LCCN 2023005765 (print) | LCCN 2023005766 (ebook) | ISBN 9781108832540 (hardback) | ISBN 9781108958646 (paperback) | ISBN 9781108961134 (epub)
SUBJECTS: LCSH: Cerebrovascular disease–History.
CLASSIFICATION: LCC RC388.5 .V34 2023 (print) | LCC RC388.5 (ebook) | DDC 616.8/ 1–dc23/eng/20230222
LC record available at https://lccn.loc.gov/2023005765
LC ebook record available at https://lccn.loc.gov/2023005766

ISBN 978-1-108-83254-0 Hardback

....

If they say beautiful Helen was abducted,
and Trojans crushed in war, take heed,
lest a very tale compels us to believe so,
when times gone by have irrevocably erased
the years of those whom the events affected.
                    Lucretius, de rerum natura 1, verses 464–8

One often unfolds the history of science as a highway leading straight from ignorance to the truth but this is wrong. It is a tangle of blind alleys where thoughts get lost and become stuck.
                    Patrick Deville (2012), p. 170

In Memory of My Teachers

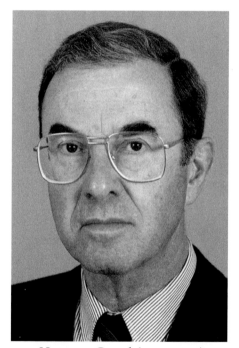

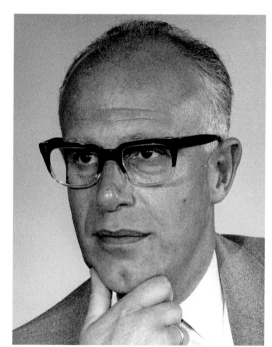

Hans van Crevel (1931–2002)   Arthur Staal (1926–2016)

CONTENTS

PREFACE

This book recounts how an ancient disease evolved into a group of diseases, sharing characteristic clinical features. At first, physicians called it 'apoplexy'; for the last half-century, the term 'stroke' has come into use.

The history of medicine can be approached from many directions, given that medicine is closely intertwined with multiple elements of society. As a result, medicine as an academic discipline is now a specialist topic for professional historians.[1] For all that, the development of medical knowledge over time remains a story deserving to be told. Doctors themselves are in the best position to tell it. Why, then, have physician–historians acquired such a poor reputation that an editor of *The Lancet* complains they produce only 'albums of colourful inventions'?[2]

Especially after my career as an academic neurologist, it began to dawn on me that two issues have often spoilt physicians' efforts, including my own, to describe the history of their discipline. The first pitfall is presentism, or reverse historiography: by looking back into the past from the present, one can only select recognizable landmarks, neglecting the circuitous routes through which these 'turning points' were reached. Such eclecticism creates a false illusion of orderly, if not triumphant, progression to the time of writing.[3] In the process, several theories, once popular, are completely neglected because, with hindsight, they proved to be blind alleys. The second problem is lack of originality. Because so many languages are represented in the medical record, there is dependence on secondary sources which mostly lean one upon another – a whispering game in which the original information risks being distorted or lost.

Restriction to primary sources, however, presents three challenges: locating them, being able to read in the original language, for medicine often Latin, and, finally, having copious amounts of time. The first condition was partly met by the collection of antiquarian medical books I could acquire over the years, thanks to my forbearing spouse. Other propitious factors were the

---

[1] Huisman (2005), Dialectics of understanding.
[2] Horton (2014), Moribund medical history.
[3] Butterfield (1950 [1931]), *The Whig Interpretation of History*.

vicinity of the Utrecht University Library and working in the digital age with ready access to the scientific heritage from the comfort of one's own desk. Retirement provided the opportunities to broaden my linguistic range and the leisure to make use of that education.

I started with ancient Greek medicine and its revival in the sixteenth century. The intervening period is not without some interest,[4] but I still lack the expertise for exploring it, especially the Arabic contributions. Whatever trail I followed from then on, it appeared again and again that no one event stands out as a moment of critical discovery. Diseases are not entities awaiting sudden revelation. Diseases are merely conventions on which most doctors agree, at least for some time; the nomenclature is constantly subject to revision, division, and oblivion.[5]

I hope this book is useful and of interest in the context of stroke. It cannot be definitive, if only because my story ends around 1975. There are at least three reasons for this caesura. First of all, new imaging techniques in the 1970s made it possible to visualize the brain and so to distinguish ischaemic from haemorrhagic brain lesions in life. This opened up – the second reason – an entirely new era: that of treatment for cerebrovascular disease, something that had been virtually non-existent before. The final reason is personal: my colleagues and I took part in some of the recent developments; it is for others to continue the story.

The book is rich in citations, allowing the past to speak for itself. Yet the choices are mine, as are the translations. I look forward to comments and emendations.

---

[4] Karenberg and Hort (1998a, b, c), Medieval descriptions and doctrines of stroke.
[5] Rosenberg (1992), *Framing Disease*, xiii.

ONE

THE VENTRICLES

Apoplexy in the Sixteenth Century

SUMMARY

Hippocratic and Galenic texts, fully rediscovered in the first half of the sixteenth century, defined apoplexy as a sudden collapse, with loss of movement and sensation, except for preserved heart action and respiration. Though this definition leaves room for divergent interpretations, early physicians who made the diagnosis rarely specified the symptoms.

Galen explained apoplexy as blockage of the cerebral ventricles by abnormal fluids, most often phlegm; animated spirits, an extremely subtle vapour, could then no longer reach the nerves. Post-mortem examination of human bodies was rare; the first inspections of the brain after apoplexy mentioned extravasated blood at its base or within the ventricles (Fernel, Duret). Varolio developed a method to remove the brain from the body and suggested that it was the substance of the brain, not its ventricles, that transported animated spirits. Two instances of hydrocephalic infants who had nevertheless shown signs of mental activity (Vesalius, Fabricius Hildanus) contributed to establishing the role of brain tissue. Physicians gradually came to use personal observation as a supplement to, or even a replacement of, written sources of knowledge.

The terms 'apoplexy' and 'stroke' have much in common, since both suggest a sudden collapse from a catastrophic illness. Yet there is a large difference. 'Apoplexy' refers to observable phenomena in patients – the manifestations of a brain disease, according to criteria developed in antiquity. By contrast, today the word 'stroke' evokes, as dictionaries testify, an anatomically defined cause: a disorder of the brain's blood vessels. This transition, from a set of clinical features to a morphological notion, is a metamorphosis many other diseases have gone through in the course of history. The difference between the two points of view, that is, what the doctor observes in the patient versus what the pathologist sees in the brain after death, explains not only why terms have changed, but also what is meant by them. As a consequence, some examples of 'apoplexy' would not be called 'stroke' today, and vice versa.

This chapter describes the earliest phase in these early developments, in the second half of the sixteenth century. During this period, the heritage of ancient Greek medicine was fully rediscovered, cleansed of Arab interpretations, and disseminated by the growing book culture.[1] Two themes dominate the chapter. The first is the definition of apoplexy as a clinical syndrome or as a set of coherent clinical features. The second theme is the theory of normal brain function and its disturbance in apoplexy. It will be necessary to switch from manifestations to explanations, and back, a few times.

APOPLEXY: AN AFFLICTION DEFINED BY ITS MANIFESTATIONS

Phenomena are recorded through observation – often, if not always, conditioned by interpretation. Readers, please discard all ideas you may have in relation to what is now called 'stroke', and open your mind to the observations and interpretations of physicians in a distant past who tried to make sense of an acute disease.

Ancient Descriptions

The cardinal feature of apoplexy, as the original term in ancient Greek implies, is that it strikes suddenly and renders the patient senseless and motionless. It is as if the victim is struck by lightning, hence the Latin synonym *morbus attonitus*, or 'stunned disease'. The disease is briefly mentioned in Babylonian texts,[2] and subsequently in Hippocratic writings. Yet the most influential author in antiquity on medical subjects was Galen (129–*c*.216) (Box 1.1). He was a prolific writer with an adventurous life.[3] Galen did not systematically deal with each disease in turn; therefore, the reader has to try and reconstruct Galenic notions from different, and sometimes contradictory, passages. Key features of the disease are found in different sentences, for example:

> When all nerves have simultaneously lost sensation and motion, the affection is called apoplexy. But when this happens on one side, the right

---

[1] Siraisi (1985), The Canon of Avicenna, 39–41; French (1985), Berengario, 66–71; Maclean (2002), *Medicine in the Renaissance*, 19–20; Wear (1995), Early modern Europe, 251–5.
[2] Reynolds and Kinnier Wilson (2004), Stroke in Babylonia.
[3] Mattern (2013), *The Prince of Medicine*; Nutton (2020), *Galen*.

Box 1.1 Claudius Galenus (129–c.216).

Galen was the son of an architect and local magistrate in the Greek community of Pergamum (now Bergama, Western coast of Turkey). He studied medicine from the age of 16, first in his home town, then in Smyrna (present-day Izmir) and Alexandria. In 157, he was back in Pergamum, as a physician for the gladiatorial school.

In 162, Galen set out to establish himself in Rome. The professional climate in the capital was highly competitive – apart from educated Greek physicians, also lay citizens or slaves offered their services to the sick. A physician's reputation depended heavily on their ability to predict the outcome of disease and also on anatomical demonstrations in live animals. Galen used pigs, goats, cattle, monkeys, cats, dogs, mice, snakes, fish, and birds. Among the spectators at such sessions was the ex-consul Flavius Boethus; he invoked Galen's help when his wife was ill and became Galen's patron when she recovered. In 166, Galen rather unexpectedly left Rome. Speculations about his motives include an epidemic of infectious disease, rivalry among colleagues, and fear of being conscripted.

He returned two years later to join the medical staff of the joint emperors Marcus Aurelius and Lucius Verus; the latter died soon afterwards. Under subsequent emperors, Galen kept this position, but he did not live in the imperial palace or join military expeditions. This arrangement allowed him to spend much of his time performing private consultations for the Roman elite – and also writing an amazing series of treatises on the structure and function of the body, illustrated with pertinent case histories. Even though, in 192, a fire destroyed his writings on pharmacology, Galen's extant collected works still take up 22 volumes in the nineteenth-century edition by Kühn.

---

or the left, it is called paralysis, of the part in which the disorder exists – sometimes the right, sometimes the left.[4]

Galen noted elsewhere that respiration was preserved in these patients, though it was laboured. He also found that the pulse of the arteries in the wrist and elsewhere continued to beat in patients with apoplexy:

> But when the respiration is affected to such an extent that [the patient] breathes as in deep sleep, then we speak of apoplexy.[5] [*And also:*] As long as the disease has not gained the upper hand, you will find [in the pulse] no change at all with regard to magnitude, force, speed, frequency and hardness.[6]

---

[4] Galenus (1625b [*c.*180]), *De Locis affectis* (C4) III, 20H; Kühn, ed. (1821–33), *Galeni Opera,* vol. VIII, 208.

[5] Galenus (1625b [*c.*180]), *De Locis affectis* (C4) IV, 22H; Kühn, ed. (1821–33), *Galeni Opera,* vol. VIII, 231.

[6] Galenus (1625a [*c.*180]), *De Causis Pulsuum* (C4) IV, 102G; Kühn, ed. (1821–33), *Galeni Opera,* vol. IX, 193.

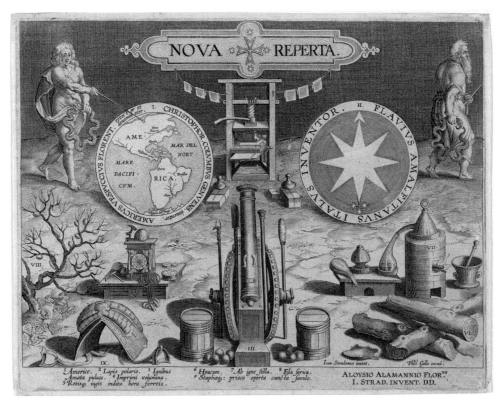

1.1 New discoveries (*Nova reperta*). A printing press is shown directly under the cartouche. On the left, a young woman with the mythical snake Ouroboros (biting its own tail) indicates the Americas. On the right side is a compass rose, with the name of its supposed inventor; an older man, again with Ouroboros, leaves the scene. In the foreground are inventions symbolizing the sixteenth century: the silkworm, a saddle and spurs, a mechanical clock, a cannon and gunpowder, medicinal bark, and an apparatus for distillation. Engraving attributed to Jan Collaert, after drawing by Jan van der Straet, c.1590. *Source:* Courtesy of Rijksmuseum, Amsterdam.

It is justified to say that, at least with regard to the definition of apoplexy, physicians in the middle of the sixteenth century started where Galen had left off more than 13 centuries ago. The term 'Renaissance' may have been coined rather recently, by nineteenth-century historians,[7] but literary humanists in the fourteenth century, such as Petrarch, already saw themselves as harbingers of a new era, after the 'dark ages'.[8] Two hundred years later, many still felt they were living in an age of discoveries (Figure 1.1). In the 'medical Renaissance' of the sixteenth century,[9] recovered and reconstituted Galenic texts came to replace medieval Latino-Arab glossaries on medicine, at a time when prices of

---

[7] Burckhardt (1860), *Die Kultur der Renaissance in Italien.*

[8] Mommsen (1942), Petrarch's conception of the Dark Ages.

[9] Wear, *et al.*, eds. (1985), *The Medical Renaissance of the Sixteenth Century.*

printed books allowed doctors to build their own library.[10] The young Jean Fernel (1497–1558), about to become an important physician, used similar terms when young: 'These disciplines and arts have clearly come to life again, after having been buried, or rather extinct and lifeless, for almost twelve hundred years.'[11] It is no surprise, therefore, to find an almost Galenic description of apoplexy in the first known treatise on diseases of the nervous system,[12] published in 1549 by Jason Pratensis (c.1486–1558; Latinized name for 'van der Velde'); he practised in Zierikzee, in the Southwest of the Low Countries:

> Apoplexy is a disease in which an affected person is deprived of motion and sensation; only breathing remains, though not intact, but abnormal in a variety of ways. Most often this illness arrives without fever, and the person suddenly tumbles down on the floor with a great fall. The collapsed person cannot be woken up by any speech, or by any shouting or poking. The numbness keeping the stricken patient down is so severe that no stimulus can overcome it. [...] And in the same way, the arteries originating from the heart are less impeded in this disorder, because they retain their pulsations, though these are much more subtle [...][13]

Thus, the standard definition of apoplexy, often repeated and essentially unchanged in the sixteenth and seventeenth centuries, and even later, consists of three main characteristics: (1) a sudden fall; (2) loss of movement and sensation; and (3) preservation of respiration and pulses, at least by and large. Still, there are some loopholes in this definition. A case report can help to clarify this – it is unique for several reasons: it dates from the middle of the sixteenth century and the patient is also the author.

A Self-Reported Case History

Conrad Wolffhart (1518–1561) (Figure 1.2) included an account of his own apoplexy – and his recovery – in a collection he edited of prodigious events spanning from pre-biblical times to the middle of the sixteenth century; his humanist name was Lycosthenes. Born in Rouffach (Alsace), Wolffhart studied philosophy in Heidelberg. In 1542, he moved to Basle where he became Deacon of the Church of St Leonard.[14] This is how he looked back on his disease episode:

> On 21 December of the year 1554, on leaving the building where I was already preparing the edition of my collection of 'Aphorisms' for the press, a horrible incapacity overwhelmed me. I suddenly collapsed on the floor and in a single moment I lost not only my voice, but also all sensation and movement on the right side, from head to heel (except sight and hearing).

[10] Jones (1995), Reading medicine, 155–6; Nutton (2005), Printing and medicine, 421–2.
[11] Fernelius (1548), De abditis Rerum Causis, 2.   [12] Pestronk (1988), The first neurology book.
[13] Pratensis (1549), De Cerebri Morbis, 121.   [14] Beyer (2012), Lycosthenes.

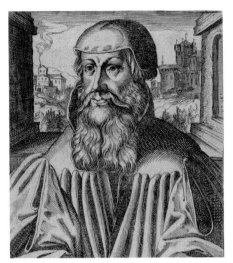

1.2 Conrad Lycosthenes (1518–1561). Etching by Simon Frisius, *c.*1610, 150 × 115 millimetres. *Source:* Courtesy of Rijksmuseum, Amsterdam.

I could not utter a single word, until 12 days later; I could not stand on my feet or move a finger for three entire months, during which period I was bed-bound. My [right] limbs seemed to be converted not into wood but into the hardest stone; the blood of the affected parts was so much frozen and hardened by the coldness of the humours and the obstruction of my nerves, that rubbing, compresses or any other measures entirely failed to warm them. At that time, owing to the humours that were disappearing from the head and the brain (it is astonishing to say), I lost all memories, to such an extent that the words of my Sunday sermon and all my knowledge of literature had vanished completely. [. . .]

My excellent friends were witnesses of my disaster. They could not understand me because I could only communicate by nodding, though I was sound of mind and reason. They held up a slate on which the letters were chalked in alphabetical order, so that I could point out the letters in their proper order with the index finger of my left hand; in this way the letters formed syllables and the syllables sounds, which they, after some mulling on my part, made me utter. But my affliction seemed to be a chronic and irreparable disease. As a result, not only I myself, but all who watched this cruel disease despaired about my life. But God in his mercy, on whose power all infirmity depends, overhearing my persistent prayers and those of his church on my behalf, restored me for the greater part, through the effort of Dr Guglielmo Gratarolo from Bergamo. Therefore, if you have possibly thought that in the part of life left to me some products of my pen have some merit for muses and profession, I would like to thank God Almighty in the first place, and thereafter Dr Gratorolo [. . .][15]

Ambiguity in the Interpretation of Clinical Symptoms

This unique case history also serves to show that the criteria for the diagnosis of apoplexy are somewhat imprecise, that is, open to different interpretations.

Consciousness. Medical treatises of the sixteenth century often distinguish between external senses (sight, hearing, touch, smell, and taste) and internal senses, viz. intellectual activities such as reasoning, imagination, and memory. So 'loss of one's senses' is practically synonymous with the modern term

[15] Lycosthenes (1557), *Prodigiorum ac Ostentorum Chronicon*, 640–1.

Box 1.2 Pieter van Foreest (1521–1597).

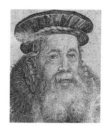

van Foreest was the third child of a wealthy couple in Alkmaar, a city north of Amsterdam. After secondary school, he studied liberal arts and medicine in Louvain (1536–1539), then made a tour of medical faculties in northern Italy. Having graduated in Bologna (1543), he also spent time in Venice, Ferrara, and Padua, made an eventful foot journey to Rome in the company of botanists (1545), and visited Paris and Orléans.

The next year, van Foreest settled in Alkmaar where he married Eva van Teylingen and established a solid reputation. Twelve years later, he accepted the post of city physician in Delft where the plague was raging. He remained in Delft for the next 37 years, a period of political turmoil, religious strife, and revolt of the United Provinces against Spanish rule. In 1574, during the siege of Leiden, he became the personal physician of William the Silent, prince of Orange and leader of the revolt.

In 1595, his wife Eva died, predeceased by their four children; van Foreest, now aged 74, decided to return to Alkmaar as a city physician. Meanwhile he had started to publish a series of books with case histories, followed by comments (*scholia*). These volumes continued to appear after his death, the last with medical subjects (no. 17) in 1606, followed by two more volumes with surgical cases. Reprints of his collected works continued to appear up to 1661.

Source: Portrait courtesy of Rijksmuseum, Amsterdam.

'unconsciousness'. But either term is based on the absence of reactions from the patient, such as speaking and moving the limbs or eyes. Since Lycosthenes, once recovered, could write about his fall and its circumstances, he must, at the time of the event, have been able to think and remember – or others must have recounted later what had happened. At any rate, the reason why a later medical compiler classified the disease as a case of apoplexy[16] must have been that the patient was unable to speak and could not signify he was sentient. Bystanders – and physicians – depend on verbal communication to find out whether someone can think and feel; at any rate, when a patient had collapsed and was speechless, with their eyes closed, it was assumed that all mental activity had been lost.

Language. If, however, a patient was mute but showed signs of awareness by other means, sixteenth-century physicians tended to diagnose 'paralysis of the tongue'. An example is found in the *Observationes et Curationes Medicinales* of Pieter van Foreest or Forestus (1521–97) (Box 1.2). This extensive work, often reprinted,[17] contains the following story in the section on apoplexy:

---

[16] Schenck von Grafenberg (1609), *Paratereseon*, 91.
[17] Breugelmans and Gnirrep (1997), Bibliografie.

> A high-born and noble young man, Mr van Cruningen, about 29 years old, was melancholical, more than fitting for his age and nature; this melancholy had increased when, long before, he had been kept in custody in Hoorn, together with Mr de Bossu. Early on the night of March 8, 1581, he suddenly sustained a fairly strong apoplexy, which quickly evolved into a paralysis of the entire right side, arm as well as leg, with impairment of the tongue, so that he could hardly speak; also, he could not properly understand.[18]

Although the report mentioned difficulty in understanding spoken language, the medical community apparently saw language as a purely motor phenomenon.

Paralysis. Van Foreest's report also shows that he designated right-sided hemiplegia after the patient had come round as 'paralysis', in keeping with the rule that apoplexy was diagnosed only if *all* movement was abolished. Yet it is difficult to be sure that a collapsed patient can move anything at all. Lycosthenes was unable to say this; had he been able to speak, his disease might have been classified as 'paralysis'. Perhaps he made no spontaneous movements with the left limbs because he was lying on this 'good' side, or because he was too frightened to stir at all. Of course, someone might have prodded or pinched him, in order to evoke some sort of response. But if this test was done on the affected side and gave no result, there was no good reason in those times to try the other side. Moreover, if a patient happened to be in deep coma, it would have made no difference. Another source of uncertainty is how violent the stimulus should be. Pratensis recommended the application of white-hot iron,[19] but probably he mentioned it only for the sake of didactic drama and never tried it himself.

Respiration. That breathing was preserved, though with some difficulty, while other movements were suspended, continued to puzzle physicians; a common explanation was that it represented 'a movement of nature, not of the will'. Van Foreest followed Galen in distinguishing four types of respiration in apoplectic patients, with different chances of survival.[20] Many authors mentioned frothy sputum around a patient's mouth as an ominous indication of outcome, a sign that goes back to the aphorisms of Hippocrates, though in the context of judicial hanging.[21] Hercules Saxonia (1551–607), appointed Professor of Practical Medicine in Padua in 1575, thought he could distinguish two kinds of sputum on the lips – if frothy and thick, with bubbles from exhalation, patients might recover; but no hope was left, he wrote, if it consisted of lung tissue liquefied by heat, with bubbles from enclosed spirit.[22]

---

[18] Forestus (1653 [1590]), *Observationes et Curationes*, vol. x, 526.
[19] Pratensis (1549), *De Cerebri Morbis*, 422.
[20] Forestus (1653 [1590]), *Observationes et Curationes*, vol. x, 510.
[21] Hippocrates (1959b [*c*.400 BCE]), Aphorisms, 119 (aphorism 43).
[22] Saxonia (1639), *Opera practica*, 39.

Differential Diagnosis. Physicians had to distinguish apoplexy from other conditions with sudden onset in which the senses were affected, for example epilepsy, paralysis, syncope, and 'suffocation by the uterus', a kind of swooning attributed to vapours rising up from the womb. Van Foreest stipulated that the distinction was difficult if the patient had already died by the time the doctor arrived. His example was the sudden death of a certain Hugo Grotius (not the famous lawyer of the same name); van Foreest ascertained that eyewitnesses had not observed any signs of breathing or of fluid emerging from the patient's mouth, so he concluded that the cause of death was not apoplexy, but syncope, a sudden cessation of heart action through loss of 'innate heat'.[23]

Apoplectic or Dead? A related problem was the distinction between severe apoplexy and death. For the detection of barely perceptible respiration, many authors described tests such as applying a piece of cotton wool or a mirror to the mouth and nose, or putting a mug full of water on the patient's chest.[24] Similarly, van Foreest warned that feeling the pulse could be misleading and even treacherous, as illustrated by horror stories of patients deemed dead and about to be buried until their miraculous recovery – hence the statutory delay of three days between apparent death by apoplexy and the burial.[25] This precautionary interval is a recurring theme in almost every text on the subject from widely different parts of Europe.

In conclusion, it was up to the physician which observations or tests were necessary in deciding whether the criteria for a diagnosis of apoplexy were met. Such details were almost never recorded, at least not until the middle of the seventeenth century – and even then, by only a minority of physicians. As a rule, the reader was supposed to accept the diagnosis on trust.

BRAIN FUNCTION: SPIRITS PERFECTED IN THE VENTRICLES

Despite the possible differences of interpretation, the written criteria for the diagnosis of apoplexy remained largely unchanged until at least the beginning of the nineteenth century. By contrast, ideas about the location of brain function began to shift at an earlier stage. The most influential ancient medical authority in the sixteenth century was Galen; he is our starting point. However, Galen's views on brain function are scattered across different texts.[26] To obtain a coherent account of how he was understood in the sixteenth century, it is best to consult a distinguished interpreter of that era.

---

[23] Forestus (1653 [1590]), *Observationes et Curationes*, vol. x, 513–14.
[24] Forestus (1653 [1590]), *Observationes et Curationes*, vol. x, 513.
[25] Forestus (1653 [1590]), *Observationes et Curationes*, vol. x, 529.
[26] Rocca (2003), *Galen on the Brain*.

Box 1.3 Jean Fernel (1497–1558).

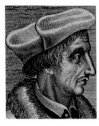 Fernel's father was a furrier and innkeeper in Montdidier (Somme); the family moved to Clermont (near Paris) when he was 12 years old. Jean's ambition to continue his education at the university was new in his family, but he got his way and became a Master of Arts at *Collège Ste Barbe* in 1519. At around that time, Fernel discovered that the spirit of the 'new times' had not yet reached the University of Paris and that his teachers had provided only medieval glossaries containing Latino-Arabic interpretations of the ancients. Besides, his Latin was 'barbaric'.

In the next five years, Fernel studied on his own – apart from Plato, Aristotle, and Cicero, he developed a keen interest in mathematics and astronomy. Having finally chosen medicine as his profession, Jean provided for his own upkeep by teaching, since his father had to support the younger children. In 1530, he graduated and obtained a licence to practise; in the meantime, he had published three folio volumes on mathematical and astronomical subjects.

After his marriage to Madeleine Tornebüe in 1531, Fernel had to give precedence to his tasks as a physician, but he continued teaching until 1550 when his medical practice had become too large. His medical lectures were probably private, because he was never officially appointed to the university, while the relations with his colleagues at the medical faculty were strained. In 1542, he was appointed physician to the Dauphin; when the latter became King Henri II in 1547, Fernel excused himself from the function of royal physician but accepted it 10 years later.

Source: Portrait courtesy of Wellcome Foundation.

Spirits and the Brain: Jean Fernel's Interpretation of Galen's Model

A didactic synthesis of Galen's ideas about brain function appeared in 1554, in a seminal book called *Medicina* by Jean Fernel (1497–1558) (Box 1.3). His erudition is the more remarkable since he was largely self-taught after his graduation in Paris;[27] unlike young physicians from well-to-do families, he could not finish his education with a tour of foreign universities.[28] The first part of Fernel's book is entitled *Physiologia*. This newly coined term means 'Laws of Nature'; the neologism caught on and eventually withstood the test of time, though its meaning evolved. Fernel's book was the first treatise of its kind after Galen's *On the Function of Body Parts* (*De Usu Partium*).

Fernel systematically represented the Galenic model of the different spirits, with minor adaptations;[29] it is schematically represented in Figure 1.3. The

---

[27] Sherrington (1946), *The Endeavour of Jean Fernel*, 1–17.

[28] Frank-van Westrienen (1983), *De groote Tour*; Cunningham (2009), *Peregrinatio medica*; de Ridder-Symoens (2009), The mobility of medical students.

[29] Fernelius (1554), *Medicina (Physiologia)*, 120–1.

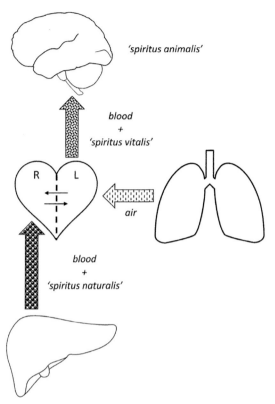

'spiritus animalis'

blood
+
'spiritus vitalis'

R   L

air

blood
+
'spiritus naturalis'

1.3 The synthesis of spirits, in three different phases. Schematic illustration of the Galenic model, according to Jean Fernel. The liver converts nutritional substances into blood and also produces a primitive form of spirit (*spiritus naturalis*). In the heart, a mixture with air and innate heat converts the spirits to a higher form (*spiritus vitalis*); the wall between the right and left ventricle is supposed to have tiny openings, not visible to the human eye. Finally, the brain produces the subtlest form of spirits (*spiritus animales*), which flow into the nerves and carry information about sensation and movement.

liver was thought to synthesize blood from digested food and also to add a vapour-like component, which Fernel and others preferred to call 'natural spirit', though Galen himself had been equivocal about its nomenclature.[30]

The second stage takes place in the heart. There, blood is thought to flow from the right to the left ventricle through small, invisible pores in the septum separating them. Famously, Andreas Vesalius (1514–1564) (Box 1.4), Professor of Anatomy and Surgery in Padua between 1537 and 1542,[31] had wondered about these invisible pores in the first edition of his seminal *Fabrica*;[32] in the second edition, 12 years later, he denied their existence.[33] At any rate, the 'invisible

[30] Rocca (2003), *Galen on the Brain*, 65–6.
[31] O'Malley (1965), *Andreas Vesalius of Brussels 1514–1564*.
[32] Vesalius (1543), *De humani Corporis Fabrica Libri septem*, 589.
[33] Vesalius (1555), *De humani Corporis Fabrica Libri septem*, 734, 746.

Box 1.4 Andreas Vesalius (1514–1564).

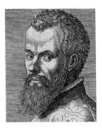 Vesalius, a teacher of surgery and anatomy in Padua between 1537 and 1542 and author of the epochal work *De Humani Corporis Fabrica* (1543), has become canonized to such an extent that it is difficult to imagine him as he was seen by his contemporaries.

His surname van Wesele was derived from the town of Wesel in the region of Cleve in Rheinland-Westfalen, at the confluence of the rivers Rhine and Lippe. Andreas' father Andries had distinguished ancestors but was an illegitimate child; he lived with his family in a somewhat inhospitable region of Brussels and was eventually employed as a pharmacist at the court of Emperor Charles V. Andreas went to a Latin school in Brussels, then took elementary university courses at Louvain; he went on to study medicine, mainly in Paris (1533–1536). After a final year in Louvain, he came to Padua, initially as a graduate student; after brilliant examinations, he was soon appointed Professor of Anatomy and Surgery.

Having completed the *Fabrica*, Vesalius became the personal physician to Emperor Charles V. In 1544, he married Anne van Hamme; they had a daughter with the same name. When Charles V abdicated in 1556, Andreas established a private practice and tried to respond to the careful and restrained comments on his anatomical work written by Gabriele Falloppio (c.1523–1562), one of his successors. In 1564, Vesalius made a pilgrimage to Jerusalem; on the return journey, he became ill on board and died on the island of Zakynthos, off the Western coast of Greece.

Source: Portrait courtesy of Wellcome Foundation.

pores' in the interventricular septum were an important element of the Galenic model. The mixture of blood and air, as well as the 'innate heat' of the heart, were supposed to transform the primitive spirits into 'vital spirit' – a subtler, energy-carrying principle that sustained all elementary functions of the body.

In the third and final stage, as the theory goes, the vital spirit is transported to the ventricles of the brain, via the choroid plexus. During this passage, it is transformed into the subtlest form of spirit, thanks to the intrinsic properties of the brain, with some contribution from air inhaled through the nose. Galen designated it as πνευμα ψυχικον, 'psychic spirit'. The Latin translation is *spiritus animalis*; the adjectival noun does not refer to beasts (*animalia*), but to *anima* or 'soul', the intrinsic principle of all living creatures, to be distinguished from 'animus', the rational faculty of mankind. The English translation 'animal spirits' is infelicitous, since it plainly refers to animals. The alternative term 'mental' excludes interaction with muscles; 'nervous' comes close, but in the sixteenth century, that designation had not yet included the brain. The best choice seems 'animated spirits'.[34] These spirits, Galen and Fernel thought,

---

[34] A suggestion of Dr Dirk van Miert.

perform all the functions of the brain, internal (reasoning, imagination, and memory) as well as external, by flowing either from the cavities of the brain into its nerves and giving rise to movement or, conversely, by mediating sensory impressions.

Since Galen had performed many dissections and experiments on animals,[35] he cleverly introduced empirical details in his writings. Yet a substantial part of his theories remained speculative and heavily influenced by Aristotelian teleology, in that Galen often explained physiological actions by their utility. The notion that the contents of the cerebral ventricles were more important than the surrounding brain tissue was not surprising, given that 'fluidism' was an important principle in ancient medicine. And, practically speaking, the main point of pouring or drinking is the fluid, whereas the can or the cup is a mere utensil. Even at the end of the eighteenth century, at least one serious anatomist still proposed the ventricles as the true 'organ of the soul'.[36]

The Rete Mirabile

An anatomical issue related to the production of animated spirits, controversial for several centuries, was Galen's description of the 'wonderful network' (*rete mirabile*) of vessels at the base of the brain. This structure is present in many kinds of sheep, oxen, and other ungulate animals, mostly outside the *dura mater* or enveloped by a duplicature of this membrane.[37] Galen assumed a similar structure in humans. In most interpretations of Galenic texts, it was this basal network of vessels that was assumed to convert vital spirits into animated spirits; in Fernel's view, we saw, most refinement of the spirits took place in the ventricles, with only a minor role for the network.[38]

An early anatomist, Berengario da Carpi (*c.*1460 to *c.*1530), from Bologna, had expressed doubts about the existence of such a vascular web at the base of the brain.[39] Vesalius initially accepted the existence of the network and even included it in a drawing,[40] but in his later *Fabrica* he made it abundantly clear that such a structure did certainly not exist in man (Figure 1.4).[41] Perhaps Fernel, a 'physiologist' rather than an anatomist, had not yet noticed Vesalius' criticism, or he had decided not to change his views.

[35] Mattern (2013), *The Prince of Medicine*, 145–55; Nutton (2020), *Galen*, 62–4.
[36] Sömmerring (1796), *Das Organ der Seele*.
[37] Gillan (1974), Blood supply to brains of ungulates with and without a rete mirabile caroticum; Rocca (2003), *Galen on the Brain*, 205–10.
[38] Fernelius (1554), *Medicina (Physiologia)*, 121.
[39] da Carpi (1530), *Isagogae breves et exactissimae in Anatomiam humani Corporis*, O5r–6r.
[40] Vesalius (1538), *Tabulae anatomicae sex*, tabula III.
[41] Vesalius (1543), *De humani Corporis Fabrica Libri septem*, 310.

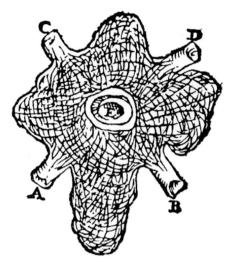

1.4 The 'miraculous network', drawn by Vesalius, though he no longer believed in its existence. His own legend reads: 'In this figure I made up the network as it must be in order to agree with the descriptions of Galen in his book *On the usefulness of the Parts*. A and B might indicate the arteries entering the skull, soon to disperse in that miraculous tangle; as C and D [I drew] the branches in which the elements of this network are assembled; they precisely correspond in size to the arteries I indicated by A and B. E represents the gland receiving the phlegm from the brain.' (Vesalius, 1543, p. 621).

The Exit for Fluid from the Ventricles

The excrements of the brain, Fernel wrote, again following Galen,[42] are a watery substance left over after the brain tissue has been nourished by blood. It is collected in the ventricles of the brain, from which it 'retains a certain cold and humid constitution' before being excreted via the base of the brain to the palate and the nose, from which it is removed by blowing one's nose or by spitting.[43]

Vesalius elaborated on this idea by regarding the most caudal extension of the third ventricle as the passage through which the waste products passed out of the skull. He therefore called this part the *infundibulum*,[44] Latin for 'funnel', 'basin', or 'cup'. He included a small drawing (Figure 1.5) to illustrate how the fluid from the ventricles might pass down to the gland below; he called it the *glandula pituitaria*, or viscous gland. Today it is known as the pituitary gland, or hypophysis, buried in the skull base and separated from extracranial structures by a thin layer of bone. Though Vesalius castigated Galen for his belief that viscous fluid from the brain could pass through the skull base more anteriorly,[45] he did

[42] Galenus (1625c [*c*.180]), *De Usu Partium* (C1) VIII, 168 B–C; Kühn, ed. (1821–33), *Claudii Galeni Opera omnia*, vol. III, *De Usu Partium*, 649–50; Rocca (2003), *Galen on the Brain*, 124–5.

[43] Fernelius (1554), *Medicina (Physiologia)*, 183, 192.

[44] Vesalius (1543), *De humani Corporis Fabrica Libri septem*, 640.

[45] Vesalius (1543), *De humani Corporis Fabrica Libri septem*, 32 and 641.

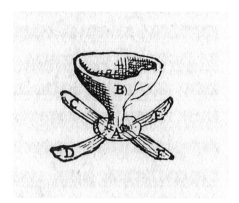

1.5 Vesalius' drawing of the exit for fluid from the ventricular system. His legend reads as follows: 'With this figure I drew the basin ('pelvis') or cup, through which the phlegm (*pituita*) of the brain drips into the gland below it. I also drew four small channels carrying phlegm through openings close to the gland. Thus, A is the gland to which the phlegm trickles down, B the basin through which it is led there; C, D, E and F are the channels fashioned to allow an easier exit for the phlegm that comes down.' (Vesalius, 1543, p. 621)

not shy away from a similar speculation himself; he even adorned his drawing with a number of channels leading away from the pituitary gland.[46]

THE PRESUMED CAUSE OF APOPLEXY: BLOCKED VENTRICLES

The clinical features of apoplexy, with the sudden cessation of all brain functions while breathing and arterial pulsation are preserved, suggested to sixteenth-century physicians a sudden disruption in the traffic of spirits between their storage sites in the brain and their flow into the nerves. They followed Galen's explanation of apoplexy as obstruction within the ventricular system. In the didactic style of Jean Fernel:

> The cause [of apoplexy] resides in the brain, the common origin of all movement and sensation. Actually, it is phlegm, too thick and too cold; for it is improbable that it can occur as a result of blood or black bile, even if these abound in the entire body. And this cold phlegm, despite forming the brain's own excrement, brings about apoplexy when it abundantly fills all its ventricles [...][47]

Different Humours Incriminated as Potential Causes of Obstruction

Despite general agreement on obstruction of the ventricles as the key event in apoplexy, opinions differed on the question of which fluid most often caused such impediment.

[46] Vesalius (1543), *De humani Corporis Fabrica Libri septem*, 641.
[47] Fernelius (1554), *Medicina (Pathologia)*, 133.

Phlegm. Fernel was rather emphatic in his opinion that phlegm was the exclusive culprit. Many others disagreed. An example is Pieter van Foreest, who determined the nature of the fluid from circumstantial evidence: phlegm if it occurred in someone with a pale complexion and a weak pulse or during cold weather, excess of blood in a plethoric person, or black bile in an individual with a melancholic disposition.[48] Other sixteenth-century physicians favoured blood or black bile as the main causative agent.

Blood. Petrus Salius Diversus (*fl.* second half of the sixteenth century), practising in Faenza, emphasized the importance of identifying blood as the cause of apoplexy. He warned that warming the head, a common treatment for apoplexy if it was attributed to an excess of cold fluids, could be disastrous in sanguineous apoplexy.[49] Felix Platter (1536–1614), Professor of Medicine in Basle, implicated blood more often than phlegm as the cause of apoplexy. He regarded haemorrhage through the nose or mouth as a sign that blood had invaded the brain,[50] a comment suggesting that such 'apoplectic states' actually resulted from trauma, not from spontaneous disease.

An excess of blood could be assumed as the cause of apoplexy not only in a person with a reddish, 'plethoric' face, but also after cessation of customary blood loss, for example menopause. It was in this manner that the German surgeon Wilhelm Fabry (1560–1634) explained apoplexy in a goldsmith from Lausanne who had suppressed his recurrent heavy nosebleeds by wearing an amulet.[51]

Black Bile. It was received knowledge that under some circumstances, accumulation of black bile or melancholy also could give rise to apoplexy. Only Fernel was a conspicuous dissenter. A completely opposite stance was that of Girolamo Cardano (Hieronymus Cardanus; 1501–1596), a philosopher, physician, astronomer, and mathematician, at one time a teacher in Padua, but often moving around because of his great talent for making enemies;[52] he postulated that practically *all* cases of apoplexy are caused by black bile.[53]

The only way to try and end the debates was by having a look.

OPENING THE SKULL

Infringing on the human body after death has always been met with apprehension and taboo. In the eyes of the public, there was – and sometimes is – no great distinction between, on the one hand, necropsy by physicians

[48] Forestus (1653 [1590]), *Observationes et Curationes*, vol. X, 514–15.
[49] Diversus (1584), *Curationes quorundam particularium Morborum*, 231.
[50] Platerus (1602), *De Functionum Laesionibus*, 27.   [51] Fabricius (1614), *Centuria tertia*, 57–8.
[52] Siraisi (1997), *Girolamo Cardano*.
[53] Cardanus (1564), *Aphorismorum Hippocratis Particulas Commentaria*, 727.

investigating the causes of disease in patients they had been trying to save, and, on the other, dissection as a method to instruct medical students in the details of anatomy.

Dissection and Disgrace

Being 'anatomized' could be the fate of criminals undergoing capital punishment, a disgrace compounded by the perceived ignominy of being denied a proper burial. Such views have largely persisted through time. A somewhat anachronistic, but irresistible, example one finds in the following passage from a well-known nineteenth-century British novel:

> Mrs Dollop became more and more convinced by her own asseveration, that Dr Lydgate meant to let the people die in the Hospital, if not to poison them, for the sake of cutting them up without saying by your leave or with your leave; for it was a known 'fac' that he had wanted to cut up Mrs Goby, as respectable a woman as any in Parley Street, who had money in trust before her marriage — a poor tale for a doctor, who if he was good for anything should know what was the matter with you before you died, and not want to pry into your inside after you were gone.[54]

The Anatomy of Disease

In fact, there are vast differences between the two procedures. Apart from the minds and aims of doctors, the locations where the dissections take place differ – anatomical theatre versus mortuary, improvised or not – and so does the very method of the procedures. It is therefore surprising that some historians make little or no distinction between these two kinds of dissection.[55] As an investigative tool for understanding disease, it is commonly called autopsy, thus with a more restricted meaning than its literal translation from Greek ('to see for oneself').

In the distant past, medical dissection of the human body after death took place only in Alexandria, and presumably only in the third century BCE.[56] The Alexandrian physician Erasistratus (c.310–250 BCE) was exceptional in that he investigated solid organs.[57] Autopsy was forbidden in all other periods of antiquity, including Galen's time. An exception is in the preparation for embalming, which was almost always carried out by servants.

[54] Eliot (2011 [1872]), *Middlemarch*, 442–3.   [55] Sawday (1995), *The Body Emblazoned.*
[56] von Staden (1992), Human dissection in ancient Greece.
[57] King and Meehan (1973), A history of the autopsy.

In the thirteenth and fourteenth centuries, dissection of cadavers occurred in northern Italy on rare occasions, mostly for legal reasons. The attitude of the Catholic Church has often been represented as antagonistic, but there are valid arguments for believing that clerical authorities have favoured, rather than opposed, post-mortem investigations in humans.[58] Autopsy even played a role in the canonisation of saints.[59] If clerical opposition did occur, it tended to be less if the purpose of dissection was scientific, and not didactic.[60] In general, resistance mainly sprang from humanitarian and aesthetic concerns. In the course of the fourteenth century, dissections were gradually introduced in medical schools, as evidenced in the earliest anatomical treatise by Mondino dei Liuzzi.[61]

As long as Galenic texts dominated medical knowledge, there was little aspiration to expand the use of dissection, as it had little relevance to medical practice; exceptions in the late fifteenth and early sixteenth century were Benedetti, Benivieni, and Massa.[62] But in the second half of the sixteenth century, physicians became more inquisitive and increasingly performed post-mortem dissections, either with permission or furtively. Felix Platter (1536–1614), Professor of Medicine in Basle, confessed to once having visited a cemetery in the dead of night and secretly dissected the body of a phthisic boy with a perforated stomach.[63]

First Glances at the Brain after Apoplexy

Thus, to open the skull of a person who had died after apoplexy was a momentous decision, given the resistance of relatives and friends. Even from a purely practical point of view, the procedure is far from easy, since it requires effort, expertise, and equipment. Physicians might have had little, if any, first-hand experience and had to rely on recollections of anatomical demonstrations from their student days; a colleague or surgeon might have assisted. Finally, physicians needed good reasons for doubting the accepted Galenic doctrine that in apoplexy, the cavities of the brain were stuffed, probably with phlegm. Most medical practitioners in the second half of the sixteenth century felt satisfied with that assumption and did not feel the need to verify the dogma and take the trouble to obtain permission and seek assistance.

Jean Fernel published in 1548, six years before his seminal *Medicina*, an example of what was probably the first autopsy report of apoplexy, in a book with the

---

[58] Cunningham (2010), *The Anatomist Anatomis'd*, 12–15.
[59] Bouley (2017), *Pious Postmortems*.   [60] Carlino (1994), *Books of the Body*, 182–6.
[61] Dei Liuzzi (1988 [1316]), *Anothomia*.   [62] Carlino (1994), *Books of the Body*, 191–3.
[63] Platerus (1614), *Observationum, Libri tres*, 407.

intriguing title *De abditis Rerum Causis*, or *About hidden Causes of Things*. Surprisingly enough, Fernel found the lesion not in the brain, but under it:

> Once I saw that a man, [previously] in perfect health, had suddenly collapsed after a rather strong punch on the left eye, in a stunned state, soon deprived of sensation and motion, with difficult breathing and snoring as well as other signs of a severe apoplexy. He could not be saved by venesection or in another manner and died after twelve hours. I thought therefore that the cause of death was worth investigating. When the head had been dissected and opened, the bone, the membranes and the substance of the brain showed nothing that was broken or bruised; yet I detected that the mere force of the blow had ruptured the internal veins of the eye. From these a volume of two spoonfuls of blood had extended to the base of the brain; having clotted, this narrowed the arteries that form the net-like structure.[64]

The sentence 'I thought therefore that the cause of death was worth investigating' sounds mundane but is, in fact, revolutionary. Fernel must have had qualms about the usual explanation that phlegm had suddenly filled the cavities of the brain, given the preceding blow. Fernel's case, though perhaps attributable to trauma, is important because later generations of physicians often cited it; also, several questions remain open, which exemplifies how difficult it was at the time to investigate the brain without knowing what to look for.

One initial problem is that the blood vessels in the eyes are enclosed in the orbits; it is not impossible to open them, but they are certainly not immediately spotted after the top of the skull has been taken off, which is the usual procedure. More important is the possible contradiction between the finding that the membranes of the brain were intact and that, on the other hand, there were about two spoonfuls of blood at the base of the brain. Was the blood found inside or outside the hard membrane (*dura mater*) surrounding the brain?

Fernel's conclusion that the pool of blood must have compressed the net-like arteries is remarkable, given that he could not have seen such a network – he just assumed it was there. On the same page, Fernel briefly mentioned that he had dissected another patient after 'apoplexy', without details; he found that a thick, viscous fluid compressed this same arterial web he deemed present at the base of the brain, but that he could not truly have seen.

Other observations of brain dissection in the sixteenth century are extremely sparse, at least in reports of individual patients; general comments such as 'After death by apoplexy one often sees ...' probably reflect opinion rather than perception. There are two more instances from the sixteenth century; in both cases, the reader has to take the diagnosis of apoplexy for granted, because no clinical information is given. One of these cases is by Louis Duret (1527–1585),

---

[64] Fernelius (1548), *De abditis Rerum Causis*, 218.

nominated Professor of Medicine in 1568 at the *Collège de France* in Paris.[65] In his commentaries on Hippocrates' *Coan Ideas*, which appeared posthumously, he briefly alluded to dissections he performed on two dignitaries who had died after apoplexy:

> The exit of animated spirit is blocked because the cavities of the brain are filled by an excessive amount of phlegm, black bile or blood. And when they are being filled, not when they are full, the symptom is that of an epileptic convulsion, which is ended by an apoplectic paralysis. I have seen this in the Bishop of Nevers and in the Tax Collector of Ballon; when they had relinquished their life, it was found that the cavities were filled with blood that had burst into them.[66]

In both patients, the site of obstruction was the ventricular system of the brain, perfectly in line with the Galenic doctrine. However, the observations were cursory, almost timid: the brain must have been cut open to arrive at the ventricles, but there is no information about a possible source of the haemorrhage elsewhere. Moreover, a single, brief sentence summarizes the findings in two different patients.

Details are also sparse in a second report by Duret's contemporary Marcellus Donatus (1538–1602), the personal physician of the Duke of Mantua;[67] he examined the body of a court dignitary:

> I was charged with dissecting the administrator of her Highness Maria Justiniana de Arrivabene [in Mantua], who had died of a severe Apoplexy. I brought with me as witnesses the gentlemen Hippolitus Genifortus from Mantua and Ludovicus Cangerla from Vicenza, both practising surgeons in our town; they were present at the dissection. We found that the entire substance of the brain was drenched and filled with an aqueous fluid, which had also flowed into the ventricles of the brain. And, which was truly remarkable, when the temporal arteries[68] had been opened, thick and black blood flowed out in such great profusion that I could hardly believe that so much could be found in the entire body.[69]

A circumstantial, but noteworthy, detail is the presence of colleagues as witnesses. Still, it seems that, in fact, the three physicians did not find very much. Fluid in the cavities of the brain, as well as in the space between the brain and its membranes, was a normal feature of anatomy, well known at the

[65] Hirsch (1884–8), *Biographisches Lexikon*, vol. II, 244.
[66] Duretus (1588), *Hippocratis Magni Coacae Praenotiones*, 366.
[67] Hirsch (1884–8), *Biographisches Lexikon*, vol. II, 202.
[68] It is uncertain whether 'temporal' refers to an extracranial or an intracranial artery.
[69] Donatus (1586), *De medica Historia mirabili Libri sex*, 59v.

time. Apparently, the amount of fluid seemed excessive, as was the volume of blood. A quantitative judgement of this kind presupposes extensive practice in dissecting brains, a level of experience that seems quite unlikely for that period.

THE ROLE OF THE VENTRICLES CHALLENGED

It was a common, and almost sacrosanct, belief that the ventricles of the brain were the production site, or at least the repository, of animated spirits and that these cavities also formed the passage through which all signals of sensation and movement flowed from or into nerves. This idea was finally challenged in the second half of the sixteenth century, on the basis of two different objections. One was based on the structure of the brain; the other was represented by two almost identical reports of infantile hydrocephalus.

A New Dissection Technique: Removing the Brain from the Body

The person who publicly questioned the role of the cerebral ventricles as the passage, if not the smithy, for animated spirits was an ambitious young anatomist from Bologna – Costanzo Varolio (1543–1575) (Box 1.5). Information about his life is regrettably scarce.[70]

Importantly, Varolio introduced a new method of dissecting the brain after the top of the skull had been removed. By carefully tilting the brain and cutting its nerves and blood vessels as they came into view near the skull base, he managed to free the organ from its attachments and remove it entirely from the skull and the rest of the body. Turning the brain upside down and removing the dura mater provided a full view of the basal structures.[71] The woodcut, based on Varolio's own drawing (Figure 1.6A), is less artistic than the corresponding illustration in Vesalius' *Fabrica* of 30 years before (Figure 1.6B), but has more accuracy of detail. Probably Vesalius' version was made at a later stage in the dissection, after most upper parts of the brain had been cut away in the usual fashion, from top to bottom. The longer the time interval between death and dissection, the softer the brain tissue became.

Removal of the brain from a cadaver had far greater implications than the mere practicality of allowing to invert the brain and study its contours in more detail. The new procedure revealed the brain as an isolated object, disengaged from the body and its identity – now a 'thing', inviting close scrutiny.

---

[70] Tubbs, *et al.* (2008), Costanzo Varolio; Zago and Meraviglia (2009), Costanzo Varolio.
[71] Varolio (1573), *De Nervis opticis*, 11r–12r.

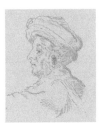

Box 1.5 Costanzo Varolio (1543–1575).

Little is known about Varolio's youth, except that he was born in Bologna, in the year that also saw the first edition of Vesalius' *Fabrica*. Coincidence or not, Varolio always admired Vesalius' work and strived to follow his example. Probably they never met. The profession of Varolio's father is unknown. Costanzo studied medicine at the University of Bologna and graduated in 1566. Anatomy was taught at the time by Julio Caesar Aranzio (1530–1589). In 1569, the senate of Bologna appointed Varolio to an extraordinary professorship of anatomy and surgery; he focused his own investigations on the structure of the brain.

Two years later, Varolio moved to Rome, probably because of the controversies his findings had stirred up in Bologna. He earned a solid reputation as a medical practitioner, especially for removal of stones from the bladder. Rumour has it that he was close to Pope Gregory XIII, but it is uncertain whether he acted as his personal physician. He died from an unknown ailment in 1575, aged 32 years.

Source: © Biblioteca Comunale di Bologna.

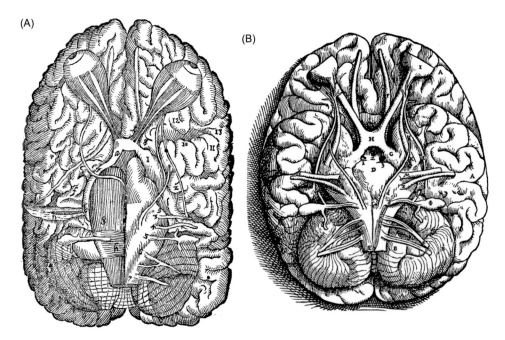

1.6 (A) View of the base of the brain after the entire brain has been detached from the skull and turned upside down (Varolio, 1573). The cranial nerves are numbered from 1 (optic nerve) to 7. A main issue on which Varolio wanted to insist was that the optic nerve continued much further backwards (to the bottom of the drawing) than had been assumed previously. Incidentally, Varolio also identified the 'bridge' (*pons*), the transversely striped structure marked 'h'. (B) The base of the brain, in Vesalius' *Fabrica*. The optic nerves, having crossed, seem to end in the medial part of the temporal lobes. The structure of the brainstem, especially the outline of the pons, is less accurately represented than in Varolio's illustration (A). Both illustrations leave out blood vessels. The pit between 'H' and 'D' indicates where the funnel-like structure drawn in Figure 1.5 is thought to excrete superfluous fluid from the brain into the pituitary gland. (Vesalius, 1543, p. 315).

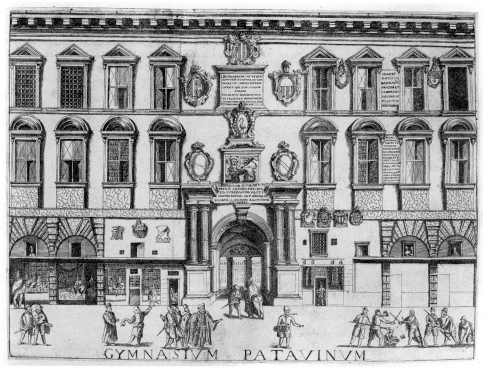

1.7 The university building (*archiginnasio*) of Padua. Engraving by Giacomo Filippo Tomaselli, 1654. *Source:* Courtesy of the Wellcome collection.

A Revolutionary Idea: Ventricles Mainly Serving as the Sewer of the Brain?

In 1572, shortly before Varolio's departure from Bologna to Rome, where he was to die three years later, he wrote a letter to Hieronimus Mercurialis (Girolamo Mercuriale; 1530–1606), who had been appointed in 1569 as Professor of Theoretical Medicine in Padua. Padua was another centre of medical learning (Figure 1.7),[72] governed by the powerful city state of Venice, and therefore less subject to ecclesiastical rule than Bologna. The Paduan university attracted the best professors from abroad, for example Vesalius for anatomy and surgery, at least between 1537 and 1542. Also, the senate of Venice allowed admission of students from all regions of Europe, including Protestants and Jews.[73]

Mercurialis enjoyed a great reputation by virtue of his expertise in ancient Greek medical texts.[74] It is clear from the tone of Varolio's letter that he regarded Mercurialis, his senior by 13 years, as a higher authority; he appealed to him as an impartial judge to whom he submitted his new findings on the

---

[72] Gallo (2001), *L'Età Medioevale.*   [73] Bylebyl (1979), The School of Padua.
[74] Hirsch (1884–8), *Biographisches Lexikon*, vol. IV, 209–10; Ongaro (2007a), Girolamo Mercuriale.

anatomy of the brain.[75] Some controversy had arisen between Varolio and his colleagues in Bologna about the structures at the base of the brain, especially the course of the optic nerves and the structure of the brainstem – findings that were in conflict with received opinion;[76] apparently, the young anatomist sought support from Mercurialis. But in the course of his argumentation, Varolio came up with a revolutionary proposition on another subject, that of the cerebral ventricles. To soften the blow, he introduced it with a polite and tentative phrase:

> Highly esteemed Mercurialis, the principal target I aim for in this work must be to be engaged with an account of [the structure of] the head, disregarding all speculations. Yet I shall not be silent on what I feel about the function of the ventricles of the brain. As you know, the common and most widespread opinion is that the ventricles of the brain are the home of the animated spirits, in the same way as the left ventricle of the heart is the home of the vital spirits. Surely, I would not dare to attack this opinion, since nobody could ever undertake this without the stigma of defiance. Yet I will propose for your consideration a single function as the main one. I should like you to think that I submit it in a doubtful manner rather than as a certainty. [. . .]
>
> Presently it is known to all that phlegm drips from the brain to the palate via the infundibulum; if one considers the arrangement of the body parts through which the phlegm passes, it will be easily understood that it is first collected in the ventricles. [. . .] Therefore, I conclude that the primary function of the ventricles of the brain is to serve as receptacles for viscous fluid that is generated in the brain and excreted via the palate. And this is not incompatible with the very common convictions of those who think they are the home of animated spirits, since (as has been said before) more functions can be assigned to a single part [of the body].[77]

Animated Spirits Conveyed by the Substance of the Brain?

Mercurialis flatly disagreed. After many compliments about Varolio's new anatomical findings, he adduced many citations from Hippocrates, Plato, and Galen, before opposing the idea of an excretory function of the ventricles in his own words:

---

[75] Varolio's letter was printed in 1573 in Padua, together with Mercurialis' response and Varolio's rejoinder; in 1591, a reprint appeared in Frankfurt.

[76] The most important novelty in Varolio's findings was that the optic 'nerves' continued much further backwards than traditionally assumed; the conventional opinion was that they ended in the thalamus – hence its full name 'thalamus opticus'.

[77] Varolio (1573), *De Nervis opticis*, 7v–9v.

By the manner in which you have used that peculiarly sharp mind of yours to explain the function of the ventricles of the brain, you have at the same time (please allow me to say this) got yourself entangled in inextricable difficulties. For how can it happen that at the same site where the most pure and subtle bodies, the spirits, are concocted and perfected, in a stove as it were - that in that same place a thick, cold, dark fluid is collected, [a fluid that is], let me say it with a single word, highly toxic for the spirits themselves? What is more, when apoplexy occurs, completed or in progress, or epilepsy, or a nightmare, all writers of medicine implicate the following as causes, that phlegm, black bile or too thick winds are retained in the ventricles. These [fluids], filling them entirely or for the largest part, strangle the spirits, as it were.[78]

Varolio reciprocated, after profuse expressions of gratitude towards Mercurialis, that he persisted in his opinion about the excretory function of the ventricles. He went as far as proposing a different medium for the transport of spirits: the tissue of the brain! He introduced a new argument, on top of his earlier proposal that excretion of waste products might be the main function of the ventricles. This was the fact, supported by Galen, that most nerves in the skull originate from the brainstem. Large-scale transport of spirits by the brainstem would be at odds with the absence of a corresponding central cavity, if ventricles indeed acted as a store room for spirits; conversely, very few nerves take their origin from the brain area with large ventricles.

Galen says in *De usu partium* (Book 8, Chapter 13) that animated spirit is contained in large amounts in the entire mass of the brain, and similarly in that of the cerebellum, which he regards as the beginning of the nerves of the entire body; he even infers from this that [the cerebellum] must necessarily be crammed with spirits. If therefore the cerebellum, though lacking any cavity, contains such an excess of spirits in its substance that these [spirits] can flow from there to all parts of the body; for what reason, I beseech you, have such large cavities been created for the sake of animated spirits for the brain, which conveys only nerves and spirits to the parts in and around the head, according to Galen? If spirit flows from the cerebellum to so many nerves, over such great distance, why does it not rather flow in the same way, without cavities and channels, from the brain to fewer and much closer parts?[79]

Normal Ventricles in Victims of Apoplexy?

One of Mercurialis' objections was that assigning the transport of animated spirits to the brain tissue itself undermined the time-honoured belief that

---

[78] Mercurialis (1573), Responsio, 23r–v.   [79] Varolio (1573), *De Nervis opticis*, 26r–v.

blocked ventricles were the cause of apoplexy and other acute brain disorders. But Varolio, recalling from Galen that apoplexy could also occur with lesions of 'the beginning of the spinal medulla' (currently called *medulla oblongata*), now came up with an astonishing fact:

> You will perhaps admit, to paraphrase Galen (*De locis affectis*, Book 3, Chapter 7) at least in part, that epilepsy and other, similar affections arise because obstruction of spirits has occurred by humours abnormally irrigating the beginning of the spinal medulla. This point of view is supported by dissections of patients who have died of Apoplexy in whom (please believe me) no greater quantity of excrements is found than one usually finds in all others.[80]

Varolio's surprising argument that post-mortem studies of patients who had died of apoplexy had shown the same quantity of fluid in the ventricles as in persons without brain disease seems important in the light of later developments. Yet it was a casual, almost offhand remark, not substantiated with details about person, time, or place, let alone supported by witnesses. By contrast, Varolio's exclamation 'please believe me' rings with such conviction that the observation was perhaps his own, not just hearsay.

Why did the striking finding that patients with fatal apoplexy had normal ventricles fail to be publicized? Presumably because the finding conflicted with received opinion – such facts were inconvenient, unwelcome, and unheard of, things one might gossip about but not openly discuss. The same cognitive distortion that caused Fernel to see a non-existent structure because he supposed it was there could have led others to deny, or at least suppress, observations that went against the grain of common tradition.

Infantile Hydrocephalus: Occluded Ventricles, Yet Sensation and Motion

Two almost identical observations cast even more doubt on the notion that brain function depended on its cavities. Both concerned a young child with progressive and ultimately fatal enlargement of the lateral ventricles; the salient point with regard to brain function was that the children had for a long time been able to move and interact.

The first report appeared in print in the middle of the sixteenth century; it did not attract immediate attention but was increasingly cited as time went on. Its author was none other than Andreas Vesalius, in the second edition of his *Fabrica*:

> In Augsburg I saw a girl of two years whose head had enlarged in about seven months to such an extent that no head of any man I have ever seen

---

[80] Varolio (1573), *De Nervis opticis*, 28r–v.

could compare with that mass. This was the affection the ancients called hydrocephalus, from water retained and gradually collected in the head. [...] Here it was in the cavity of the brain itself, in fact in the right and left ventricle; their volume and width had enlarged to such an extent, and the brain itself was so much stretched that they contained – so help me God – almost nine pounds of water, or three Augsburg measures of wine. As a result, the brain at the top of the head was thin like a sheet and somehow continuous with its tender membrane. The skull also was quite soft; only the lower part was bony, corresponding to the width of the girl's skull before her head had expanded abnormally. [...] In conclusion, I was exceptionally astonished – with the Physicians who were present – that such a mass of water had for such a long time been collected in the ventricles of the brain without major symptoms. [...] Until her death the girl has been in complete command of her senses.[81]

The second record is in the writings of the surgeon Wilhelm Fabry or Guilhelmus Fabricius (1560–1634) (Box 1.6);[82] he had also contributed the case of the goldsmith and his suppressed nosebleeds. The sad story of the young child had occurred in 1594:

In a neighbourhood of Cologne called *Ehrestrasse* I saw several times a boy, son of parents in robust health. [...] His head started to grow enormously when he had barely reached the age of seven months. No disease had preceded this; yet the rest of the body was poorly developed. Within 30 months the head increased to the size I indicated. In the end he lapsed into a lethargic sopor and died not much later, on February 19, 1594. When the head was dissected, in the presence of the very learned physicians *Joannes Slotanus* and *Henricus Pallantius*, we found water in the two anterior ventricles, clearer than crystal, with a volume of 18 Cologne pounds. This [fluid] stretched not only the ventricles, but also the substance of the brain, to such an extent that the entire brain (with the exception of the cerebellum) was as thin as the cloth of a bag. [...]

Indeed, he had eaten, drunk, excreted and slept like a normal [child]; only proper growth had been lacking, for his entire body (with the exception of the head) remained quite small and diminutive, as appears from the picture drawn true to life that I have at home.[83]

Several aspects of these case histories are noteworthy. To begin with, it is a vital piece of information that both infants had moved and interacted with their parents long after enlargement of the ventricles had started to occur. A second peculiarity is the very fact of the autopsies, for which the children's parents must have given their permission. As intimated above, it was an uncommon

[81] Vesalius (1555), *De humani Corporis Fabrica Libri septem*, 24.
[82] Jones (1960), Fabricius Hildanus. The addition 'Hildanus' refers to Fabry's birthplace Hilden.
[83] Fabricius (1606), *Observationum & Curationum chirurgicarum Centuriae*, 60–1.

Box 1.6 Guilhelmus Fabricius (1560–1634).

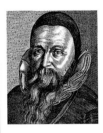

Wilhelm Fabry, the 'father of German surgery', was born in Hilden, Nordrhein-Westphalia, where now a bust of him overlooks a central square. His father, a court clerk, died when Wilhelm was still young; his mother remarried but was soon widowed again. At school, Wilhelm showed great talents; he might have gone to university, had not the Thirty Years War caused a complete upheaval of normal life. Eventually Fabry had to give up his ambition of being a doctor.

Instead, he became an apprentice to several surgeons; one of them was Cosmas Slotanus, a surgeon at the ducal court in Düsseldorf and a pupil of Vesalius. Wilhelm not only was introduced to modern anatomy, but also learnt much from the physicians at the palace.

When Slotanus died in 1585, Fabry began a wandering existence. At first, he practised in Metz and Geneva, where he married Marie Colinet, herself a surgeon and an obstetrician. Further peregrinations included Cologne and Lausanne. As his fame increased, he travelled far and wide to wherever patients lived. From 1598 onwards, he published his case histories, one hundred at a time (*centuriae*). Several editions followed, in Latin and in vernacular language. In 1615, Fabry finally settled in Berne, as a surgeon to the town and canton. His later years were troubled by gout. On his death in 1634, Fabry left a wife and a son Johann, also a surgeon; seven other children did not survive him.

Source: Portrait courtesy of Wellcome Foundation.

---

event for physicians to dissect a cadaver. Fabry was an exception; he provided more examples of autopsy in his reports.[84]

Finally, both physicians enhanced the trustworthiness of their observations by inviting other physicians to attend and perhaps to participate; Vesalius only hints at the presence of colleagues, whereas Fabry even recorded their names. This is an early example of establishing 'matters of fact' by engaging witnesses of appropriate social stature to confirm new observations. This practice in medicine predates similar approaches to the advancement of knowledge by the experimentalists of the Royal Society a century later.[85] What is more, Fabry preserved some of the evidence by keeping the bony part of the skull and a drawing of the patient's body as exhibits in the 'Museum' at his home.

THE BRAIN SUBSTANCE VINDICATED AS THE SITE OF APOPLEXY

A few years after the Varolio–Mercurialis correspondence, the French-Swiss medical student Gaspard Bauhin, or Caspar Bauhinus, (1560–1634) (Box 1.7)

---

[84] Fabricius (1606), *Observationum & Curationum chirurgicarum Centuriae*, 132, 139–40, 197–9.
[85] Shapin (1994), *The Social History of Truth*, 212–32.

Box 1.7 Gaspard Bauhin (1560–1632).

Gaspard Bauhin was born in Basle as the second son of the physician Jean Bauhin. The father had studied in Paris under Sylvius (Jacques Dubois) and became a successful practitioner in the French capital, until 1532 when persecution of Protestant citizens forced the elder Bauhin to seek refuge in England. On his return, three years later, he narrowly escaped death on the pyre, thanks to the intervention of the princesses he had previously treated. Eventually father Jean settled in Basle.

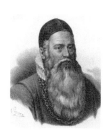

  Gaspard also studied medicine, first in Basle, then in Padua (1577–1579), and two more years in Montpellier; he settled in his home town in 1581. In addition to his medical practice, he taught anatomy and botany. In 1582, Bauhin also became Professor of Greek at the University of Basle. Seven years later, the same university appointed him Professor of Anatomy and Botany and, finally, in 1614, chair of Practical Medicine as the successor to Felix Platter. In 1623, Bauhin published *Pinax Theatri Botanici*, in which he described thousands of plants, with a simplified nomenclature predating the binomial system of Linnaeus. His elder brother Jean was also a botanist.

Source: Portrait courtesy of *Bibliothèque interuniversitaire de Santé*, Paris.

---

visited the universities of Northern Italy. Among the many books Bauhin published later in his career, the best known is his textbook of anatomy *Theatrum Anatomicum*, first published in 1605.[86]

  The contents of the *Theatrum* make it abundantly clear that a printed version of the correspondence between Varolio and Mercurialis must have come to Bauhin's attention. He copied large portions of text, including Mercurialis' objections and also Varolio's woodcuts.[87] Nowadays it seems strange that Bauhin failed to cite Varolio, apart from casual acknowledgements elsewhere in the text, but laws or conventions for authorship and copyright were non-existent. Bauhin included parts of Varolio's argumentation not yet cited above; an example is Varolio's appeal to common sense in favour of his proposal that the fluid in the ventricles represents waste products from the brain:

> Indeed, we see before our eyes that if someone is voluntarily spitting, he first grates and grunts, as it were [to clear] the upper parts of the palate, [then] collects the portion of excrement in the cavity of his mouth and finally discharges it. If he immediately wants to spit again, he produces a smaller portion of sputum, and if he tries this once more without delay, he produces even less, so that soon a stage is reached where he comes up with nothing to spit out, although he forcibly clears his palate. But after

---

[86] Hirsch (1884–8), *Biographisches Lexikon*, vol. VI, 460–1.
[87] Bauhinus (1605), *Theatrum anatomicum*, 687.

some time has elapsed, the excrement again easily descends into the oral cavity. This is a most obvious sign that the material is collected in some quantity before it is expelled, as we see with urine and faeces.[88]

At the end of the paragraph on the cerebral ventricles, Bauhin addressed the main issue: the location of animated spirits within the brain tissue. There he reproduced another argument of Varolio. Spirits do not take up space, Varolio reasoned; not even the cerebellum, which Galen supposed to be crammed with spirits, has discernible channels. Therefore, spirits do not require visible space either:

> Since Galen showed that animated spirit can flow and reflow without any discernible channel, [...] why can't we therefore assign it to the substance of the brain, [only] because some people assign it to the ventricles, which they have not properly studied?[89]

Later authors mostly cited Bauhin on this issue, instead of Varolio, who had first proposed it. Probably the original text had a modest circulation, in contrast to Bauhin's anatomy book, which became popular and was reprinted in 1621.[90]

The Seat of Apoplexy: Ideas Change Slowly

Bauhin, once back in Basle, must have disseminated the Varolian idea that animated spirits travelled via the tissue of the brain. Such relocation of the seat of movement and sensation to the substance of the brain did not fail to change ideas about the location of brain lesions causing apoplexy. At any rate, one finds this new opinion in the textbook written by Bauhin's older colleague and Professor of Medicine in Basle Felix Platter, or Platerus (1534–1614) (Box 1.8), whom Bauhin later succeeded. In Platter's explanation of apoplexy, he categorically and boldly located animated spirits in brain tissue, though partly retaining the traditional theory by his suggestion that abnormal fluids could affect brain tissue also indirectly, by inundation of its surface or by overfilling of the ventricles.

> If [phlegm] persistently inundates the brain substance to such an extent that the great mass of the brain is made too soft and too slack, it suddenly dissolves and collapses. [Then] it presses on the beginning of the nerves at the base of the skull, blocks the transit of the animated spirit, and gives

---

[88] Bauhinus (1605), *Theatrum anatomicum*, 696 (corresponding to Varolio (1573), *De Nervis opticis*, 31r–v).

[89] Bauhinus (1605), *Theatrum anatomicum*, 698 (corresponding to Varolio (1573), *De Nervis opticis*, 26v–27r).

[90] Bauhinus (1621), *Theatrum anatomicum*.

Box 1.8 Felix Platter (1536–1614).

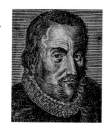

Felix Platter was born in Basle. His father Thomas, a humanist and self-educated teacher of Latin, Greek, and Hebrew, was headmaster of the local gymnasium and also functioned as printer and publisher. In 1552, Felix departed on horseback to study medicine in Montpellier, in the company of a friend. On his return, five years later, he extensively travelled in France before graduating in Basle and marrying Madlen Jekermann, the daughter of a local surgeon.

In 1562, Platter became Professor of Anatomy at the University of Basle, and in 1571 a city physician and Professor of Practical Medicine. Among the conditions he described were two affections now called 'meningioma' and 'Dupuytren's disease'. Felix Platter kept an accurate diary of his life as a student, which has been preserved.

Source: Portrait courtesy of Wellcome Foundation.

---

rise to severe apoplexy. Of course, when phlegm suddenly fills the ventricles or cavities of the brain it can also cause apoplexy, [but] not through obstruction, since the animated spirit has its seat not in these [ventricles] but everywhere in the substance of the brain and in the nerves, and since [the phlegm] does not pass via the ventricles, but by compressing the base of the brain in the same manner.[91]

On the same page, Platter briefly referred to the autopsy he had witnessed as a student at the University of Montpellier;[92] in the 1550s; he used a few more words to describe the event in a book with medical observations, published later in 1614, the year he died:

> An old woman from Montpellier suddenly died after she had been struck by apoplexy. When I opened her skull in the monastery before she was buried, I found that her brain within the thick membrane fluctuated on both sides. When the hard membrane had been cut and opened, some rather thick and whitish fluid resembling porridge flowed down over her entire face and was scattered over the cloth on both sides.[93]

Platter's report clearly indicates that the abnormality was found in the substance of the brain, but leaves most other questions unanswered. As in earlier examples, the clinical features that led to the diagnosis of apoplexy are unknown. Especially important is the time course of the disease: did the word 'sudden' apply to her death or to the apoplexy? If the brain tissue was actually

---

[91] Platerus (1602), *De Functionum Laesionibus*, 24.
[92] Platter chronicled his *grand tour*: Le Roy Ladurie (1995), *Le Mendiant et le Professeur*.
[93] Platerus (1614), *Observationum, Libri tres*, 14–15.

'dissolved', one might think of inflammatory disease, or of decay owing to a delay between death and autopsy. Moreover, the description of the abnormal texture of the brain is global, without distinction between its parts.

Bauhin's anatomical compendium and Platter's textbook on diseases did not influence physicians until the early seventeenth century; even then, it took some 50 more years before the traditional interpretation of Galenic physiology had faded. For example, as late as in 1641, a few years after Bauhin's death, an academic thesis on apoplexy defended in Basle still mentioned the ventricles, as well as the substance of the brain, as the site where the flow of animated spirits could be interrupted.[94] But as the sixteenth century drew to a close, more and more physicians became used to the idea that the science of medicine was incomplete and ancient writings no longer sufficed. Practical physicians like Pieter van Foreest paid much attention to new observations recorded by colleagues, in letters or books; one-third of the hundreds of citations in his text on apoplexy refers to contemporaries. Also, younger physicians were less fettered by tradition, whereas the prestige of university professors still depended on literary expertise. 'Research' as an academic activity was not just non-existent; it was entirely unknown.

All in all, the 'ventricular hypothesis' died a slow death, even in northern Italy. In the account of apoplexy by Alexander Massaria (1510–1598), appointed in 1587 to succeed Mercurialis as Professor of Theoretical Medicine in Padua,[95] he assigned a prominent role not only to the ventricles, but also to the *rete mirabile*:

> [...] the heart continuously provides [the brain] with heat and vital spirit, mediated by those vessels forming a considerable network, commonly called the miraculous net, by which the animated spirit, very subtle and easily soluble, can be continuously regenerated and stored. If, therefore, the arteries forming this network happen to be obstructed and impeded, so that less vital spirit can be transported to the ventricles of the brain, then necessarily also the vital spirit will be destroyed and wanting, since it lacks its nourishment. Through this deficiency the actions of the brain necessarily desist, the person is deprived of sensation and motion, and apoplexy occurs.[96]

In contrast, Ercole Sassonia (Hercules Saxonia; 1551–1607), Professor of Practical Medicine in Padua during the 1570s,[97] firmly located apoplexy in the tissue of the brain: 'Its immediate site (no matter what others say), is the substance of the brain.'[98]

[94] Falkhusius (1641), *De Apoplexia Positiones*, thesis VIII.
[95] Hirsch (1884–8), *Biographisches Lexikon*, vol. IV, 161.
[96] Massaria (1601), *Practica medica*, 80.   [97] Hirsch (1884–8), *Biographisches Lexikon*, vol. V, 182.
[98] Saxonia (1610), *Prognoseon Practicarum*, 53.

Still, at the dawn of the seventeenth century, there was no firm evidence that apoplexy could be caused by lesions of brain tissue itself. A few post-mortem dissections had been carried out, but they had been performed, or at least described, in a cursory fashion, while the clinical features that had led to the diagnosis of apoplexy remained unspecified. That theories dominated medical thinking is not very different from today, but a vital difference was the inflexibility of the theory. Eyes had to be taught to see what there actually was, instead of what ought to be seen. This is what caused Varolio to write, when he had been met not only with disbelief, but also with accusations of cheating when he had demonstrated that basal structures of the brain differed from ancient descriptions:[99]

> Indeed, so great is the power of established opinion of men, that many even seemed to be in doubt while they were beholding the very truth with their own eyes.[100]

Observation as a source of knowledge, instead of scriptures, required a routine that had to be learnt.

THE ART OF OBSERVATION

The distinction between observation and interpretation is never sharp, not even today,[101] not even in particle physics where some conclusions are based on the interpretation of photographs of events in bubble chambers.[102] Seeing is always, to some extent, believing; visual impressions are often selective or fraught with meaning. Medicine is no exception; this applies not only to clinical features of illness, such as the interpretation of a reflex,[103] but also to pathological–anatomical observations after death.

It is therefore appropriate to review the advance of medical knowledge in the second half of the sixteenth century from a somewhat broader perspective than that of a particular disease. Several writings, not exclusively in medicine, emanated a presentiment that nature had not yet revealed all her secrets. Accordingly, there was a slow transition from recognition of known patterns to attempts at learning. The process of observation, to see what is in front of one's eyes, to use Varolio's expression, was a key element.

Clinical Observations

In recording clinical phenomena of disease, the word 'observation' did not always have the same connotation. 'To observe' may also imply a form of

---

[99] Varolio (1573), *De Nervis opticis*, 13v.   [100] Varolio (1573), *De Nervis opticis*, 11r.
[101] Hanson (1958), *Patterns of Discovery*, 4–30.
[102] Pickering (1984), Against putting the phenomena first.
[103] van Gijn and Bonke (1977), Interpretation of plantar reflexes.

obeisance, or 'observance', in the sense of acknowledgement, recognition, and confirmation of something already known and perhaps even expected. Gianna Pomata has argued that in the period between 1500 and 1650, 'observation' gradually evolved from a prescriptive to a descriptive meaning and so came to represent a new epistemic genre, of facts on their own – especially in astronomy and medicine.[104] It is in the modern sense of the word that *observationes* became popular in the medical world of the late sixteenth century: case records of patients, with clinical phenomena; the corresponding theories were relegated to a sequel with explanatory notes (*scholia*). This method of presentation, first applied in northern Italy, became the template of published case records. But it was not easy to disengage perceptions from preconceptions; theoretical notions invariably tended to creep in.

Looking inside the Head

The very decision to try and have a look at the brain of a patient who succumbed after apoplexy was a momentous step, given the practical and moral obstacles. Up to the middle of the sixteenth century, doubt about causes of disease was scarce.[105] Physicians were generally satisfied with interpretations of the clinical phenomena of apoplexy in Galenic terms: phlegm overfilling the cerebral cavities. Though early post-mortem investigations were sometimes prompted by judicial arguments, doubt must have been the driving force in at least some of them.

Questioning Galen was indeed a bold step. Around 1550, physicians like Fernel felt they were part of a medical Renaissance: their art had come to life again, thanks to the restoration of ancient Greek wisdom, purged from barbarisms. These ancient medical texts, almost matching the Bible in age and peremptory style, had a status far outstripping the bare fact that they were actually based on observations, and, what is more, observations anybody could repeat and check. Even so, their contents were almost universally regarded as inviolate truths, defying the capacity of the senses, in the same way as in ancient times the rules of mathematics were felt to surpass the physical reality of material objects or of visual representations by means of lines and angles.[106] In addition, the synthesis between Aristotelian natural philosophy and Christian theology, crafted by Thomas of Aquino and other theologians in the thirteenth century, endowed the Greek heritage with an

---

[104] Pomata (2011), Observation rising.
[105] Gulczynski, *et al.* (2009), Short history of the autopsy.
[106] Dijksterhuis (1961), *The Mechanisation of the World Picture*, 50–3.

almost religious supremacy.[107] Any censure or objection might be felt to border on heresy.

As we saw, the first reports in which physicians inspected the brain of victims of apoplexy were not very informative. The lack of detail proved the inspection could not have been more than a quick peek: blood or phlegm at the base of the brain, compressing a fictitious network of vessels, or ventricles of the brain filled with blood or aqueous fluid.

Similarly, Varolio's almost casual comment that he had witnessed dissections of patients with apoplexy where the ventricles contained 'no greater quantity of excrements than one usually finds in all others' was not supported by information on identities or on the patients' symptoms before death. This finding, in fact great news in medicine, was apparently muffled because it did not agree with ancient theory.

Handling and Exploring the Brain as an Object

Varolio's name is remembered by medical students solely – if at all, because eponyms are going out of fashion – by his description of a prominent structure at the base of the brain he called 'the bridge' (pons; Figure 1.6A). He deserves to be remembered for more. First of these is the technique he developed for removing the brain from the rest of the corpse. Though acknowledged by early historians of medicine,[108] this feat has become obliterated; one finds it only in historical compendia of brain anatomy.[109] The psychological, almost metaphysical consequences of the Varolian technique far outshine the practical advantages. Until then, the brain, considered the seat of reason, but also of morality, had remained part of the corpse as a whole and represented almost the very core of the person. But by entirely removing the brain from the rest of the body, like the heart, the lungs, the spleen, or other organs, Varolio opened the way to the exploration of not only its inner structure, but also its diseases.

Finally, perhaps his most important feat, Varolio proposed that the substance of the brain, not its cavities, was the location of 'animated spirits'. He derived this premise from his observation that most nerves originated near the part of the ventricular system with the smallest cavity. His additional, teleological argument that a storage site was needed for secretions from the nose and throat was eventually to be disproved.

---

[107] Dijksterhuis (1961), *The Mechanisation of the World Picture* 128–35.
[108] Sprengel (1821–8), *Geschichte der Arzneykunde*, vol. III, 126; Neuburger (1897), *Entwicklung der experimentellen Gehirn-und Rückenmarksphysiologie*, 125.
[109] Clarke and O'Malley (1996), *The Human Brain and Spinal Cord*, 820–3.

The Combination of Brain Dissection and Clinical Signs and Symptoms

Vesalius and Fabry had each dissected an infant with exceedingly large ventricles. Both children had died at the age of around two and a half years. Sparse, but vital pieces of clinical information attested that each child had made limb movements and had manifested 'sensation' in the sense of interaction with the parents, even at a stage of enormous expansion of the cerebral ventricles. These two case reports were often cited by contemporaries and later generations because they removed the last foothold in the notion that the cerebral ventricles were essential for the production and transport of animated spirits. The resulting conceptual turn, in which the 'signals of thought' were relocated in the substance of the brain instead of in its watery cavities, was an indispensable step in the understanding of apoplexy.

In conclusion, recording clinical facts was an art that had to be developed, not in a single physician's lifetime, but in the course of several generations. The same applied to recording changes in the brain of patients who had died of apoplexy – the anatomy of disease. In the sixteenth century, this started with fragmentary information on manifestations of disease and anatomical changes. Only the combination of clinical and pathological characteristics allowed further understanding of brain disease.

TWO

THE FORCE OF BLOOD

Apoplexy in the Seventeenth Century

SUMMARY

Harvey's description of the circulation of blood slowly replaced Galen's theory. The ancient model had taught that the liver synthesized new blood, to be subsequently consumed by body organs; the liver also transported the blood to abdominal organs, and the heart supplied mainly the chest and all muscles.

Wepfer performed brain dissection in four patients with apoplexy; the brain was damaged or compressed by extravasated blood in three of them. Though the fourth patient had become unconscious in the course of protracted illness, Wepfer still diagnosed 'apoplexy', but as a variant with excess of 'serum' in the brain. Later physicians also applied the diagnosis to some cases with gradual onset or with external causes, if an 'apoplectic state' was the key symptom, with preservation of breathing and heart action.

Whether or not interruption of blood flow to the brain could cause apoplexy remained a contentious issue – Wepfer thought it was possible but could not cite examples; Willis excluded it, given the arterial interconnections. To explain apoplexy without brain haemorrhage, some physicians invoked inactivation of spirits by chemical reactions (Willis) or congelation of the blood flow (Bayle, Cortnumm). Overflow or obstruction dominated most explanations, while anatomical proofs remained scarce.

In the early seventeenth century, the medical world agreed that brain lesions causing apoplexy interfered with the transport of 'animated spirits': an imperceptible, ethereal, almost immaterial matter, supposed to flow from the brain into nerves, and vice versa. It transmitted impressions from sense organs, created thought and memory, and made muscles move.

An important question was: in what part of the brain does this interruption take place? Some physicians, following Varolio, had become convinced that it was in the substance of the brain tissue itself rather than in the ventricles, as Galen had it. Others, perhaps the majority of physicians, held on to the traditional belief. It was in the seventeenth century that pathological anatomy began to change ideas on apoplexy and other brain diseases.

Before that time, the diseased brain had not yet been closely inspected and the diagnosis of apoplexy was not supported by depictions of the clinical features. This paucity of both clinical and pathological details was to change in the course of the seventeenth century, when the 'anatomy of illness' started to emerge.

A FIRST SPOTLIGHT ON BLOOD VESSELS

In 1629, a monograph about apoplexy appeared in Wittenberg, a small university town halfway between Leipzig and Berlin, made famous by Luther. One year before, a publisher in Frankfurt had printed the now famous book by William Harvey about the circulation of blood. Harvey's theory was fated to overturn medical thoughts, also on apoplexy, but the author of the book on apoplexy, Gregor Nymmann, or Nymmanus (1592–1638) (Box 2.1),[1] was not yet aware of it. He was Professor of Medicine in Wittenberg; it had taken him much time to rework his doctoral thesis of 1619 into a treatise, a problem compounded by delays at the printer. In the dedication of his book to the worthies of Saxony, he evinced a modern mind by intimating that existing knowledge was incomplete:

> Someone entrusted with a sum of money who only hoarded it in a piece of cloth at home, instead of making a profit by business, is reproved and called a useless slave. We all deserve the same reproof if we are merely content with the art as it has been left to use by our predecessors and do not add anything to it and strive to supply what is still missing to it.[2]

Channels at the Back of the Head

Nymmann provided an extensive review and criticism of previous explanations of apoplexy, and praised Varolio for his method of removing the brain

---

[1] Friedensburg (1917), *Geschichte der Universität Wittenburg*, 461.
[2] Nymmanus (1629), *Tractatus de Apoplexia*, iii–iv.

Box 2.1 Gregor Nymmann (1592–1638).

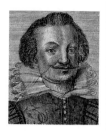

When Nymmann (Nymmanus) was two years old, he lost his father, Professor of Medicine at the University of Wittenberg. He was raised by his mother Sibylla (née Strauch) and his stepfather Tobias Tandler, a physician and mathematician. The young Gregor Nymmann studied philosophy and medicine in his home town, obtaining his licence as physician in 1618; a year later, he became Doctor of Medicine with a disputation on the subject of apoplexy. At the age of 26, he was appointed Professor of Botany in Wittenberg. In 1626, he succeeded Wolfgang Schaller as the junior professor of medicine, and in 1637, Daniel Sennert as the senior. Having survived the plague in Wittenberg, he died a year later from 'a chronic disease of the spleen'. In 1628, a year before the appearance of his book *De apoplexia*, an expanded version of his doctoral thesis, he published *De vita foetus in utero*; in this work, he proposed that if a pregnant woman was about to die, the child might be salvaged by caesarean section.

Source: Portrait courtesy of Wellcome Foundation.

---

from the skull. He then reported his own attempts at finding a single site in the brain where obstruction might cause all the impressive symptoms of apoplexy:

> I confidently conclude that a very severe disease of such kind cannot evolve unless the vessels and channels that carry the vital spirit and distribute it through the brain are occluded, . . .[3]

Thus, Nymmann, perhaps unwittingly, took up an earlier suggestion of Jean Fernel, some 80 years before, that obstruction of the blood flow to the brain might cause apoplexy by depriving the organ from vital spirits, about to be elaborated into animated spirits. Fernel's suggestion involved a 'miraculous network' of vessels at the base of the brain that proved fictional, at least in man, but the principle was the same. Nymmann continued:

> At the end of the day, however, when I looked into the matter a little deeper and carefully contemplated the vessels of the brain one by one, I came upon a site, which I have shown in all my public and private dissections, from the time when I first proposed this, ten years ago, until today. From this site blood and spirit are distributed to the brain like from a wellspring; by its occlusion the brain can be at once deprived if not from all, at least from most of its spirits. This is the confluence of all sinuses of the thick membrane (which some people have called the Wine press or *Torcular*, because blood from veins and arteries that has flowed to

---

[3] Nymmanus (1629), *Tractatus de Apoplexia*, 96.

those channels is pressed into the entire substance of the brain, like from a wine press).[4]

Nymmann's reasoning critically depended on the traditional, pre-Harveian concept of the movement of blood. Although arteries and veins had been distinguished according to differences in the structure of their walls, blood was thought to move more or less to and fro, depending on the needs of organs. Nymmann thought venous sinuses transported blood towards, not away from, the brain. He therefore regarded the point where the four sinuses converge, now still called the *torcular (Herophili)* or wine press, as the site from where blood entered the brain. As a consequence, he reasoned that obstruction at this point might prevent all access of spirits to the brain and so cause apoplexy. He even suggested some evidence:

> It can easily happen that this is occluded; indeed, also in some cadavers after a violent death I found around this region a thick sanguineous fluid, often also mixed with viscous phlegm, solidified and quite compact, very suitable for obstructing it. [. . .] [Because of this obstruction] no blood or spirits can be discharged into the third and fourth sinus; the brain, bereft from the largest supply of spirits, is deprived of all its functions and Apoplexy necessarily follows.[5]

Nymmann cited evidence from autopsies here, but still casually; no report by him is known with clinical details about the illness leading to 'viscous phlegm'. Later on, he mentioned black bile and blood clots as other potentially obstructive substances.[6]

A Collapsing Brain

Yet, Nymmann considered, obstruction of the torcular was not sufficient in itself to explain the full-blown apoplectic syndrome; he went on to present it as a two-stage process:

> No small contribution to this occlusion of vessels and channels is also made by the collapse of the brain. For since this organ is vaulted over and is characterised by certain arches and, as long as it is enriched and made light by the vital spirits, [it is] extended and stretched; its cavities are dilated and much larger than they appear in the dead. However, as soon as the source of spirits is closed off, and the point of confluence of all sinuses is occluded, having been despoiled of the greatest part of the spirits that sustained it, [the brain] does not have the intrinsic power exerted by the spirits and it caves in; once collapsed, it compresses not

[4] Nymmanus (1629), *Tractatus de Apoplexia*, 103.
[5] Nymmanus (1629), *Tractatus de Apoplexia*, 103–4.
[6] Nymmanus (1629), *Tractatus de Apoplexia*, 120–8.

only the cavities and pores, but also the channels of the vessels, including the lower cervical arteries that are otherwise hiding below its base. [...]

From all this it is clear that in the first place by an obstructed and occluded confluence of sinuses, as the primary cause, and in the second place, thereafter and depending on this, by sagging of the brain, which in my opinion always occurs too, as the secondary cause, all sense and mental actions are arrested and abolished in Apoplectics.[7]

In other words, Nymmann assumed that spirits not only have a signalling function, exerted via nerves, but also sustain the scaffolding of the brain, as gas in a balloon. Interestingly, in order to bolster his point of view, he adduced a clinical observation that has failed to be confirmed, if only because his explanation again assumed that veins – of the neck, this time – transported blood towards the brain:

This opinion of mine is in keeping with the swelling of the jugular vessels in the neck of Apoplectics. When these cannot discharge themselves into the sinuses of the brain, the blood and spirits contained in them go back and distend and inflate them.[8]

This is a nice example of how theory can influence observation: a chance observation serves to support an emerging theory and is generalized.[9]

ENTER HARVEY

Praxagoras (*fl.* *c.*300 BCE) had introduced the convention that all vessels attached to the right half of the heart were called 'veins', and those attached to the left half 'arteries'. To solve the problem that the 'artery' between the lungs and the left ventricle had a thin wall, his pupil Herophilus (*c.*325 to *c.*285 BCE) called it the 'vein-like artery'; conversely, the thick-walled vessel between the right ventricle and the lungs was designated as the 'artery-like vein'.[10]

Some five centuries later, Galen already knew the structure and function of the four valves in the heart. Also, he opposed Herophilus' contemporary Erasistratus by claiming that arteries transported not just air, but also blood.[11] Galen's views on the movement of blood, however, rested on four assumptions that have not withstood the test of time.

---

[7] Nymmanus (1629), *Tractatus de Apoplexia*, 105–6.
[8] Nymmanus (1629), *Tractatus de Apoplexia*, 107.
[9] This has been called *Gestaltsehen* (Fleck (1980 [1935]), *Entstehung einer Tatsache*, 121).
[10] Harris (1973), *The Heart*, 179.   [11] Harris (1973), *The Heart*, 342–3.

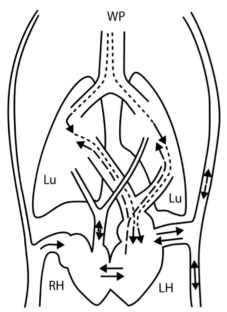

2.1 Directions in which blood and air move in the chest, according to Galen. WP = windpipe; Lu = lungs; RH and LH = right and left chamber of the heart (after van den Berg, 1965).

The Galenic Model of Blood Flow

A first assumption was that air from the lungs enters the left chamber of the heart, via the large 'vein-like artery' (Figure 2.1). Air and blood were then thought to be mixed in the heart, passing between both chambers via 'invisible pores' in the wall (*septum*) between them;[12] from this mixture, intrinsic heat produced the 'vital spirits'. Blood from the right ventricle provided nutrition and cooling to the lungs, whereas the left ventricle supplied especially muscles.

Secondly, Galen situated the origin of all veins in the liver, where he assumed all blood was produced, after preliminary digestion of foodstuffs by the stomach and bowels. Via these veins, the liver carried blood to all the abdominal organs and even to the diaphragm and lower part of the chest.[13]

Thirdly, he supposed that organs and muscles consumed all blood distributed to them by the heart and liver. All that remained, in this idea, was waste material – 'soot'. Its volatile part was eliminated from the left chamber to the lungs via the same route as the incoming air; as black bile, it went to the spleen, and as yellow bile to the large ('hollow') abdominal vein or to the gall bladder; superfluous fluids were excreted via the kidneys.[14]

The fourth difficulty in Galen's version is the 'hydrodynamic' aspect of the movement of blood. Galen only partly used mechanical explanations, such as

[12] Harris (1973), *The Heart*, 305, 308, 334.   [13] Harris (1973), *The Heart*, 325–9.
[14] Harris (1973), *The Heart*, 306, 366.

Box 2.2 William Harvey (1578–1657).

Harvey was the eldest son of a merchant and landowner in Folkestone.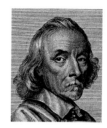
He went to grammar school in Canterbury and received a bursary to
study medicine in Cambridge. In 1599, he went for further studies to
Padua, where he obtained a doctorate three years later. On his return,
he established himself as a private practitioner in London; in the course
of time, he also became a physician on the staff of St Bartholomew's
Hospital (1609) and he was appointed Lecturer in Anatomy at the
Royal College of Physicians (1615). From 1618, he served as one of the
physicians to the king (James I, and after 1625, Charles I) and he carried out diplomatic
missions. Harvey followed King Charles during the civil war between 1642 and 1646;
during the reign of Protestant republicans, he was allowed to resume his anatomical
teaching, but his political role had ended. Harvey died before the restoration of the
monarchy in 1660. Apart from his famous book about circulation (1628), Harvey also
published a treatise on the reproduction of animals (1651).

Source: Portrait courtesy of Wellcome Foundation.

---

heaviness or *horror vacui* – in the same way as suction through a straw replaces
air by fluid, the left chamber of the heart was supposed to suck air from the
lungs via the 'vein-like artery', in the expansion phase of heart action. Yet, for
the most part, the movements of blood in the Galenic model were defined not
in a physical, but in a teleological manner: each organ withdrew specific
components from blood according to its needs.[15] Viewed in this way, it is
the balance between supply and demand that determined the direction of
blood flow in many vessels; unavoidably this implied, to some extent, a back-
and-forth movement (Figure 2.1),[16] or even a two-way traffic.[17]

Experimental Medicine

William Harvey (1578–1657) (Box 2.2) was well aware – as was Galen before
him – that the movement of blood could only be studied in living creatures.
However, his observations in animals led him to a reverse conclusion on the
stages of heart action. The phase in which the heart becomes smaller and more
compact, as well as paler, represented for Harvey the active phase (*systole*), in
which it is emptied. The 'auricles' (upper chambers, now called *atria*, at the
time not regarded part of the heart) contracted slightly earlier than the
ventricles, as in the act of swallowing. Also, the arteries expanded when the

---

[15] Harris (1973), *The Heart*, 329–30.
[16] van den Berg (1965), *Het menselijk Lichaam*, opposite to 40.
[17] Harris (1973), *The Heart*, 367–74, 393–6.

heart contracted.[18] The liver, however, did not move at all.[19] Harvey also performed experiments with a tourniquet in animals: if the vena cava was tied below the heart, the part between the ligature and the heart emptied, while the heart became pale. Conversely, ligation of large arteries resulted in dilatation of not only the artery, but also the heart itself, while it assumed a purple colour.[20]

A pump function of the heart does not necessarily imply circulation, but Harvey had other strings to his bow, perhaps inspired by earlier findings. In fact, some investigators had established, as far as we know independently, that the septum of the heart is impermeable and that blood is forced from the right chamber (ventricle) of the heart into the lungs, where it is mixed with air and subsequently returns to the left ventricle. The first of these was Ibn-al-Nafis from Damascus (thirteenth century);[21] later proponents were the Spanish humanist Michael Servetus (1511–1553) and Realdo Colombo (1515–1559), the successor of Andreas Vesalius in Padua.[22] In addition, Andrea Cesalpino (1525–1603), Professor of Medicine and Botany in Pisa, had argued that the liver should be dethroned as the source of all veins.[23]

Harvey's key argument for his theory of circulation was the amount of blood leaving the heart, by simple calculations. He started by assuming 1000 heartbeats in half an hour (corresponding to a pulse rate of about 33 per minute) and an outflow per heartbeat of between 1 dram (almost 4 grams) and an ounce (about 31 grams). Then the quantity of ejected blood in each half hour would range between more than 10 British pounds weight (almost 4 kilograms) and more than 83 pounds (or about 31 kilograms). It was simply not possible for the liver, Harvey pointed out, to produce such quantities of blood in so short a time.[24] In fact, even the upper margin of Harvey's estimate is conservative: an expelled volume per beat of about 70 ml, with a pulse rate at rest of about 72, corresponds to more than 150 litres per half hour – or about as many kilograms, to follow Harvey's measure of weight.

Another finding in favour of Harvey's theory was that the flow in the superficial veins in the human arm was exclusively directed towards the heart. To demonstrate this phenomenon, Harvey used the discovery of the valves in veins by Fabricius ab Aquapendente (1537–1619), former Professor of Anatomy

[18] Harveius (1628), *De Motu Cordis et Sanguinis*, 22–30.
[19] Harveius (1628), *De Motu Cordis et Sanguinis*, 37.
[20] Harveius (1628), *De Motu Cordis et Sanguinis*, 47–8.
[21] Pagel (1967), *Harvey's Biological Ideas*, 149–50.
[22] Pagel (1967), *Harvey's Biological Ideas*, 137–45, 154–5. Servetus regarded the mixing of blood and air as a metaphor for divine inspiration (O'Malley (1953), *Michael Servetus*, 200–8).
[23] Pagel (1967), *Harvey's Biological Ideas*, 169–89, 200–9.
[24] Harveius (1628), *De Motu Cordis et Sanguinis*, 44–5.

TABLE 2.1 *Professors of anatomy and surgery at the University of Padua, 1537–650*

Name	Lifespan	Tenure
Andries van Wesele (Vesalius)	1514–1564	1537–43
Realdo Colombo	*c.*1515–1559	1544–51
Gabrielle Faloppio	1523–1565	1551–62
Girolamo Fabrici d'Aquapendente	1537–1619	1565–1609
Giulio Casseri	1552–1615	1609–15
Adriaen van den Spiegel (Spigelius)	1578–1625	1616–25
Johann Wesling (Veslingius)	1598–1649	1632–49

in Padua (Table 2.1). By applying a tourniquet to the arm in such a way that it occluded the superficial veins, but not the deeper arteries, he showed that the examiner's finger could move the contents of the swollen veins beyond a valve only in the direction of the shoulder, but not towards the hand. His illustration (Figure 2.2) was the same as that of Fabricius. Yet the Paduan professor had not attributed any other functions to his 'little doors' (*osteoli*) than that of preventing stagnation of blood in the hands and feet.[25] Harvey used it to strengthen his argument that all venous blood eventually returned to the heart.

In his outlook on nature, Harvey was as much an Aristotelian thinker as an experimentalist; he was in search of a complete and, especially purposeful, system:

> Thus, the heart deserves to be called the origin of life and the sun of the Microcosm, in the same way as, on another scale, the sun deserves to be called the Heart of the world. By its power and pulse blood is moved, perfected, invigorated and protected against decay and clotting. That faithful hearth fulfils its function by nourishing, warming and invigorating the entire body. But more about this elsewhere, when I will elaborate on the cause defined as purpose (*causa finalis*) of this movement.[26]

Reception of the Circulation Theory

Reactions to Harvey's *Exercitatio Anatomica* ranged between wary acceptance and militant rejection. Also, other controversial issues compounded the discussion. One was the lingering debate of whether or not the septum of the heart contained pores.[27] Another wrangle was the function of the recently

---

[25] Fabricius ab Aquapendente (1603), *De Venarum Ostiolis*, 1.
[26] Harveius (1628), *De Motu Cordis et Sanguinis*, 42. 'Hearth': Harvey wrote *lar* (household god, fireside).
[27] Maire, ed. (1647), *Disceptationes de Motu Cordis*.

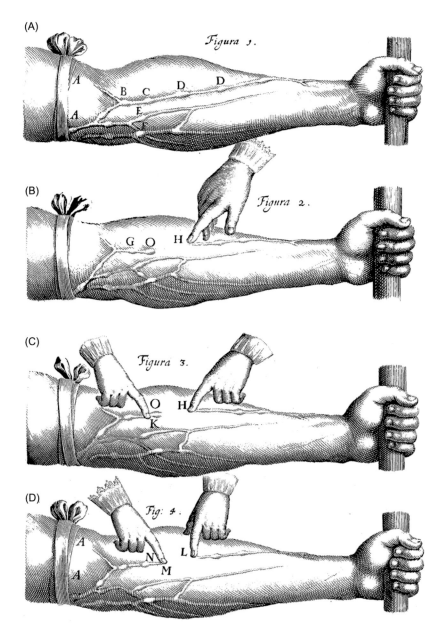

2.2   Illustration of venous blood flowing to the heart, in Harvey's *De Motu Cordis et Sanguinis*. The test person forcefully clenches his fist; a tourniquet (A) has been applied to the upper arm, sufficiently tight to compress the local veins and cause the veins between the tourniquet and the hand to distend, but not so much that the arteries of the upper arm are compressed as well. (A) The sites where the veins are somewhat broader correspond to valves (BCDDEF). (B) The examiner moves his index finger from H beyond O, with gentle pressure; this part of the vein remains empty after the finger returns to H. (C) It is not possible for the finger at K to move blood beyond O in the direction of the hand. (D) If the vein has been emptied from L to M, the vessel refills only by removing the finger at L, not by removing the finger at M.

discovered 'lactic vessels' (lymph vessels).[28] At several universities, professors whose careers had been built on teaching Galenic medicine felt that not only medical tradition was at stake, but also their personal reputation.

Also, the matter became mixed up with religious controversies, especially in the United Provinces. Descartes supported the circulation theory, albeit in a modified form. He thought the intrinsic heat in the heart (*feu sans lumière*) rarefied blood entering the heart and caused the heart to expand. Thus, he saw dilatation (*diastole*) as the active phase of heart action, as in an explosion motor.[29] A struggle between factions of Protestantism resulted in a ban of Cartesian philosophy at the University of Leiden and that of Utrecht.[30] The tone of the debates was often caustic, for example when adherents of Harvey's theory were called *circulatores*,[31] Latin for 'peddlers' or 'mountebanks'.

A full tale of the theory's reception is told elsewhere,[32] but the briefest of summaries might be as follows. Early adopters, apart from members of the Royal College of Physicians of London, were Franciscus Deleboë or Sylvius (1614–1672; Leiden), Jacobus de Back (*c.*1594–1658; Rotterdam), and, after initial hesitations, Johannes Walaeus (1604–1649; Leiden). Others were more gradually won over, for example Vopiscus Fortunatus Plemp (1601–1671; Louvain) and Thomas Bartholinus (1616–1680; Copenhagen). Inveterate adversaries were Emilo Parigiano (1567–1643; Venice), the indefatigable pamphleteer James Primrose (1600–1659; Hull),[33] and the authoritarian Parisian professor Jean Riolan Jr (1577–1657; the only one whose criticisms Harvey deigned worthy of a reply). The debate was to continue until almost the end of the century.

Apoplexy in the Eyes of a Non-believer

Caspar Hofmann (1572–1648) was among those unconvinced by the theory of circulation, even after William Harvey, in 1636, had paid a visit to Altdorf, where Hofmann was Professor of Medicine; the two had been friends as students in Padua.[34] Hofmann remained faithful to some other ancient views, but not to the location of spirits in the ventricles of the brain. In his *Institutiones Medicae*, published in 1645, he wrote the following comments about apoplexy:

> What is its cause? A single one, or several? I have always distinguished a single (proximal) one: obstruction. [...] With regard to the ventricles, something the majority of Physicians believes in, this falls to pieces as a mere phantasy if it is proved that they are not the production site of the

[28] Aselli (1627), *De Lactibus sive lacteis Venis*.
[29] Descartes (1664), *L'Homme et un Traitté de la Formation du Foetus*, 4.
[30] French (1989), Harvey in Holland.
[31] Primirosius (1644), *Antidotum adversus Henrici Regii venenatam Spongiam*, 30.
[32] French (1994), *William Harvey's Natural Philosophy*, 114–285.
[33] Maire, ed. (1647), *Disceptationes de Motu Cordis*.   [34] Wright (2012), *Circulation*, xv–xix.

spirits. Since this has been done before me by great men, [. . .], there is no need of others here. Perhaps only this. Before [the writings of] G. Nymmanus had come into my hands, I regarded the channels of the brain, as our Anatomists call them, as the site that was directly affected. Therefore, although I was first at a distance from him [in opinion], I now see eye to eye with him, and I totally embrace the *Torcular* he put forward.[35]

APOPLEXY AND THE CIRCULATION: A SYNTHESIS

It is time to turn to explanations of apoplexy in which Harvey's idea of the circulation was not merely acknowledged but actually applied, in the sense that the movement of blood is not seen as the passive result of the needs of each organ, but as a separate, continuous force, imposing its impetus on other structures in the body. In 1658, almost thirty years after Nymmann's treatise, when the battles in medical circles about the revolutionary theory were still raging, another book on apoplexy appeared in Schaffhausen, under the title *Anatomical Observations from the Corpses of Persons taken away by Apoplexy, with a Discourse about its Site of Affection.*[36] The book's author, who was to have considerable influence on interpretations of apoplexy in subsequent generations of physicians, was Johann Jakob Wepfer (1620–1695) (Box 2.3), a city physician of Schaffhausen.[37]

After a dedication to the Council of Senators of the Republic of Schaffhausen and a preface to the readership, Wepfer began by recounting four case histories of patients. Of each patient, he gave full clinical details up to the time of death, followed by his personal observations at autopsy. Only then did he present his conclusions about the causes of apoplexy; he explicitly related them to the circulation of blood, comparing his opinions with those of earlier authors. His extensive treatise (over 300 pages in octavo) is styled as a continuous narrative, without partition in chapters; it almost seems as if Wepfer was developing his arguments as he wrote. The only 'signposting' is the use of larger type for some main issues. Nevertheless, it is possible to distinguish five main sections in his text, despite occasional overlaps.

In the first section of the book, Wepfer rides roughshod over the rearguard of believers in the Galenic model of brain function and apoplexy; he then presents a detailed anatomical study of the arterial system of the brain. In each of the three later parts, he discusses a different type of apoplexy. For all three

---

[35] Hofmann (1645), *Institutionum medicarum Libri sex,* 431.
[36] Wepfer (1658), *Observationes anatomicae.*   [37] Eichenberger (1969), *Johann Jakob Wepfer.*

Box 2.3 Johann Jakob Wepfer (1620–1695).

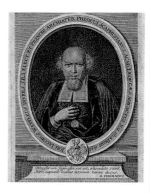

Wepfer was born in 1620, in Schaffhausen, Switzerland, as the eldest child of the judge Georg Michael Wepfer; his mother's maiden name was Stokar. Johann studied medicine in Strasbourg and Basle, graduating in 1644. He spent the following three years in Italy, mainly in Padua; his tutors included Johannes Wesling (1598–1649) from Minden and Thomas Bartholinus (1616–1680) from Copenhagen.

On his return, Wepfer obtained in 1647 his doctorate, at the University of Basle, with a thesis on palpitations of the heart. Soon afterwards, he was appointed physician to the city of Schaffhausen. This office, shared with one or two colleagues, involved medical care for the citizens of the city, at home or in the local hospital, and also for the convents in a larger area. Other tasks included giving advice to the court of justice on medical matters, examining candidate surgeons, overseeing pharmacists, and, importantly, performing autopsies. In 1650, he married Barbara Rink; they had eight children, five of whom survived to adulthood. As Wepfer's reputation increased, he was consulted by the aristocracy of the independent counties in what is now southwestern Germany. A spirited advocate of post-mortem dissection as a means to increase medical knowledge, he stipulated that his own body should also be dissected after his death. The posthumous edition of his *Observationes* (1727) recorded his terminal illness – heart failure – and the findings at autopsy, with an engraving of his diseased aorta.

Wepfer systematically recorded case histories. His correspondence and manuscripts amount to almost 12,000 handwritten pages. These were bought in 1774 by the University of Leiden, where they are still archived. Wepfer is especially famous for his two books on apoplexy (1658 and 1675). During his lifetime, he also published a book on the use and abuse of hemlock (1679); other collections appeared posthumously.

Source: Portrait courtesy of Wellcome Foundation.

---

forms, he offers dynamic explanations, with blood and blood vessels as the main factors; there is no longer a place in his thinking for phlegm or bile.[38]

Driving out the Ghost of Galen

The turmoil of opinion following upon William Harvey's new theory makes clear that traditional interpretations of Galen's texts were still common in Wepfer's time. An indirect measure of the popularity of the old model is the vigorous and often sarcastic phrasing Wepfer used in castigating time-honoured assumptions. Three notions he attacked in particular. Foremost was the *rete mirabile*, the alleged network of blood vessels at the base of the brain, where the vital spirits from the heart were believed to be honed into

---

[38] Wepfer (1658), *Observationes anatomicae*, 274–7.

animated spirits. Secondly, according to ancient doctrine, the cerebral ventricles drew these animated spirits from the network and further perfected or at least stored them. Thirdly, the ventricles were regarded as the pathway through which the animated spirits reached the nerves at the base of the brain and the spinal cord.

It is not necessary to pile Pelion upon Ossa and reproduce the multitude of arguments with which Wepfer demolished these beliefs.[39] He was happy to find support for his criticisms in the writings of his former fellow student Caspar Hofmann,[40] despite their disagreement about the circulation of blood. The favourite target in Wepfer's attacks on the old guard was Jean Riolan the younger (1577–1657), a highly influential Professor of Medicine in Paris and staunch Galenist. Apart from didactic texts, such as his own textbook of anatomy,[41] Riolan had published a volume with criticisms of seven other anatomists and physicians, among whom were Bauhin, Bartholinus, and Hofmann.[42] In the following passage, Wepfer counters Riolan's argument against Hofmann's opinion that the animated spirits travelled to the nerves via the brain tissue, and not via the ventricles:

> For he [Hofmann] stumbled particularly over the issue how in fact the animated spirits, dissolved in the pool of the ventricles, can pass into the nerves? A problem Riolanus thinks to have solved by questioning Hofmann on how the animated spirits produced from the vital ones are diffused in the substance of the brain and subsequently pass into the nerves? But what if someone would question Riolanus about the manner in which the animated spirits are distributed through all the nerves – faster than the spoken word? The matter would be concluded. For it is certain that something can be dispersed in a moment from the brain to the nerves, whether spirits or whatever kind of ray, somehow related to rays from the sun. If passage is permitted through nerves [that are] denser than the brain, why not also through the brain? And what can impede its diffusion through the brain when nothing delays it in healthy nerves? If therefore nothing impedes their diffusion through the substance of the brain, why can't they be propagated from the brain to the nerves and to the entire body? After all, the nerves are continuations of the brain; together they even form a single organ.[43]

The discussion is speculative on both sides, but one cannot help admiring Wepfer for the emphasis he puts on the lightning speed of the signals travelling through the brain and nerves.

---

[39] Wepfer (1658), *Observationes anatomicae*, 20–86, 44–7, and 141–4.
[40] Hofmann (1645), *Institutionum medicarum Libri sex*, 146–50.
[41] Riolan (1649a), *Encheiridium anatomicum et pathologicum*.
[42] Riolan (1649b), *Opuscula anatomica nova*.   [43] Wepfer (1658), *Observationes anatomicae*, 131.

Apoplexy and Extravasated Blood: The First Clinico-anatomical Reports

Here follows one of Wepfer's four case histories. The translation is unabridged, to do justice to the accuracy of his reporting. The other three patients follow later, in abridged form.

> *Barbara Zuberin,* fairly close to seventy years of age, spent almost the entire course of her life as a servant; she had married in old age and had somehow got through life. Widowed, she was admitted to the Hospital. She was of average build, and as far as I know she had not been much stricken by disease, except that for some years her eyesight had begun to deteriorate; at some stage she was almost completely deprived of vision, yet she regained it to some extent, almost without medical assistance; then the malady further deteriorated. However, she never became totally blind. In both eyes obvious early signs of grey cataract could be seen. For several months the people around her had already observed forewarnings of apoplexy, when her speech repeatedly halted; yet this defect of language soon disappeared.
>
> On January 10 of the year 1657, on a day of full moon, at three o'clock in the afternoon, while she was spinning wool with her companions in a healthy state, as they believed, she suddenly lost the use of speech and was seen to lean forward. She was soon taken to her bed by helpers; during that walk it was noticed that on the right side she still moved her foot, lifted her hand to her head and produced some words, though barely comprehensible. Suddenly, however, she lost all sensation and purposeful movement, with preservation of respiration (though soon afterwards this became laboured) and of the pulse; her face had a red colour. Few remedies were administered, because after the attack she was no longer able to swallow. She expired on the same day, at six in the afternoon.[44]

The style of this story may not sound unusual to modern physicians. Yet it is striking how much Wepfer's account differs from most, if not all, such reports in the previous century. Even in Wepfer's time, however, physicians used to jump to conclusions. This great variety in the reporting of clinical features is confirmed by a vast collection of dissection reports, entitled *Sepulchretum*, appearing in 1679. The editor Théophile Bonet (1620–1689) had become confined to his writing desk in Geneva by progressive hearing loss; he collected autopsy reports, on many of which he wrote commentaries (*scholia*). Wepfer's stories stand out, whereas, for example, Charles Drelincourt (1633–1697), Professor of Medicine in Leiden, did not use more than a single sentence for each of his two cases of apoplexy.[45]

Wepfer's report is even more detailed with regard to dissection of the brain. After describing *in extenso* how he had adopted Varolio's method of removing

---

[44] Wepfer (1658), *Observationes anatomicae*, 5–6.   [45] Bonetus (1679), *Sepulchretum*, 86.

the brain from the cadaver, he went further than all his predecessors by examining its inner structures, searching for an explanation of apoplexy:

> Having taken out the brain, I removed the thick membrane that was still covering it: it appeared that the right half of the brain was entirely covered with blood, on its upper, posterior, inferior – but not as far as the base – and anterior surface, to the front. The brain was soft in these places and some fluctuating kind of fluid could be distinctly detected by palpation. The process of removal had produced a tear on this side, from which a clot of pitch-black blood protruded, with the size of a nutmeg. Having inserted my finger, I gradually widened the tear with a small knife. I found a wide cavity, in front almost to the forepart, upwards almost to the falciform body and the third sinus;[46] at the back it extended to the midline, at a lower level even beyond it. The length of this cavity or abnormal hole exceeded eight inches,[47] the breadth four, and the depth two-and-a-half inches. It contained a blood clot resembling a hen's egg, apart from other smaller clots and fluid blood, in weight about eight ounces, or almost an entire pound. At first, we thought this was the lateral ventricle; but by searching more accurately we found that this cavity was not the ventricle, or some portion of it, but separate and abnormal, created by blood that had burst outside its vessels. [It originated] from some branch that had ruptured, a twig from a large branch of the anterior division of the carotid artery. [...]
>
> Quite a few of its branches clearly entered the substance of the brain, in more than one place. And that indeed one or more branches of this artery had ruptured in this place we could observe clearly and without doubt, for when we investigated its course on this side, we found that the primary branch and its ramifications, at its origin as well as in the entire remaining course, was completely depleted of blood; all other arteries looked different, the posterior arteries on this side as well as some anterior [vessels] not originating from this branch.[48]

The Impulse of the Blood

When Wepfer's depiction of the abnormalities in the brain of Barbara Zuberin had arrived at the vessel he presumed to have ruptured, and before adding his findings on other parts of the brain, he could no longer suppress the urge to explain how this extravasation was related to the circulation of blood, a theory he firmly believed in and for which he even used an abbreviation (CS, for *circulatio sanguinis*):

> Therefore, I recognised that by the continuous pressure of blood, after one or two of these arteries had ruptured, and blood had gushed into a

---

[46] Now called the superior sagittal sinus.
[47] The Roman '*uncia*' ('twelfth part') corresponds to about 2.5 centimetres.
[48] Wepfer (1658), *Observationes anatomicae*, 6–11.

deeper convolution, more and more space in the convolution had been taken up, just as one wave is pushed forward by another. And while the deeper part of the convolutions was pressed down by the continuous pulse of invading blood, the tissue elsewhere, tender, delicate and soft as it was, gave way to the impulse of the blood, was destroyed and easily gave way to this extent, not unlike what happens in an aneurysm, except that such a cavity is formed faster in the brain, because of its softness, than in any other part [of the body]. The outer surface of the convolutions remained intact, since the *pia mater* preserved it, by securing it and holding it together, so to speak. Also, the bottom of this cavity was not ruptured, by the presence of the roof or rather fornix of the right ventricle, which is more like marrow and firmer than the more flaccid tissue of the convolutions in the cerebral cortex, as Dr Bartholinus calls it.[49]

Wepfer also addressed the question of why arteries could burst. One category of causes, he proposed, in agreement with existing beliefs, was the condition of the blood. To begin with, its overall quantity might be excessive; among the examples he cited were women who stopped menstruating, or the patient described by Fabry (see Chapter 1) who fell victim to apoplexy when he no longer had nosebleeds. Alternatively, the blood might be too thin, for example in persons who ingested too much fluids and too little solid food. Apart from the properties of blood, a vessel might give way by lively heart action, in turn resulting from, for instance, physical exercise or mental agitation, or the heart forcefully beating to overcome an obstruction in a small artery of the brain. Finally, Wepfer supposed, the vessel wall might sometimes be damaged by corrosive fluids or by smallpox.[50]

Three More Clinico-anatomical Observations

Barbara Zuberin's fatal haemorrhage within the substance of the brain was to become a milestone in the history of neurology. It supported Varolio's still contested opinion that animated spirits reach the nerves via the brain tissue, not via its ventricles. Her case was the second of the four histories constituting the beginning of Wepfer's book, though the most recent to have occurred. All four dissections took place within a period of eighteen months,[51] a remarkable coincidence, given the scarcity of autopsies in general, let alone in patients who had died of apoplexy. It is no wonder that Wepfer was fascinated by the subject. The three other case histories follow below, in shortened form.

---

[49] Wepfer (1658), *Observationes anatomicae*, 9–10. Thomas Bartholinus (Bertelsen; 1616–1680) had been one of Wepfer's teachers in Padua.

[50] Wepfer (1658), *Observationes anatomicae*, 236–40.

[51] Wepfer (1658), *Observationes anatomicae*, 1–19.

Johann-Jakob Kenzingâ-Brisgojus (patient 1), approximately 45 years of age, was a monk at the monastery of Freiburg; as an adolescent, he had fled from the ravages of the Thirty Years War. Apart from chronic gout, he was healthy, though it was said he preferred wine to solid food. On a November morning, having assisted the abbot at mass, he retired to his cell; a few hours later, he was found on the floor, completely senseless; Wepfer was called, but despite interventions, he died the following afternoon. At autopsy, Wepfer detected no wounds on the skull, even after shaving. After incision of the hard membrane, he found much sanguineous fluid around the brain, as well as a large collection of blood at the base of the brain and in all ventricles.

Anna Baltherin (patient 3), well over 60 years of age and a mother, had from childhood worked in the local vineyards, before functioning as a midwife and wise woman. One evening in July, she had gone out to collect lightwood but failed to return. The next day, she was found dead near a hedge in the woods, with a superficial wound at the left temple. The local authorities asked Wepfer to perform a dissection, which he carried out in the presence of his younger brother Johann, also a physician.[52] It turned out that the wound had not even penetrated the skin. The brain looked normal on first inspection, but after it had been taken out, it transpired that its base was covered with blood, mostly on the right side; the ventricles were filled with yellowish serum.

The fourth patient with apoplexy showed abnormalities other than haemorrhage.

BRAIN HAEMORRHAGE AND APOPLEXY ARE NOT SYNONYMOUS

'Serous Apoplexy'

The fourth patient *Jakob Reutinger Viterdinga* was exceptional on two counts. The first peculiarity was the finding on dissection of the brain. The abnormality consisted of an excess of serum, not of blood. Wepfer's interpretation, 'serous apoplexy', was to be taken up by many other generations of physicians before it disappeared from the nosological classification, some 150 years later. This new diagnosis will be the main subject of a later chapter, with the complete case history and comparable observations of later physicians.

The other exceptional aspect of Jakob Reutinger's story is clinical: the mode of onset. As will be told in detail later, Reutinger had already been severely ill when he lapsed into an 'apoplectic state' – in other words, a sequence of events that nowadays would not have been classified as a 'stroke'. Why did Wepfer

[52] Eichenberger (1969), *Johann Jakob Wepfer*, 12.

decide to apply the diagnosis of apoplexy, despite the fact that it occurred in the course of a protracted illness?

Stretching the Diagnosis, through Reversal of Reasoning

Beyond doubt, Wepfer would not have applied the term 'apoplexy' to other progressive illnesses, for example patients with fever whose consciousness became more and more clouded in the course of days and then died. His diagnosis must be traced to the local changes in the brain that had caused an illness to change into a state of unresponsiveness.

This conceptual turn is important, because it heralded subsequent developments in the definition of apoplexy. According to Galen's ancient definition, apoplexy consisted of a set of three phenomena: sudden collapse, loss of sensation and motion, and preservation of breathing and heart action. Wepfer investigated the brain of Barbara Zuberin, who had shown all three features, and found haemorrhage in the substance of the brain. He also found blood at the surface of the brain in two other patients who had died after the same set of phenomena. Then he found a different abnormality, that is an excess of serum, in the brain of Jakob Reutinger, who had also shown loss of sensation and motion with preserved respiration and pulse, but without collapsing out of the blue.

Thus, Wepfer must have reasoned, apoplexy was a more complex disease than just haemorrhage, since even in the absence of a sudden onset, an excessive amount of serum could apparently cause loss of sensation and motion, while respiration and pulse continued. By drawing this conclusion, he had reversed the direction of reasoning. What had started as a question of how a set of phenomena could be explained by lesions in the brain had become the reverse process, at least partly: how lesions in the brain defined the clinical features.

Two factors probably contributed to Wepfer's 'reverse thinking'. To begin with, an excess of serum is akin to the ancient notion of viscous phlegm. 'Serum' was a term that could be applied to any fluid that was more or less clear; later the term proved interchangeable with 'water' and 'lymph'. Secondly, no less important, 'loss of sensation and movement' in a person who still showed breathing and heart action apparently was, for some at least, the pivotal element in the phenomenological definition of apoplexy.

Loss of Sensation as the Key Feature

How absence of sensation and movement should be defined or ascertained was not strictly clear and resulted in ambiguous interpretations, as discussed in Chapter 1. What was actually implied in this definition was the absence of reactions, that is, absence of movements signifying that the patient could feel, see, or hear. Similarly implied was the absence of 'internal sensation', or thinking, which connected external sensation with movement. Terms like 'complete loss of sensation' and 'senselessness' were used to indicate this cardinal feature of apoplexy. Previously in this book, the more modern, but equally imprecise, term 'unconsciousness' has been used.

In reality, the absence of wakefulness was – and is – not an all-or-nothing phenomenon. The recognition of this problem led to the introduction of new terms to describe the degree in which the 'flame of consciousness' had been reduced: carus, coma, lethargy, somnolence, stupor, etc. In medical textbooks from the seventeenth century, some of these states were distinguished from the loss of sensation in apoplexy, but the difference was more theoretical than practical. Medicine kept struggling with abstractions of this kind until the end of the twentieth century, as we shall see later. In seventeenth-century practice, the term 'loss of sensation', for patients who responded very little or not at all to whatever stimuli, falsely implied that it was self-explanatory, whereas in fact the expression escaped definition.

Wepfer must have been intrigued by the question of what part of the brain was the seat of awareness. He was not the only one. The same problem intrigued his contemporary Thomas Willis (1621–1675), working in Oxford and later in London. Willis, who will reappear later in this chapter (Box 2.4), regarded the corpus callosum as the central structure where all animated spirits converged and from where they were again distributed.[53]

It remained an enigma for Wepfer why *all* mental functions had been abolished in Barbara Zuberin, whereas the haemorrhage had affected only part of the brain. He found this easier to understand when haemorrhage occurred at the base of the brain, near the origin of the nerves, as had happened in his first and third cases.

> From the second case history [*Barbara Zuberin*] it is obvious that a rather extensive excretion of blood within the anterior convolution has produced apoplexy. [. . .] It deserves further study why abolition of all animated actions ensued, very quickly causing death, although the other part of the brain and the cerebellum appeared healthy on inspection. [. . .] I cannot extricate myself in any other way than by saying that, given the severe lesion of the deeper and nobler parts of the brain, also the other, admittedly unharmed [half] becomes immediately affected in concert. However, I am well aware that in apoplexies that are lethal as well as in those that end up in complete or at least some degree of health only one of the two sides is occupied by the proximal cause, since these usually begin with hemiplegia. [. . .] Now, in which way this concurrence [of the

---

[53] Willis (1664), *Cerebri Anatome*, 128–9.

Box 2.4 Thomas Willis (1621–1775).

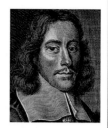

Willis was born in Wiltshire, as the first child of a farmer and steward, after whom he was named. Several more boys and girls were to follow. Around 1630, the family moved to a village near Oxford, where his mother Rachel Howell had inherited a small estate; she died soon afterwards. Thomas Junior received a solid classical education at a private school in Oxford; at the age of 16, he matriculated at the university. Soon after his graduation as Master of Arts in 1642, the Civil War broke out and his father and stepmother succumbed to epidemic fever. Willis became responsible for two farms, as well as for his siblings and stepbrothers. After two years in the Royalist army, which was eventually defeated in 1646, Willis returned to university. At the end of that same year, he became a Bachelor in Medicine, with a licence to practise after merely a few months of training.

Willis started by touring the markets of neighbouring villages. He read much and became aware that his knowledge was insufficient. He felt inspired by the chemical writings of the Flemish physician Joan Batista van Helmont (1579–1644). Despite some shyness and a stammer, Willis became involved with an informal group of academics dedicated to 'experimental philosophy', including the flamboyant physician William Petty (1623–1687) and the young Christopher Wren (1632–1723); later members were Robert Hooke (1635–1703), Richard Lower (1631–1691), and Robert Boyle (1627–1691). When Willis' practice had sufficiently grown, he married Mary Fell in 1655. After the restoration of the monarchy in 1660, he was nominated as Professor of Natural Philosophy at the University of Oxford. He was among the founding members of the Royal Society in London. With Richard Lower, he performed dissections of the brains of humans and of several animal species; he published extensively. After the Great Fire of London (1666), he moved to the capital; his advice was much sought, and his practice no longer allowed him to participate in scientific activities. He died at the age of 54 and was buried in Westminster Cathedral.

---

two symptoms] occurs is something about which I suspend my judgement for the time. A more conscientious study and the work of others will perhaps disclose the truth for me.[54]

So Wepfer remained puzzled over why some patients with hemiplegia subsequently became 'apoplectic' and others did not. At any rate, by distinguishing between hemiplegia and apoplexy, he made it clear once more that he regarded loss of consciousness as the essential feature of apoplexy.

Apoplexy Defined by Unconsciousness

Once the term apoplexy can be applied to every more or less unexpected episode of unconsciousness, regardless of whether the patient had already been

---

[54] Wepfer (1658), *Observationes anatomicae*, 231–3.

ill before, the diagnostic spectrum is considerably expanded. This is indeed what happened, to judge from several case series after Wepfer's initial publication of 1658. These included not only rapid worsening of long-standing illnesses, but also external causes such as toxic fumes and head injuries by blows, bullets, or falls from a height or down stairs.

A reprint of Wepfer's book appeared in 1675. It also contained 17 new histories, all with fatal outcome and followed by dissection. Several of these observations were borrowed from colleagues, but Wepfer added his own comments after each report.[55] Of the seventeen new cases, the cause of the 'apoplectic state' was head injury in eleven; in the remaining six, it represented an exacerbation of a pre-existing illness. In this subgroup of six, three patients were categorized as 'serous apoplexy' – to be discussed later.

A few years later, Théophile Bonet, introduced above, published his vast compendium of post-mortem investigations, in two folio volumes.[56] The diseases included all parts of the body. After Bonet's death, Jean Manget published a new edition in 1700, with fresh additions.[57] Lastly, at least as far as Wepfer's work is concerned, two posthumous publications appeared in the early eighteenth century. The first, in 1724, was another reprint of the 1658 treatise, supplemented with almost 40 newly collected cases of apoplexy from 'renowned physicians', as well as most examples of apoplexy already listed by Bonet and Manget.[58] Finally, in 1727, Wepfer's descendants published his unpublished observations on a variety of diseases of the head, including 10 cases of apoplexy, with or without dissection.[59]

Table 2.2 shows all the cases of apoplexy that have been listed in Wepfer's two books and in the four later collections. A quick look at the top row suffices to understand that cases of 'spontaneous apoplexy', without preceding illness, followed by death and autopsy, make up only a small minority. The authors of a recent article on apoplexy in the Bonet/Manget collection were understandably baffled by the 'inclusiveness contributing to the great variety of pathologic findings in those deemed to have died of apoplexy'.[60]

The table also shows how unique Wepfer's first series of four patients actually was. An important factor is Wepfer's persistence in obtaining permission for dissection, 'with entreaty and bribery' (*prece et pretio*).[61] He made good use of his influence among the nobility and clergy; also he had the good fortune to be backed by the senate of Schaffhausen, to whom he expressed profuse thanks in the preface of his first book:

[55] Wepfer (1675), *Observationes anatomicae, cum Auctuario*.   [56] Bonetus (1679), *Sepulchretum*.
[57] Mangetus (1700), *Theophili Boneti Sepulchretum*.
[58] Wepfer (1724), *Historiae Apoplecticorum*.
[59] Wepfer (1727), *Observationes de Affectibus Capitis*.
[60] Schutta and Howe (2006), Seventeenth century concepts of 'apoplexy'.
[61] Wepfer (1675), *Observationes anatomicae, cum Auctuario*, 397.

TABLE 2.2 *Published reports of apoplexy in the seventeenth century (repetitions omitted)*

	Wepfer 1658	Wepfer 1675	Bonet 1679[a]	Manget 1700	'Wepfer' 1724	'Wepfer' 1727
Spontaneous apoplexy; autopsy	3		4 (4)	2	1[b]	
Spontaneous apoplexy, death; no autopsy			4[c](1)	3	10	3
Sudden death				2		
Apoplexy, survival					10	4
Head injury, drowning, lightning		11	14 (4)	3	2	1
Intoxication			1 (0)			
History complicated or unclear	1	6	24 (0)	3	5	2
General comment (no specific cases)			9 (4)		11	

[a] Between brackets: number from the sixteenth century (also included in total).
[b] Performed early in the eighteenth century.
[c] Including one autopsy in which the issue was absence of apoplexy.

Anatomists bestow even more glittering honour on this dwelling of the divine image and abode of the Holy Ghost,[62] when they openly display a part of our body by skilful dissection. In doing so they admire the indescribable wisdom and immeasurable goodness of God. At the same time, they teach in which way the health of those alive (by far the most important of all benefits that humans can obtain in this world) can be preserved – or restored if it has been lost. It seems as if this good fortune to entire Mankind is begrudged them by those who, led by whatever religion, maliciously proclaim that any Corpse must be buried intact, while they themselves are destined to become food for worms. They exert themselves as much as they can to forbid it, so that people who were good for nothing during life are also of no use when they are dead. The task may be foul and for some it may seem repulsive to drench one's hands in blood and gore, but this filth can be rinsed off with a little water. More repulsive and despicable than anatomical material is ignorance, which breeds a disgrace to Physicians and Surgeons that neither the Rhine nor the Ocean can wash away.[63]

Brain Haemorrhage, but No Apoplexy

Given that Wepfer, and others after him, regarded the loss of mental actions as the key feature of apoplexy, not only necessary but sometimes even sufficient

---

[62] Refers to the *Heiliggeistspital* in Schaffhausen.
[63] Wepfer (1658), *Observationes anatomicae*, 5–6.

for the diagnosis, the corollary is to rule out patients with 'only' sudden hemiplegia while consciousness remained. Many physicians therefore classified such events as 'paralysis', not as 'apoplexy'. Among them was Wepfer's contemporary Thomas Willis, who described an episode of cerebral haemorrhage without unresponsiveness:

> A young Englishman with a sanguineous temperament, generally quite fit, was sitting in an armchair after a rather copious meal and overindulgent wine drinking, when he experienced numbness of the right hand; because of this he dropped the glove he happened to be holding. Subsequently raising himself and trying to walk, he felt weakness of the upper and lower leg on the same side. Soon afterwards he lapsed in some sort of mental dullness and sluggishness, but without apoplexy; for he stayed always alert, properly responded to questions, though slowly and hesitating, and obeyed commands.[64]

The patient eventually died. On dissection, Willis confirmed the relation between hemiplegia and certain brain regions, especially the *corpus striatum*, or 'striped body', the area of grey matter between the insular cortex and the thalamus. In earlier publications, he had noted that the structures he called 'striped bodies' (*corpora striata*) connected the brain with the brainstem, through ascending pathways to convey sensory impressions and through descending pathways to communicate with muscles.[65] Also he confirmed his view of the brain substance, and particularly the *corpus callosum*, as the medium of mental activity:

> When the head was opened, the anterior cavity of the brain was filled with blood, partly fluid and partly solidified and in clumps, together with an excess of serum. Hence, it was easy to understand that this overflow, by compressing the *corpus striatum* and narrowing its pores and openings, impeded the flow of spirits into the nervous extension on that side, resulting in weakness of the corresponding limbs. Since the *thalamus opticus* was also compressed where it joins the corpus striatum, the eye on that side was deprived of sight. Moreover, the *corpus callosum*, vaulting over that cavity, was somewhat wedged; this explains the dullness and sluggishness of the main functions of the mind, yet without overturning or disordering them at all. From this example it seems plain that disturbances of that kind result from damage inflicted on the *substance of the brain* and its inherent spirits, and hardly at all from filling of the ventricles, as I have often indicated elsewhere.[66]

---

[64] Willis (1672), *De Anima Brutorum*, 301.

[65] Willis (1664), *Cerebri Anatome*, 156–8; Meyer and Hierons (1964), Willis' views on the corpus striatum.

[66] Willis (1672), *De Anima Brutorum*, 301.

Attentive readers will have noticed that Willis did not use the terms 'left' and 'right', perhaps to dodge the issue of 'crossed paralysis', a subject to be discussed further below. Another brief digression on the causes of paralysis is unavoidable, because it sheds light on later insights. Willis had noted before, in his book on brain anatomy, that sudden paralysis could be associated with non-haemorrhagic changes of the *corpus striatum*:

> [The function] seems to be established with even more certainty by some observations about these striate bodies, from the manner in which they are affected in 'Paralytic Disease'. For several times, when I dissected the bodies of people who had passed away after long-standing paralysis and severe inactivity of nerves, I always found these bodies less firm than other regions, and coloured like the dregs of olive oil.[67]

Before a discussion of other potential causes of apoplexy, especially since illnesses with a gradual onset became included, there follows a selection of the most relevant and informative case reports of haemorrhagic apoplexy in the remainder of the seventeenth century; these are all represented in the first row of Table 2.2.

MORE REPORTS OF APOPLEXY BY INTRACEREBRAL HAEMORRHAGE

Brain Haemorrhage and Nervous Complaints

Thirty years after the publication of Wepfer's first treatise, another example of apoplexy with intracerebral haemorrhage appeared in the *Philosophical Transactions of the Royal Society*, recorded by Bristol's William Cole.[68] The event had occurred six years before; later the author identified the patient as Lady Pakington:[69]

> A most distinguished Woman [... *description of her nobility and virtue*] had suffered for many years past of hypochondriac (as they are commonly called) and hysterical symptoms. In recent years bleeding from the nose had been added to these [symptoms], sometimes so profuse that her life was almost in danger. In order to avert the danger of diseases and of haemorrhage, she had, among other things, frequently taken recourse to venesection (I do not know whether through advice of herself or of physicians). [*More episodes of nose bleeding, the last on the day before she died.*]
>
> After she had gone to bed in the evening, she was suddenly seized by immense headache; because of this she gave orders (while her speech

---

[67] Willis (1664), *Cerebri Anatome*, 158–9.
[68] Hirsch (1884–8), *Biographisches Lexikon*, vol. II, 53.
[69] Cole (1689), *The Late Frequency of Apoplexies*, 36.

started to falter) that a surgeon should be summoned immediately, in order to draw blood. However, he lived a thousand passes away and could not call before the very Noble woman had departed from the living.

Charged with the dissection of the body, I invited the company of the most learned Dr Tomkyns. [... *The internal organs showed no relevant abnormalities*] When the skull was opened, the cause of the sudden calamity plainly presented itself. For the blood vessels running along the membranes (especially the *tender* one) of the right half of the brain were much swollen with blood; when these had been cut off from this part of the brain, a large amount of serous blood flowed out. When this had been evacuated and the substance of the brain had been incised with a knife, a large clot of coagulated blood presented itself; it weighed one and a half ounces and at this site it had inevitably produced a wide cavity.[70]

Incidentally, though Dr Cole and his colleague identified the cause of death, they were somewhat surprised not to have found an explanation for the noble lady's long-standing nervous symptoms; they decided her nervous fluids must have been corrupted in a way that escaped the eye. The phrase about the swollen vessels reflects the notion of 'fullness' that was to pervade many explanations of apoplexy; this same idea generated the practice of venesection, as a curative or preventive measure, in all classes of society.[71]

Two Episodes in the Same Patient

In 1685, the year of Cole's report, a related observation was made in the German-speaking countries; nine years later, it appeared in print, in the annals of the 'Imperial Leopoldine Academy', a continental equivalent of the insular *Philosophical Transactions*. Manget included the case in the second edition of Bonet's *Sepulchretum*, as one of the few instances of spontaneous brain disease (Table 2.2).[72] Its author was Johann Conrad Brunner (1653–1727). Having studied in Strasbourg and Paris, Brunner settled in Dießenhofen, near Schaffhausen; in 1686, he became Professor of Medicine in Heidelberg and a personal physician of the local aristocracy.[73] But perhaps the most memorable peculiarity is that he was Wepfer's son-in-law.

Anna Oberhäuser, wife of a carpenter and fellow-citizen of ours, 47 years of age, of normal stature, full posture, pale face and sanguineous-phlegmatic constitution, used to take great care of her skin. After marriage, she had triplets in her first childbed (one of them still survives);

[70] Cole (1685), *Phaenomena in cadavere*.   [71] Wepfer (1658), *Observationes anatomicae*, 12.
[72] Mangetus (1700), *Theophili Boneti Sepulchretum*, 139–43.
[73] Sträuli (1979), *Die Ärztefamilie Brunner aus Diessenhofen*.

thereafter she had twelve more children. The confinement was often difficult, and the discharges after childbirth very persistent. She managed her household properly, was virtuous and attentive, while she was not very bright and means at home were modest. In December 1680 she suffered a severe apoplectic attack: she was speechless and her entire right side was deprived of sensation and motion.

[*The story continues with Brunner's treatment and the partial recovery of her right hemiplegia; yet she became negligent and wasteful, and given to drink. One morning, five years after the initial apoplexy, she collapsed on the stairs and did not respond to her children.*] I was called and was soon present. Her limbs shuddered and shook as if by cold; her respiration was irregular, with grunting. She could not be stimulated by shouting or pinching to give a sign of feeling or understanding; when I pinched her more powerfully, she moved the limb I had pinched in a disorderly manner, on the right as well as on the left side. The pulse was rather fast at the beginning, soon slow and sparse, finally weak and languid. Also, the respiration seemed to be constrained. [*She died about one hour after this new attack.*]

Dr Brunner, though permitted to perform an autopsy in the evening of the same day, must have had some misgivings about the opportunity to examine the brain in detail:

In order not to be bothered or disturbed by unwelcome anxieties of the relatives I cut the brain loose from its nerves and arteries, which were all normal, took it out, enveloped by the pia mater, and secretly gave orders to those present that it should be brought to my home. [*There, having noted that the surface of the brain was intact, he tied the stump of one carotid and injected green wax via the other, which allowed him a clear view of the arterial system. He then started cutting the brain, piecemeal.*] In the hind part above the right ventricle, I hit upon an oblong, narrow cavity with the size of a nutmeg, in which some fluid stagnated. The adjoining brain substance showed a dark, yellowish colour, difficult to cut; it seemed to have hardened into this firm consistency some time ago. In the same hemisphere I found another small cavity, at the site where the carotid separates into different branches; in this one also some watery fluid stagnated and it was somewhat difficult to cut, like parchment. A third small cavity, similar to the other two, was found under the *corpus striatum* on the same side; this one was closed and was already sticking together by glue in between, but I could still easily separate [the walls] again; this one was yellow and again difficult to cut.

The right ventricle was full of serous blood, while the left one also overflowed with it. The site from where it erupted was halfway between the *thalamus opticus* and the *corpus striatum* in the right hemisphere, where it had made a tear. Indeed, I found in the substance of the thalamus itself a wide hiatus or fissure, produced by the force and impetus of blood, and inside it a blood clot with the size of the egg of a dove or a chicken. When the clot had been washed away, the substance of the brain was

lacerated all around it as well as torn and disrupted down to the bifurcation of the optic nerves.[74]

Interlude: The Crossing of Motor and Sensory Pathways

The reader may have noticed a strange disparity in Brunner's dissection
protocol: all abnormalities were found in the right hemisphere – a recent,
egg-sized clot and three older cavities, whereas the symptoms five years before
had consisted of right hemiplegia, with loss of speech.

Somewhere there must have been an error. Brunner was not the only one
who seemed to have confused right and left. In December 1694, Giorgio
Baglivi (1668–1707), Professor of Anatomy in Rome,[75] performed an autopsy
on the body of none other than Marcello Malpighi (1628–1694), his one-time
teacher in Bologna. Malpighi had founded microscopical anatomy. Among his
many discoveries was, in 1661, the existence of connections between tiny
arterioles and venules in the lung vesicles of the frog, the last missing piece of
evidence for Harvey's circulation theory.[76] Baglivi reported the symptoms
leading to Malpighi's death:

> In the course of the preceding several years he had been liable, owing to
> severe mental exertions, firstly to vomiting and bilious excretions, then,
> after these had been suppressed, to palpitations of the heart, stones of the
> kidneys and the bladder, blood-stained urine and attacks of gout. At last,
> on July 25 of the year 1694, preceded by rather great concerns and griefs
> on his mind, he was seized by apoplexy, at almost mid-day; this was
> accompanied by paralysis of the entire right side of the body, with his
> mouth as well as his eye awry on the right. [... *Some recovery of the
> paralysis.*] Nevertheless, because diseases are wont to infiltrate more
> widely, as a result of the preceding disease the memory and reasoning
> of this very learned Man remained affected for a large part; he burst into
> tears by the most insignificant event and suffered from lack of appetite,
> indigestion of the stomach and sudden jerks. In the end he miserably
> struggled with these and other symptoms until the morning of the 29th
> of November of the same year, while in the five preceding days severe
> spells of dizziness had worsened, with a stone of the bladder; after the
> injection of the customary enema, he was seized by a newly occurring
> Apoplexy. This was so fierce, that in spite of whatever remedies he died
> on the same day, four hours after the attack.

---

[74] Brunner (1694), *De apoplexia, post quinquennium recurrens.*
[75] Hirsch (1884–8), *Biographisches Lexikon*, vol. VI, 438–9.
[76] Malpigius (1683 [1661]), De pulmonibus epistola II.

At autopsy, parts of the lung were adherent to the chest wall or had collapsed; the heart was enlarged, as was the pelvis of the left kidney. About the brain, Baglivi wrote:

> When the head had been opened, and subsequently the right ventricle of the brain was incised, I detected in its cavity about two pounds of extravasated black and clotted blood; indeed, this abnormal outpouring of blood is commonly regarded as the principal cause of this apoplexy. In the left ventricle of the brain yellowish fluid was present, with a weight of half an ounce; some very small grains were mixed with it, in moderate amount. The vessels of the brain were varicose everywhere. The entire dura mater was strongly and abnormally stuck to the skull.[77]

Given the right-sided hemiplegia, the absence of a corresponding structural lesion in the left hemisphere is puzzling, as a nineteenth-century writer also noted.[78] Of course, a small, strategical lesion of motor pathways may have been overlooked, but the point is that Baglivi failed to see the problem. His commentary (*scholium*) was limited to the high incidence of apoplexy in those years, for which he blamed earthquakes and extreme changes in climate.

Probably, Brunner, as well as Baglivi, assumed that brain lesions should be located on the same side as the resulting hemiplegia and that, believing they had erred in their initial impressions in which the two phenomena occurred on different sides, they changed one or the other and so made them 'fit'. In the previous century, one can find similar beliefs in 'homolaterality' between brain lesions and hemiplegia: Pieter van Foreest (1521–1597), writing about a patient with right-sided hemiplegia, commented that the right ventricle must have been overfilled.[79] Although Hippocrates (460–370 BC) had pointed out the crossed relationship between brain and body half with regard to convulsions, as well as to paralysis,[80] and Aretaeus of Cappadocia (second century CE) had more fully explained this principle,[81] this interchange of sides may have been too paradoxical for general acceptance in the heyday of the medical Renaissance.

In retrospect, one may wonder whether the great Wepfer, when he wrote (as cited above) that his patient *Barbara Zuberin*, at the onset of what eventually proved to be a haemorrhage in the substance of the right hemisphere, 'on the right side still (*adhuc*) moved her foot, lifted her hand to her head and produced some words', did not actually intend to suggest that she was about to lose all

---

[77] Mangetus (1700), *Theophili Boneti Sepulchretum*, 143–4.
[78] Serres (1819), Nouvelle division des apoplexies, 330.
[79] Forestus (1653 [1590]), *Observationes et Curationes*, vol. X, 530.
[80] Hippocrates (1959a [c.400 BCE]), On wounds in the head; Hippocrates (1994 [c.400 BCE]), Epidemics 7, 338.
[81] Aretaeus (1735 [c.150]), *De Causis et Signis Morborum*, 34.

movement on the right side, instead of implying that she was already paralysed on the left, as a modern reader might conclude. Indeed, elsewhere Wepfer wrote about another patient, with progressive left-sided hemiplegia, that he supposed fluid had collected over the left hemisphere – a hypothesis he could not verify, since the patient's wife refused to give permission for autopsy.[82] On the other hand, among the new – but often spurious – cases of apoplexy Wepfer added in the reprint of his book almost two decades later, there are two examples with hemiplegia and brain lesion on different sides. In the first case, Wepfer reserves his judgement with regard to the explanation,[83] but in the second, he explicitly comments:

> I have observed, with many others, that with affections of one side [of the brain] the opposite side becomes paralysed.[84]

The definitive change in medical opinion on crossed paralysis was to take place in the early eighteenth century, with Antonio Valsalva (1666–1723) and his pupil Giovanni Battista Morgagni (1682–1771) as the main protagonists (Chapter 3, p. 100).

APOPLEXY BY BLOCKED INFLOW OF BLOOD?

The Galenic notion of apoplexy as obstruction of 'animated spirits' within the brain was still fully alive throughout the entire seventeenth century, though ideas about the site of the obstruction had shifted from the cavities of the brain to its substance. Wepfer's reports had an important role in this transition. Yet an alternative explanation, rather obvious to many, was that the vital spirits, or rather the blood carrying them, might be obstructed on their way towards the brain. Jean Fernel had suggested this more than a century before,[85] even though the site of obstruction he proposed was the fictitious *rete mirabilis* at the base of the brain.[86]

After Harvey, this explanation of apoplexy could be applied only to arteries, not to venous structures, as Nymmann had suggested. In discussing this possibility, Wepfer agreed with Harvey that the brain needs a continuous, uninterrupted flow of arterial blood instead of a supply 'on demand'; he referred to episodes of fainting (*leipothymia*) to underline this view. Most importantly, he pointed out the flaw in Galen's contention that the functions of an animal remained unharmed despite 'interruption of the blood stream' by ligation of both carotid arteries; Wepfer explained that the vertebral arteries,

---

[82] Wepfer (1658), *Observationes anatomicae*, 288–9.
[83] Wepfer (1675), *Observationes anatomicae, cum Auctuario*, 336.
[84] Wepfer (1675), *Observationes anatomicae, cum Auctuario*, 402.
[85] Fernelius (1554), *Medicina*, 133.   [86] Fernelius (1548), *De abditis Causis*, 218.

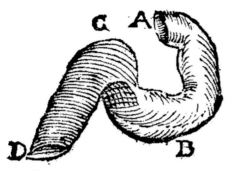

2.3 The internal carotid artery as it courses through the skull base (from Wepfer, 1658, p. 38). At D, it is still outside the skull base; at A, it is about to perforate the hard membrane around the brain. No branches take off anywhere in this section of the artery.

situated deeper in the neck, still carried blood to the brain.[87] In addition, Wepfer meticulously investigated and described the anatomy of the arterial system.

Four Interconnected Arteries

While once more dismissing the 'wonderful net' to the realm of fairy tales, Wepfer emphasized that the internal carotid artery, after its origin in the neck, did not give off any branches before or during its passage through the skull base; he even provided an illustration, the only one in the entire book (Figure 2.3). He then described the course of the four arteries entering the skull: the paired carotid arteries in front, and both vertebral arteries at the back.[88]

In addition, Wepfer described the connections between the carotid and vertebral systems, as well as – in the following manner – the junction between the right and left anterior arteries:

> The remaining part of the foremost arterial branch at the base of the brain courses further forwards, towards the *crista galli*. Where the brain is divided in two parts, the right branch is joined with the left one; in some I verified with an inserted probe that the branches were joined; however, soon afterwards they are again separated and, close together, both of them course separately to the *crista galli*, with which they are in close contact.[89]

Thus, Wepfer depicted in words the structure that came to be called the 'circle of Willis', because of the accurate illustration appearing a few years later in Willis' anatomical treatise (see below).

---

[87] Wepfer (1658), *Observationes anatomicae*, 174–80.
[88] Wepfer (1658), *Observationes anatomicae*, 99–114.
[89] Wepfer (1658), *Observationes anatomicae*, 109.

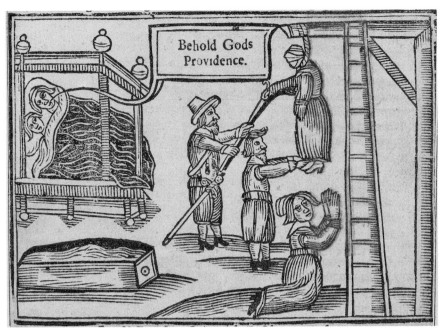

2.4 The story of Anne Greene: the hanging (friends pulling at her feet to relieve her suffering), the casket, and the bed in which she was put, and the other woman at her side to warm her (pamphlet by W. Burdet, 1651). *Source:* © Bodleian Library, Oxford.

Apoplexy by Occlusion of Arteries Still Possible?

Despite the surplus of arteries to the brain and their mutual interconnections, Wepfer did not dismiss the possibility that multiple occlusions might still cause apoplexy. As a potential example, he extensively recounted and discussed the miraculous history of 22-year-old Anne Greene from Oxford.[90] He had read, Wepfer wrote, a German translation of a popular account in English.[91] In 1650, Anne was accused of infanticide and sentenced to death by hanging (Figure 2.4); after the execution, her body was transported to a nearby building in order to be dissected later on. The physicians who first examined the body were William Petty (1623–1687) and Thomas Willis. When these physicians opened the casket and heard faint breathing, they applied all kinds of measures to revive her spirits. Their attempts were successful – Ann Greene was pardoned and eventually returned home. Wepfer attributed her apoplectic state largely to a 'lack of arterial blood and spirits'.[92]

Wepfer could not cite convincing examples of apoplexy by arterial obstruction from personal experience. But he had sometimes found polypous, friable bodies in the ventricles of the heart, and so had others, for example the

---

[90] Wepfer (1658), *Observationes anatomicae*, 181–6.
[91] Burdet (1651), *A wonder of wonders*; Watkins (1651), *The Miraculous Deliverance of Anne Greene*.
[92] Wepfer (1658), *Observationes anatomicae*, 186–94.

Amsterdam physician Nicolaas Tulp (1593–1674);[93] it is not difficult to imagine, Wepfer suggested, that part of these bodies can break off and get stuck at the point where an artery enters the skull base.[94]

Other possible sites of arterial obstruction, Wepfer figured, were the smaller arterial branches of the brain, if mucous substances accumulated on their walls. He did not provide examples in humans, but, thinking especially of small arterioles, he drew an analogy with incrustations in watermills:

> If blood repeatedly passes through these vessels perforating the medullary substance and is mixed with very many viscous and gluey particles, gradually some small portions of this kind will begin to adhere. Similarly in hot spring resorts, where stony patches develop in the pipes through which water flows repeatedly and very rapidly. In the vicinity of Abano [*this must have been during Wepfer's time as a student in Padua*] I saw a water mill that had its wheel turned by water from hot springs, very clear and pure to the senses; within a short time, it became everywhere incrusted with a very dense and shining layer of stone, two thumbs in thickness. The millers were forced to polish it every other month, which delayed its operation. Thus, albeit these arterioles or the pores through which the vital spirits are distributed to the medullary substance are not immediately and completely obstructed by such gluey humours, yet they are surely predisposed to step-wise occlusion.[95]

If this occurred on one side, Wepfer reasoned, the result was hemiplegia or loss of speech; but if it occurred on both sides simultaneously, true apoplexy would strike the patient. As treatment, particularly with occlusion of one or only a few arterioles within the brain, he recommended venesection, citing several instances with favourable outcome. This treatment displaced obstructive material, he explained, still reasoning in a time-honoured, teleological mode:

> For first of all venesection counteracts the abnormal impulse of the blood, which often provides an opportunity for this obstruction. It rushes in smaller quantity to the brain, when, after blood has been drawn, from the brachial vein for example, a sizeable portion makes for the arms in order to refill what was lost through venesection. Subsequently blood from the rest of the body and from the brain paces without delay to the heart, deprived as it is through that venesection, in order to assist the impoverished [organ]. The heart, liberated from the load that oppressed it before and during the paroxysm itself, propels the blood flowing back to it with greater alacrity, in a more proper order and in a quantity that will be wholesome for the brain.[96]

[93] Tulpius (1641), *Observationum medicarum Libri tres*, 54–8.
[94] Wepfer (1658), *Observationes anatomicae*, 195–205.
[95] Wepfer (1658), *Observationes anatomicae*, 207–8.
[96] Wepfer (1658), *Observationes anatomicae*, 219.

As further support for the role of displacement, Wepfer cited the example of a woman with apoplexy who began to improve as soon as her friends had started to shake her body and move her around.[97]

SUPPORT FOR WEPFER, FROM THOMAS WILLIS

Thomas Willis (1621–1675) (Box 2.4) made brief appearances earlier in the chapter. In 1672, he published the book *On the Soul of non-thinking Creatures* (*De Anima Brutorum*), with extrapolations to diseases of humankind. In the chapter on apoplexy, he extensively cited and approved Wepfer's opinions.[98] Willis' own investigations had also been predominantly on the brain, covering many aspects other than apoplexy. Eventually he became very influential, though his chemical explanations of bodily processes were not universally accepted.[99] The subtitle of the new book was 'which in man is the vital and sensitive [principle]'. So the term *anima* should not be understood in a moral or religious sense, but as the vital principle that keeps the machinery of living creatures going or, in his own words, as the 'corporeal soul', to be distinguished from the 'rational soul'.[100]

Anatomical Research and Experiments

In his now famous book on the anatomy of the brain published previously (1664), Willis had paid special attention to the interconnections between the basal cerebral arteries, skilfully drawn by Christopher Wren (Figure 2.5).[101] The anatomist Giulio Casseri (1552–1616) in Padua had provided an earlier, but incomplete illustration,[102] as had Johann Vesling (Veslingius; 1598–1649) (Figure 2.6), one of Casseri's successors.[103] Willis was more explicit than Wepfer in pointing out the importance of these 'communicating arteries', as they are called nowadays:

> These vessels have many possibilities to connect with each other; of course, in order to ensure that for blood on its way to the different regions of the brain there is more than one pathway open for each of them; this is safer. For if one or the other access is closed off, another one

---

[97] Wepfer (1658), *Observationes anatomicae*, 209–15.
[98] Willis (1672), *De Anima Brutorum*, 264–5.
[99] Compston (2021), '*All Manner of Ingenuity and Industry*', 601–13.
[100] Willis (1672), *De Anima Brutorum*, A6–7 (preface).
[101] The actual engraving might have been performed by someone else (Compston (2021), '*All Manner of Ingenuity and Industry*', 188–90).
[102] Casserius and Bucretius (1627), *Tabulae anatomicae LXXIIX*, 93.
[103] Vesling (1647), *Syntagma anatomicum*, 195.

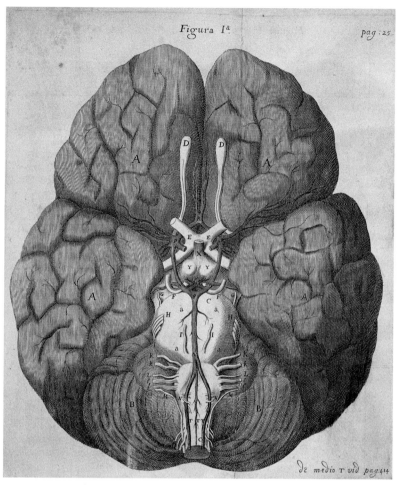

2.5 Engraving of the base of the brain (from Willis (1664), *Cerebri Anatome*). The drawing on which the engraving is based was made by Christopher Wren (1632–723), the later architect. The two vertebral arteries (bottom of figure; dark) first join and then separate again. On each side, one branch goes sideways to the hind part of the brain. The other division moves forward to connect with the carotid artery (the small stumps), on each side of the optic chiasm. The carotid artery divides into a large branch going sideways between the two lobes of the brain, further dividing in its course, and into an anterior branch, which crosses above the optic nerve and connects with its counterpart. Thus, the arteries form a circle, now named after Willis. The letter 'X' indicates the infundibulum.

is easily found in its place. If, for example, the carotid system is obstructed on one side, the vessels on the other side supply both territories. Even if both carotids are blocked, their duties are taken over by the vertebral [arteries]; vice versa, the carotids make up for deficits of occluded vertebral arteries. In this way the extraordinary construction acts as a safety measure to ensure that there is no shortfall in the blood supply anywhere, in whatever part of the brain or its appendages within the skull. If it has happened by chance that three of them are occluded, it will be through only a single [artery] that the provided [quantity of] blood immediately

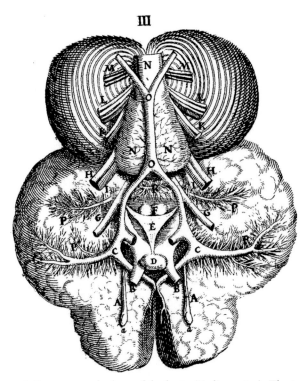

2.6 Structures at the base of the brain (Vesling, 1647). The two vertebral arteries join into a single vessel O–O, to be split again into two vessels, which join the carotid system. Vesling omitted the posterior cerebral arteries and explains the fictitious system P–P–P–P–P as 'minute arterial branches, which some call the *rete mirabile*'. The carotid arteries (cut off; stumps pointing towards D) divide at C into a large lateral branch and a small anterior branch. The anterior branches seem to touch each other in the midline, but it is not clear whether they are connected. The structure marked E is the infundibulum (Vesalius' 'funnel') in a purely diagrammatic form; D is the pituitary gland.

> supplies all channels and twigs of all other [arteries], since there are four separate entries for this fluid, at some distance from each other.[104]

Willis even provided experimental evidence:

> I have proved this by experiment, quite often performed, not without admiration and the greatest satisfaction. Indeed, as often as I injected fluid that was mixed with ink into one or the other carotid artery, the ramifications on either side were immediately stained with the same colour – even the main branches of the vertebral arteries. What is more, if such an injection through a single [vessel of] entry was repeated at different times, the vessels running to any nook and corner of the brain and cerebellum were stained with the same colour.[105]

Willis' experimental technique was in keeping with the tradition that had developed in the circle of his friends in Oxford. In 1660, under the patronage

[104] Willis (1664), *Cerebri Anatome*, 93–4.   [105] Willis (1664), *Cerebri Anatome*, 94.

of restored monarchy, this group of natural philosophers, later called 'scientists',[106] was transformed into the 'Royal Society'. Willis interpreted the results of his experiments with dye as proof of the hypothesis he had formulated on the basis of his (and Wepfer's) anatomical observations of the arterial system. Support for the functional importance of interconnections between major brain arteries was the chance finding of an occluded carotid artery in a patient who had died of a disease unrelated to the brain:

> Not so long ago I dissected the corpse of a deceased person who had succumbed to a giant tumour of the bowels, which had eventually ulcerated. When I had opened his skull and reviewed the brain and its connections, I found that the right carotid artery, as it entered the skull, was plainly bone-like or rather stone-like, while its cavity was almost entirely occluded. Because the inflow of blood along this route was closed off, I therefore wondered why the patient had not previously died of Apoplexy. However, this was not at all the case, since he had full command over his mind and intellectual function up to the last moments of his life. Indeed, nature had made provisions for a quite useful remedy against that danger of Apoplexy.[107]

To his disappointment, Willis had not been permitted to dissect the brain in even a single case of what he regarded as apoplexy.[108] As mentioned above, he had classified the cerebral haemorrhage of a 'young Englishman' with sudden hemiplegia as 'paralysis', since not all 'senses' had been lost at onset. Therefore, in Willis' chapter on apoplexy in *On the Soul of Brutes*, he had to rely on Wepfer's observations. Nothing should be altered in the writings of his colleague abroad, Willis wrote, apart from a few additions, such as apoplexy by rupture of a brain abscess.[109] Also, apoplexy could manifest itself not only as an unexpected and catastrophic event, Willis proposed, but also as a more gradual form.[110] To explain this type, he left the realm of observations and developed his own hypothesis. He was not the only one in the last quarter of the seventeenth century.

HYPOTHETICAL EXPLANATIONS OF APOPLEXY

Willis' 'Habitual' Form of Apoplexy

Willis proposed that in some patients, a certain predisposition to apoplexy builds up in a stuttering form: they are 'at first bothered by skirmishes (*velitationes*) of a rather mild sort, later by more serious attacks, with shorter intervals'.

---

[106] William Whewell (1794–866) is credited with coining the term 'scientist' (Ross (1962), Scientist: the story of a word).
[107] Willis (1664), *Cerebri Anatome*, 95.   [108] Willis (1672), *De Anima Brutorum*, 275–6.
[109] Willis (1672), *De Anima Brutorum*, 265–8.   [110] Willis (1672), *De Anima Brutorum*, 269–71.

> It is permitted to suppose that during the onset of the Apoplectic parox-
> ysm some material that has been accumulated and distributed earlier at
> the *periphery of the brain* goes down to its centre; there it assaults all spirits
> and suppresses and inactivates them at the very source of their effusion.
> Yet it is not entirely clear whether they bring this about only by *overfilling*
> *the pores of the medulla* or by *destruction of the spirits themselves* and by making
> them inactive; yet it is probable that it occurs in both ways. And
> I maintain that the pores in the medulla of the brain are somewhat
> obstructed, because the same matter that at first caused speechlessness
> by occupying the *corpus callosum*, has then moved down into the *corpus*
> *striatum* and, subsequently overfilling its pores, commonly gives rise to
> hemiplegia.[111]

A peculiarity in Willis' model of brain function was that he attributed the
conscious perceptions and actions to the brain (*cerebrum*), especially to the *corpus
callosum* and other medullary parts, but 'automatic' functions, such as breathing
and beating of the heart, to the cerebellum.[112] He even went as far as supposing
that attacks with sudden cessation of respiration and heart action might result
from an apoplexy of the cerebellum.[113]

In trying to explain how these 'alien particles' inactivated the animated
spirits in the medulla of the brain, Willis used a chemical metaphor. To
understand his reasoning, a brief review of the budding relationship between
chemistry and medicine is necessary.

Iatrochemistry

The foundation of 'chemical medicine' is traditionally attributed to the colourful figure of Philippus Aureolus Theophrastus Bombastus von Hohenheim
(1493–1541). He adopted the name Paracelsus, or 'on a par with Celsus' (the
original Celsus, *c.*25 BCE to 50, was a Roman encyclopaedist who also wrote
on medicine). Paracelsus' attempts to put medicine, and natural philosophy in
general, on a completely new footing were highly unsystematic, if not chaotic,
as is the story of his life.[114] His view on apoplexy, written in a mixture of
German and Latin, is representative:

> *Gutta* (paralysis, *apoplexia*) is any part that loses its own power, such as
> [with] gonorrhoea, similarly with a defect of speech, or sight, or hearing.
> And the disease is nothing else than that a body part can no longer
> perform its *officium*. There is no defect in the stomach or in nutriments.
> It also involves paralysis in the heart and the spleen. The cause is that

---

[111] Willis (1672), *De Anima Brutorum*, 269.   [112] Willis (1672), *De Anima Brutorum*, 263.
[113] Willis (1672), *De Anima Brutorum*, 266–7.   [114] Ball (2006), *The Devil's Doctor*.

synovia is separated from its body part; for there is no body part or it has *synovia*, like in joints.[115]

Paracelsus' term *gutta*, Latin for 'drop', refers to the wise woman's tale that a drop of blood falling from the head to the heart can stop its action and so cause apoplexy.[116] Nowadays, the term 'synovia' denotes the membranes lining joints; Paracelsus probably had a kind of lubricant in mind. Somewhat later in the text, he used the German word *Altenwachs* for it.

The seventeenth-century Flemish physician Joan Baptista van Helmont (1577–1644) took up Paracelsus' approach in a modified fashion; he worked in isolation, having been put under house arrest during the Spanish Inquisition.[117] van Helmont regarded water and air as the main constituents of matter, instead of Paracelsus' salt, sulphur, and quicksilver; earth, in van Helmont's view, served as a kind of skeleton. His work represents a curious combination of quantitative and experimental analysis with vitalist and almost anti-rational ideas.[118] He coined the term 'gas' but did not use it in its current material sense, but to indicate a specific, almost metaphysical essence that remained after a substance had been burnt.[119] van Helmont also drew attention to the acidity of gastric fluid and its role in the process of digestion; he warned that it could be harmful outside the stomach.[120]

Whereas Paracelsus and van Helmont had been outsiders, some more traditional physicians also tried to integrate chemical principles in the existing corpus of medical knowledge. Examples were Daniel Sennert (1572–1637), Professor of Medicine in Wittenberg and predecessor of Gregor Nymmann, and furthermore Thomas Willis,[121] Michael Ettmüller (1644–1683), Professor of Surgery and Anatomy in Leipzig, and Franciscus de le Boë (Sylvius) in Leiden. Sylvius' student Reinier de Graef proved by means of experiments in dogs and calves that pancreatic juice was not a waste product, as often believed, but a useful substance.[122]

Otto Tacke (Tachenius; 1610–1680), born in Westphalia, a student in Padua and practising physician in Venice, followed Sylvius' lead by conceiving a dualistic model not only for digestion, but also for health and disease in

---

[115] Sudhoff, ed. (1931), *Paracelsus, Sämtliche Werke,* vol. v, 244.
[116] Nymmanus (1629), *Tractatus de Apoplexia,* 6.   [117] Pagel (1982), *Joan Baptista van Helmont.*
[118] Brock (1992), *The Norton History of Chemistry,* 49–51.
[119] van Helmont (1648), *Ortus Medicinae,* 73–81.
[120] van Helmont (1648), *Ortus Medicinae,* 294.
[121] Dewhurst (1980), *Willis's Oxford Lectures,* 154; Compston (2021), '*All Manner of Ingenuity and Industry*', 560–78.
[122] de Graef (1664), *De Succi pancreatici,* 22–33. In the end, pancreatic juice did not prove to be acidic, as Sylvius expected, hoped, and found, but alkaline or lye-like (*lixivus*).

general. He saw the body as the battleground between two substances – one acidic and the other 'alkaline' – his newly coined term.[123]

Nitre, Sulphur, and Saline

Willis postulated chemical factors to explain not only apoplexy, but also some normal body functions. He regarded the intrinsic warmth of the body as a continuous, dynamic reaction in the blood, for which he used the term 'fermentation', in a rather metaphorical sense.[124] One source of energy for this reaction was formed by particles in air, called 'nitre'; these were thought indispensable to animal life, as well as necessary to keep candles burning. The other source for the dynamic reaction, in Willis' view, consisted of 'sulphurous' particles in the blood, a term reminiscent of Paracelsus and van Helmont. When air and blood combined, they produced 'nitro-sulphurous' particles, as well as heat. In turn, these nitro-sulphurous particles activated the 'animated spirits' in the brain, thought to be 'spirituous-saline' in nature.[125]

Now, what happened in the 'habitual form' of apoplexy, Willis thought, was first of all that the blood contained some 'accumulated material':

> It occurs in the same way as in most other afflictions of the brain, that is, also *the blood* is at fault, because it imposes alien particles on the brain, either locally producing them or getting hold of them elsewhere; these are very inimical and one might say pestilent to the cohesion or structure of the animated spirits.[126]

When this foreign material eventually inundated the pores of the medullary substance in the brain, his theory went, it counteracted the animated spirits. Willis' 'alien particles' were poisonous, because they were not nitro-sulphurous, but 'vitriolic'. He compared the noxious particles to a disease of trees – blight, in which case the wind transmits morbific agents. Therefore, the animated spirits are not abnormally activated, as happens in convulsive disorders, but, conversely, they are inactivated through a kind of chemical reaction.[127]

> If the question is about the *morbid character*, or the nature of this *material*, it is fair to suspect that in *Apoplexy* the animated spirits are afflicted in a quite different fashion than in *convulsive passions*, that is, that persons liable to *the stunned disease* acquire a coupling antithetical to *explosive*, in other words *vitriolic* rather than *nitro-sulphurous;* subsequently their *spirituous-*

[123] Tachenius (1666), *Hippocrates Chymicus*.
[124] Compston (2021), *'All Manner of Ingenuity and Industry'*, 559–61.
[125] Eadie (2003), A pathology of the animal spirits.
[126] Willis (1672), *De Anima Brutorum*, 270.   [127] Willis (1672), *De Anima Brutorum*, 283–4.

> *saline* particles will be completely fettered by it and kept from initiating movements, or explosions of any kind.[128]

Despite these hypotheses, Thomas Willis was fully committed to observations, and occasionally to experiments, as a trusted source of knowledge; he is therefore deservedly regarded as a medical counterpart of the developments in physics and astronomy later labelled as the 'Scientific Revolution'.[129]

By contrast, other physicians sought refuge, as of old, in the authority of the ancients, especially in the scriptures of Hippocrates. Galen's hold might be on the wane, especially now that his dogma about the ventricular system had been disproved, but the ambiguity of Hippocratic aphorisms and other writings left ample room for hypotheses that could be adorned with his authority (Figure 2.7). Particularly irresistible was the temptation to couple the Father of Medicine with the impressive lore of chemistry, as Tachenius did by entitling his book *Hippocrates Chymicus*.

Coagulation by Acidity of Black Bile

François Bayle (1622–1709),[130] Professor of Medicine in Toulouse, even more prominently linked Hippocrates with the chemical doctrine. In his book on apoplexy, first published in 1677, in small octavo format, he used many pages to discuss, and subsequently dismiss, previous hypotheses about the events leading to apoplexy, by reinterpreting the observations of Wepfer and others.[131] He then brought Hippocrates on the stage, with extensive quotations to prove that the Father of Medicine regarded stoppage of the bloodstream as a primary cause of apoplexy.[132] Finally, collaring the association of apoplexy with black bile in the Hippocratic writings, he proposed the acidity of black bile as the key factor; this, Bayle suggested, led to a process of generalized clotting, eventually extending to the brain:

> The main quality of black bile, from which its activity depends most of all, is acidity. When it is moderate, its force lends a moderate consistency to the blood. [Its consistency] is immoderate, however, if its quantity is excessive and its acidity is made more acute, especially if it additionally has harshness, or acerbity; for in that case, it has considerable power to halt the blood. Indeed, this is testified by experience: blood outside vessels on which acid has been poured, congeals more easily; also, serum

---

[128] Willis (1672), *De Anima Brutorum*, 270.   [129] Shapin (1996), *The Scientific Revolution.*
[130] Hirsch (1884–8), *Biographisches Lexikon*, vol. VI, 464.
[131] Bayle (1677), *Tractatus de Apoplexia*, 14–55.
[132] Bayle (1677), *Tractatus de Apoplexia*, 56–70.

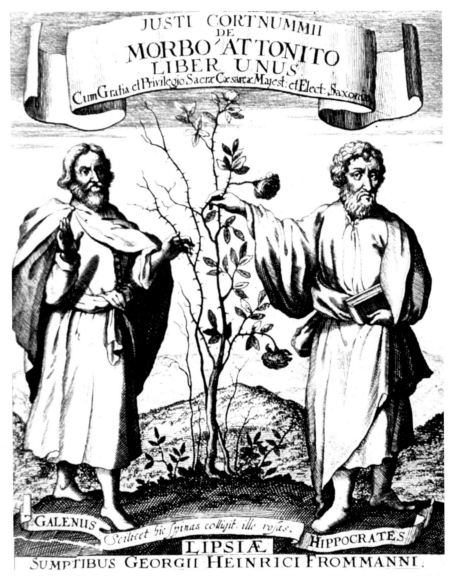

JUSTI CORTNUMMII
DE
MORBO ATTONITO
LIBER UNUS
Cum Gratia et Privilegio Sacræ Cæsareæ Majest: et Elect: Saxoniæ

GALENUS   Scilicet hic spinas colligit ille rosas.   HIPPOCRATES

LIPSIÆ
SUMPTIBUS GEORGII HEINRICI FROMMANNI.

2.7 Allegorical engraving of Galen and Hippocrates adjoining the tree of wisdom. While Hippocrates reaped fleshy leaves, Galen picked only thorns. Frontispiece of *The Stunned Disease* by Julius Cortnumm, 1677.

that has been separated from blood, [being] liquid and clear like water, coagulates in the same way if acid is poured on it. But the same clotting can be brought about if acid fluids are discharged inside vessels. Since acids obtain that power, it is therefore obvious that black bile, if collected in some body part and made too acid, is moved out and passes into the mass of blood, can cause local coagulation, repress the movement of spirits and impede their production. If that collection of too acid black bile and its effusion in blood takes place in the brain, the production and inflow of spirits there will necessarily diminish or be entirely barred, depending on whether the quantity was greater or smaller and the acidity or harshness more or less intense.[133]

Extravasated blood in or around the brain was not the cause of apoplexy, Bayle maintained. Instead, stagnation of blood was the primary event, causing apoplexy and sometimes also extravasation, but only as a sequel:

> One can understand how seriously in error people are who think that an outpouring of blood at the base of the brain is a cause of Apoplexy, because Apoplexy actually precedes the effusion of blood – or at least both depend on the same cause. From the same [facts] it can be easily understood why the brain of most Apoplectics appears saturated with blood: through the great effort of the heart, blood is transported to the brain via arteries, it cannot return through veins, so it exudes into the substance of the brain if the occlusion is moderate or it ruptures its vessels if their occlusion is extensive.[134]

Obstruction and Hippocrates

In 1677, when Bayle's treatise saw the light in Toulouse, a printer in Leipzig produced another book 'The stunned disease' (morbus attonitus). Its author had died two years before; his name was Julius Cortnumm (1621–1675), Professor and Dean of the Academy in Sorau, Saxony (now Zary, Western Poland). Like Bayle, Cortnumm leant heavily on Hippocrates, but his allusions to chemistry were less explicit than those of his colleague in the West.

Cortnumm savaged the explanations of apoplexy by Fernel, Platter, and 'the Chemists' (Paracelsus and van Helmont), as well as Sennert's attempts at a synthesis of the different opinions ('a three-headed hell-hound');[135] Wepfer's work he hardly acknowledged. His own explanation of apoplexy rested entirely on the writings of Hippocrates. Like Bayle, he interpreted these as caused by an interruption in blood flow ('haemostasis').[136] He was also quite assured of where this occurred:

> Thus, the spirit, coming from the heart and heading via the carotid arteries to the brain and nerves, in which mental function, i.e. sensation and voluntary movement must take place by the will of the mind, is held back there, obstructed, so that it is prevented from flowing any further. For that obstruction must be sought in the vessels and nowhere else; we have learned this from the fact that the spirit never leaves them, as long as it is directed by the soul. Yet this is never in the vessels of the neck, nor on the outer side of the hard membrane (for in that case a cardiac syncope

---

[133] Bayle (1677), *Tractatus de Apoplexia*, 80–1.   [134] Bayle (1677), *Tractatus de Apoplexia*, 88
[135] Cortnumm (1677), *De Morbo attonito*, 55–63.
[136] Cortnumm (1677), *De Morbo attonito*, 65.

would occur, or nutrition would be withheld from all parts of the brain, which is contradicted by the circulation of blood and remaining life in stricken patients), but at the site where it leaves off, separating itself from blood, that is, in the inner branch of the carotid, beyond the hard membrane, where, close to the pituitary gland, it is divided in two branches on their way to the substance of the brain.[137]

In a separate chapter, Cortnumm explained what part of blood actually caused obstruction:

> Because it has thus been clearly demonstrated above that all those are in error who keep their thoughts on the filth of harmful or excremental fluids obstructing the ventricles of the brain, or its net-like complex of vessels, or the beginning of nerves, or whatever other part of the body, one should expressly wish that 'May at last the blindness be gone, [...] [*a few more verses of Prudentius follow*]'.
>
> We clearly perceive that the blame for this malady can be put nowhere but on blood alone; however, not on the blood that already obstructs, when it is a material part of the disease, but on the blood that is on its way to the brain and is about to become obstructive. When I say blood, I mean the mixture of fluids that is normally contained in veins, arteries and channels. But not the best part of that mixture, but the part that is kept apart from all other parts and that is truly and only alimentary, and properly named chymus, [...][138]

In other words, Cortnumm put the blame on nutritive elements in blood; having been resorbed via the alimentary system, they were supposed to cause obstruction once these arrived in cerebral arteries of smaller calibre.

APOPLEXY AROUND 1700: EXTRAVASATION OR OBSTRUCTION

The story in this chapter has especially highlighted two influential pioneers: Wepfer and Willis. Wepfer defined two types of apoplexy – haemorrhagic and serous, while also still entertaining the possibility that the supply of blood and spirits to the brain might be cut off, despite the richness of arterial byways. Willis accepted extravasation as a cause but had been critical of obstruction of arterial pathways to the brain; he also posited a separate and more gradual 'poisonous' category.

As Bayle and Cortnumm exemplified, these new ideas by no means met with rapid adoption by physicians across Europe. Despite the fame of Wepfer and Willis, and despite the gradual acceptance of Harvey's theory in the second

---

[137] Cortnumm (1677), *De Morbo attonito*, 48.   [138] Cortnumm (1677), *De Morbo attonito*, 81.

half of the seventeenth century, even physicians who had the opportunity to read books about apoplexy did not limit their views to these few categories.

Echoes of Wepfer and Willis

An example is William Cole from Bristol; he appeared earlier with a description of brain haemorrhage in a noble lady. In a book entitled *A Physico-medical Essay Concerning the Late Frequency of Apoplexies*, written not in Latin, but in English, Cole proposed cold as an important factor undermining the firmness of the brain. Yet, with regard to the 'immediate cause' of apoplexy, he went mostly along with Wepfer and Willis:

> [...] most usually (when unavoidably fatal) an *effusion of Bloud* out of its vessels upon the *substance of the Brain*, though I conceive a bare *distension of the arteries* there may occasion it, as also may perhaps a *congestion of viscous or serous matter*, when it comes to a considerable degree, and becomes freshly *excited*; or else *Polypous concretions*, or (if we can suppose it) *any other* obstructing matter deposited in it [...][139]

So, apart from haemorrhages in the brain tissue, we have encountered serum (to be discussed in a later chapter), occlusion by polyps, Bayle's 'generalized clotting by the acidity of black bile', Cortnumm's hypothesis of food elements occluding brain arteries, and also Cole's 'congestion' and 'viscosity', echoes from ancient times.

'Fluidism' Still Dominant

The new findings of extravasated blood or serum in the brain tissue modified, rather than replaced, existing notions about the pathogenesis of apoplexy; they were incorporated into the familiar scheme as examples of material causes capable of interrupting the course of animated spirits. Indeed, extravasation of blood (or serum) in the brain substance of Wepfer's patients confirmed, rather than disturbed, existing notions of ancient origin: excess of fluids, be it blood, phlegm, or other.

Undeniably, the discovery of the circulation of blood, together with the emerging practice of post-mortem dissection, gradually resulted in a preference for detailed observation of particulars above all-embracing theories. As a result, medicine adopted some causal notions associated with changes in the organs of the body. But these beginnings far from dispelled the dominant, humoral doctrine of health, based on ancient writings and in harmony with the

[139] Cole (1689), *The Late Frequency of Apoplexies*, 43–4.

formalism and rigid causality of the late Middle Ages.[140] The remedies physicians applied in patients with impending or established apoplexy reflected
these ideas: removal of fluids from the head by blistering poultices, scarifica-
tion, or cupping glasses, or from the body in general by venesection, emetics,
and enemas, and – in the case of suspected phlegm – warming of the head.

[140] Huizinga (1922), *The Waning of the Middle Ages*, 228–43.

THREE

CONGESTION

Apoplexy in the 'Long Eighteenth Century'

SUMMARY

In the eighteenth century, most diseases were still ill-defined and explained by local or remote causes. The diagnosis of 'apoplexy' was applied in a broad sense, with unresponsiveness as the cardinal symptom and overfilling of the skull or its vessels as the key event. Its purported causes included not only primary changes in or around the brain (Boerhaave), but also the general constitution and external circumstances. Thus, two doctrines of attributing causality more or less coexisted in the 'long eighteenth century', up to the 1820s. One was the morphological approach, practised in Vienna (de Haen) and Bologna (Valsalva), and especially in Padua (Morgagni distinguished three kinds of apoplexy: haemorrhagic, serous, and 'other'). The other doctrine, related to Galen's 'fluidism' and only slowly losing ground, implicated mainly external factors as the cause of fullness in the head (Portal).

In modern times, the prevailing concept of disease is one of discrete entities, with more or less uniform manifestations and, if possible, with single or at least identifiable causes. Measles is an example, or lung cancer. But in the eighteenth century, the criteria for apoplexy were flexible – some medical writers included patients in whom sensation and movement were partly preserved, as long as the onset of the episode had been sudden, whereas others made the diagnosis even in an illness with gradual onset, provided the final stage was characterized by unresponsiveness. Moreover, some of its purported causes were also implicated in the explanation of other diseases. It is useful, therefore, to review briefly the fluidity of what constituted a 'disease' and its 'cause' before the story again reverts to apoplexy.

DISEASES AND THEIR CAUSES

'Disease': An Elastic Notion

Apoplexy was far from unique in being defined by its manifestations. This happens even today – think of migraine. Physicians of the eighteenth century often defined disorders of internal organs by their symptoms. Examples abound in the 'Aphorisms' of Herman Boerhaave (1668–1738) (Box 3.1),[1] published in 1709; by borrowing his title from Hippocrates, the young professor plainly staked his claims. One finds categories based on symptoms, such as 'fevers', 'convulsions', 'angina', and 'hydrops', next to localized illnesses such as 'pulmonary phthisis', 'nephritis', and 'dysentery'.[2] Thomas Sydenham (1624–1689), practising in London at around the same time as Willis – their views differed on both politics and medicine – had been singularly optimistic about physicians' observational powers of symptoms as a means of distinguishing one disease from another. In the preface to the third edition of his book on acute diseases, mainly dealing with fevers, Sydenham wrote:

> For in what manner one can more advantageously, or in what manner at all, can one obtain the means to face the morbid cause or to find indications about a cure, other than by the certain and distinct perception of characteristic symptoms? For no circumstance is so mild or so insignificant that it does not contribute to either of these two. Indeed, though I admit that a certain variety originates from the constitution of individuals and the method of treatment, the regularity of Nature in producing diseases is nevertheless so uniform and repetitive everywhere, that in different bodies one mostly finds the same symptoms of the same disease. [...] In the same way all known plants spread themselves without a single exception according to the manner of the species in question. Someone, for example, who will have described a violet with regard to its colour, taste, smell, form and other properties, will easily note that this story fits most if not all violets in the world.[3]

The expectation that diseases could be neatly distinguished and categorised, as in the world of plants, was widely shared in the eighteenth century. François Boissier de Sauvauges de Lacroix (1706–1767), a botanist and physician in Montpellier, and also the Scottish Professor of Medicine William Cullen

---

[1] Lindeboom (1984b), *Herman Boerhaave: The Man and His Work.*
[2] Boerhaave (1709), *Aphorismi.*
[3] Sydenham (1676), *Circa Morborum acutorum Historiam et Curationem,* a5r–v.

Box 3.1 Herman Boerhaave (1668–1738).

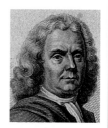

Herman was the son of Hagar Daalders and Jakob Boerhaave, Protestant minister in Voorhout. After his study of medicine at the university of close-by Leiden and a doctoral degree in Harderwijk, Boerhaave became, in 1709, Professor of Botany in Leiden. In 1714, he was appointed to hold the chair of Medicine, and in 1719 also the chair of Chemistry. Boerhaave not only continued the tradition of bedside teaching for medical students, established by his predecessors Otto van Heurne (1577–1652) and Franciscus De le Boë (Sylvius), but also raised this art to legendary heights, thanks to his didactic qualities and warm personality. He also introduced thermometry in medicine, with the help of Gabriel Fahrenheit (1686–1736). Boerhaave was a captivating speaker, rather than a prolific writer; this explains why a major part of the countless editions of his books are unauthorized lecture notes or pirate publications.

When, in 1729, near the end of his career and after a few episodes of illness, he had given up the chairs of Botany and Chemistry, Boerhaave started a course on diseases of the nervous system, delivering 206 lectures between 1730 and 1735. The content of these lectures can be more or less accurately retrieved from two sources. The best known is the posthumous edition, in 1761, by the Leiden physician Jacobus van Eems, who used his own lecture notes from more than 25 years before and compared them with those of his colleagues J. Hovius and Gerard van Swieten. The other source for the content of the lectures is Boerhaave's own manuscript, used as the basis for his teaching. Though more authoritative, the manuscript is also more succinct than the transcriptions by his former students. It now resides with all his other papers in the Kirov Institute for military medicine in St Petersburg. The reason is that after Boerhaave's death, all his papers and instruments went to his two nephews Herman and Abraham Kaau, both physicians, who moved to St Petersburg a few years after their uncle's death.

The hospital where Boerhaave made his rounds in Leiden, the 'St Caecilia Gasthuis', is now a museum of science, named after him.

Source: Portrait by courtesy of Wellcome Foundation.

(1710–1790) expressed ideas similar to Sydenham's 'flora' of diseases. Nevertheless, since apoplexy was a 'state', for want of more specific characteristics, the diagnosis was open to different interpretations and subject to preconceived ideas.

Causality

On top of the fuzziness surrounding the notion of 'apoplexy', 'causation' is an extremely contentious issue. Few physicians assumed apoplexy had a single cause. To give but one example, Cardanus had attributed all apoplexies to black bile, and Piso to serum. In fact, the notion of 'one disease – one cause' was a novelty introduced in the nineteenth century when a growing group of scientists, led by the examples of Pasteur and Koch, discovered the agents responsible for different types of infectious disease. But when Wepfer found blood clots or serous effusions in patients who had died of apoplexy, he did not regard this as *the* cause, in the sense that no further explanations were necessary. In fact, as recounted in the previous chapter, he considered the force and continuous impulse of arterial blood as the cause of the morbid changes in the brain.

Nowadays 'cerebral haemorrhage' is a familiar nosological category, and seemingly self-explanatory. The term creates the illusion of a logical explanation, although it describes only the effect of disease – a nice example of circular reasoning.[4] But to follow the chain of events backward is difficult – even now. Many physicians in the past preferred to implicate an obstructed flow of 'animated spirits' as the final and true cause, rather than extravasation of blood or serum.

Before the nineteenth century, physicians generally tried to make sense of causes of disease by assuming an interaction between many different causal factors. In attempts to allot them different places in the sequence of events leading to illness, they made a distinction between 'proximate' causes and more remote factors. Often the remote factors were, in turn, separated into 'exciting' and 'predisposing' causes, a distinction that tends to end up in a quagmire of scholastic definitions and contradictions.[5]

Interaction of Causal Factors: Constitution and 'Non-naturals'

To avoid getting lost in a maze of specific causes based on their presumed sequence or role, it is more practical to take a wider view of the factors physicians and others implicated to explain disease. The two main categories are internal and external. The internal factor is 'constitution', a more or less stable mixture of nature and nurture – hereditary factors and the multitude of influences to which the body has been exposed up to the time of illness. Stature and build are examples of the former; few early authors writing on apoplexy dared to omit a short neck as a 'risk factor' (to use a modern term). The external categories can be summarized as 'the six non-naturals': surroundings and climate (corresponding to the Hippocratic 'Airs, Waters, and Places'); food and drink; exercise and rest; sleeping and waking; excretion and retention; and emotions.[6]

---

[4] Carter (2003), *The Rise of Causal Concepts of Disease*, 106–7.
[5] Carter (2003), *The Rise of Causal Concepts of Disease*, 14–16.
[6] Knoeff, ed. (2017), *Histories of Healthy Ageing*.

These external factors formed an important, if not exclusive, element in the questions physicians put to their patients, to judge from reports from this period. A single example, out of many possibilities, is the approach of Maximilian Stoll (1742–1787), whom we shall meet again later on. He published a series of books with case records from his private practice, as well as from the *Heiliggeistspital* ('Trinity Hospital') in Vienna. The following story of apoplexy dates from the late 1770s; it is typical of the importance physicians attached to the mix of constitution and circumstances, at least until the first decades of the nineteenth century.

> A widow of 74 years, formerly wife of an army official, had for many years been in excellent health, stout and well-coloured. On August 12, cheerful as usual, she dined a bit more sumptuously and partook between courses of stronger and more wine than she used to on other occasions; she retired to bed in perfect health. The next morning, when she had not appeared for breakfast at the usual time, servants found her in bed, speechless and paralysed on the right side. The remains of yesterday's meal were soiling the bed and the floor, no doubt ejected by vomiting during the night. A physician was alerted, cut a vein in the left foot and applied three blistering plasters. On the 14th she was carried around midnight to the Hospital. [. . .] She died late at night on the 16th. [. . .]
>
> The apoplexy in a brain predisposed in this manner can be easily explained by the vomiting as a result of the gormandizing the day before. Vomiting is clearly dangerous in the aged, as anything that increases the blood flow to the brain: a rich meal, undiluted wine, straining at stools, sneezing, etc.[7]

What Stoll saw in the brain will follow later; what matters here are his thoughts about causes. If physicians of his time enquired about excretions, questions used to include common haemorrhages such as menstruation, haemorrhoids, or nosebleeds. The responses often guided the diagnosis and treatment. Another example is a case history recorded by Giovanni Maria Lancisi (1654–1720),[8] who studied and worked in his native Rome and acted as a personal physician to three popes. The second of these, Clement XI, had asked Lancisi to investigate the many sudden deaths that had befallen Rome in 1705 and 1706. Lancisi's report contained, among others, the fatal illness of a certain bishop Spada.[9]

The story begins with a description of the bishop's body: tall stature, lean body, and a sunken sternum. About one year before symptoms appeared, there had been a change in habitual discharges: bleeding from haemorrhoids had

---

[7] Stoll (1786), *Ratio medendi*, vol. 1, 135–7.
[8] Fantini (2007), Giovanni Maria Lancisi, vol. 3, 766–8.
[9] Lancisius (1707), *De Mortibus subitaneis*, 101–17.

diminished, and a pungent nasal catarrh had completely disappeared, possibly, Lancisi wrote, because of emanations from a freshly chalked wall near the prelate's bed. The first symptoms of disease were 'rheumatic outflow', 'erratic fever', and abdominal pains; then came a period with high fever and a variety of aches in different body parts. Eventually the bishop was seized by apoplexy, with paralysis of his right side and halting speech. The weakness and speech disorder persisted for the last seven months of his life, albeit intermittently, while also the level of consciousness fluctuated. The day before his death, epileptic seizures occurred on the left side. At autopsy, Lancisi, assisted by two colleagues, found some minor abnormalities in the brain and very unusual changes in the valves of the heart. In Lancisi's reconstruction of the disease, he started with implying some constitutional predispositions, but then he put most of the blame on external factors:

> I think the defects that were added to this in the course of the illness have been in the blend of fluids, that is, a mixture far too sharp, pungent and almost poisonous, from the suppression of phlegm via the nose, together with the ingestion of particles of fresh chalk. This could happen only by a gradual communication with nervous fluid or other secondary fluids.[10]

Throughout the eighteenth century, one finds a host of factors implicated as having prepared the ground for apoplexy, alone or in concert. This was not new; many sixteenth- and seventeenth-century physicians, Wepfer not excepted, were fond of reconstructing case histories in such a way that all known circumstances were rearranged until they produced some kind of logical course of events. Environmental factors, especially the 'non-naturals', figured prominently. Intemperance of any kind often topped the list. Heavy drinking, gluttony, venery, and smoking tobacco were obvious culprits, but physical exertion or strong emotions had important roles as well. Similar aetiological considerations dominated a late seventeenth-century essay by William Cole (1714–1782),[11] but as late as 1812, an author might still devote well over 10 pages to such reasoning.[12] Therefore, observation-free theorizing about the causes of apoplexy will receive some more attention below, whereas the last part of this chapter will especially highlight findings on dissection.

APOPLEXY: A MULTITUDE OF CAUSES

Two developments help to explain the impressive list of substances or circumstances that became associated with apoplexy. One, mainly through Wepfer's

---

[10] Lancisius (1707), *De Mortibus subitaneis*, 111.
[11] Cole (1689), *The Late Frequency of Apoplexies*.
[12] Cheyne (1812), *Cases of Apoplexy and Lethargy*, 144–57.

work, was the addition of intracerebral haemorrhage and effusion of serum to the list of morbid fluids already implicated by sixteenth-century physicians who followed Galen's lead. The second was inclusiveness of the term 'apoplexy' in any situation where unresponsiveness was the key feature, whether or not its onset had been sudden.

Yet there was a common theme. It seems fair to say that in the eighteenth-century congestion, overfilling of the skull, by whatever substance and in whatever part, was commonly regarded as the 'final common pathway' in the evolution of apoplexy. A notable exception is the presumption of 'poisonous' factors, as with Lancisi's patient above. The notion of fullness was most poignantly expressed by Jacques Lazerme (1676–1756),[13] Professor of Medicine in Montpellier, who, in his book on diseases of the head, encapsulated the effect of the many causes of apoplexy in the word '*infarctus*',[14] Latin for 'stuffing'. Paradoxically, and perhaps unfortunately, the term 'infarction' has a completely different ring today. The idea of 'stuffing' especially related to the amount of blood contained within brain vessels. Autopsy reports from this era almost invariably emphasized the degree of distension and congestion of blood vessels in the meninges and at the surface of the brain, quite apart from the question of whether or not this was accompanied by extravasation of fluids.

Boerhaave's List

In 1709, the year of his first professorial appointment in Leiden, Herman Boerhaave published his book of aphorisms mentioned earlier. It was a summary of the art of diagnosis and treatment in medicine. Boerhaave had gradually adapted his heuristic approach; starting with a firm belief in reasoning from first principles, he had gradually acquired a conviction that progress of science depended on information from the senses.[15]

In the chapter on apoplexy, Boerhaave began by reciting the phenomena, by now familiar, on which the diagnosis was based and by confirming the notion that the ultimate cause could not but be an interruption in the traffic of animated spirits within the brain. He then went on to list the observable material causes that could be responsible for such a blockade; Table 3.1 reproduces his categories, in abridged form.[16] It is no surprise that his first category consists of certain physical attributes representing constitutional, rather than external, factors. Boerhaave had limited experience in autopsy,[17]

---

[13] Hirsch (1884–8), *Biographisches Lexikon*, vol. III, 633.
[14] Lazerme (1748), *Tractatus de Morbis internis Capitis*, 33.
[15] Cook (2007), *Matters of Exchange*, 383–96.   [16] Boerhaave (1709), *Aphorismi*, 249–52.
[17] Boerhaave (1724), *Atrocis Morbi Historia*.

TABLE 3.1 *Material causes of apoplexy listed by Herman Boerhaave (1709)*

1. The structure of the body: a large head; a short neck; a vast and obese body; a plethoric constitution in combination with a phlegmatic disposition
2. Whatever changes blood, lymph, or the substance of spirits in such a way that they cannot freely travel through the arteries of the brain but get stuck:
    a. Polypous concretions in the carotid or vertebral arteries, or in the heart
    b. Inflammatory thickness of blood
    c. A nature of the whole blood that is thick, glutinous, phlegmatic, and slack
3. Whatever compresses the arteries themselves or the nervous channels of the brain in such a way that the blood and spirits cannot pass:
    a. Plethora: overfilling by constitution, exercise, or heat
    b. Any kind of tumour, inflammation, or abscess
    c. Too great a velocity of blood, such as by blockage of arteries downstream
    d. Factors outside the skull compressing the venous outflow
    e. Effusion of fluids outside the membranes of the brain
4. Everything that dissolves the arterial, venous, or lymphatic vessels at the inside of the brain in such a way that the fluid passes out, accumulates, and through its pressure damages the origins of the cranial nerves. Such fluids are: serum in patients with dropsy or a dropsical diathesis; blood in plethoric patients; and acid black bile in melancholic patients, scorbutic patients, or those with gout

Subcategories for the causes listed under (2) and (3) have been abridged. Also, the symptoms, signs, or circumstances corresponding to each of the causes in question have been omitted. Boerhaave also included a fifth category of poisonous vapours, but then again dismissed it because these acted either through other items on the list or via the lungs.

and none in patients with apoplexy. In his view, it was only rarely a sudden event, for example by rupture of a vessel. Mostly he regarded it as the last stage of a gradual process of compression in the skull, from whatever cause. In other words, Boerhaave joined the ranks of physicians who regarded loss of sensation and movement as the cardinal feature of apoplexy, regardless of the mode of onset:

> Sometimes rupture occurs, owing to great impetus [of blood]; but most often the vessels are merely stuffed, for the reason I already mentioned, that is, the skull forms a hard boundary no matter how it is compressed from the inside. Therefore, arteries rupture a hundred times in the nose against not even once in the skull; yet if the force is very strong this can at last occur.
>
> For this reason, if indeed a collection [of fluid] starts to form, vertigo occurs; if the trouble continues, reeling, stumbling, rotation of the background, anaesthesia, falls and finally apoplexy. The cause is the same, but merely more and more enhanced.[18]

---

[18] Boerhaave and van Eems (1761), *Praelectiones academicae*, 667–8.

Boerhaave agreed that apoplexy could also be caused by black bile – an old problem, already debated in the two previous centuries:

> Certainly, we often see that in melancholic patients, so little of life is left that they are on the brink of death, pulse and respiration being barely present. They are hardly warm, they hardly eat, drink, or sleep, but remain as if in the same state; they often become apoplectics. I have often thought, since these patients often remain stunned, as if struck by lightning, and given that in Catalepsy, that wondrous disease, [patients] freeze like a statue and yet later return to life, whether in these patients blood might not degenerate into similar black and sticky material, which does not contain or release that spiritual something; as a result, the cortex of the brain becomes vapid and varicose by blood that is too thick, resulting in Catalepsy, which later easily ends in Apoplexy.[19]

Apart from the notion that changes in the nature or consistency of circulating blood may prohibit the 'spirits' from reaching the brain, the cited passage shows that physicians at the time could assume a close relationship between apoplexy and other diseases of the brain, such as catalepsy, but also epilepsy, paralysis, or agitated forms of madness. Like many others, Boerhaave thought also paralysis was closely related to apoplexy, at least when its cause was in the brain.[20]

Boerhaave's Disciples in Vienna

Gerard van Swieten (1700–1772),[21] a one-time student of Boerhaave, wrote extensive commentaries on his former teacher's slim octavo volume of aphorisms. In the end, these annotations amounted to five volumes in large quarto, appearing between 1742 and 1772. The work thus became a complete handbook of medicine; it brought the author much fame and was reprinted several times. Initially, van Swieten combined his practice in Leiden with private lessons; he never obtained a formal university appointment because of his Roman Catholic faith. In 1745, he gave in to repeated invitations from Austria's Empress Maria Theresia (1717–1780) not only to become her personal physician, but also to modernize the University of Vienna, especially its medical faculty. In the chapter on apoplexy, which takes up 60 pages,[22] van Swieten dutifully expanded Boerhaave's list of possible causes through which 'fullness of the skull' could result in apoplexy. In his extensive comment, van Swieten cited not only ancient, but also modern authors (Wepfer, Willis, and Baglivi).

---

[19] Boerhaave and van Eems (1761), *Praelectiones academicae*, 651.
[20] Boerhaave and van Eems (1761), *Praelectiones academicae*, 686 and 696–7.
[21] Sigerist (1933), *The Great Doctors*, 205–18; van der Korst (2003), *Gerard van Swieten*.
[22] van Swieten (1755), *Commentaria*, vol. III, 250–310.

Van Swieten referred only indirectly to autopsies in his chapter. However, Anton de Haen (1704–1776) (Box 12.1, p. 369),[23] Chief Physician of the *Bürgerspital* in Vienna, having moved from Leiden ten years after van Swieten, performed four dissections on patients with apoplexy. He recorded them in the fourth instalment of an annual medical report.[24] In cases where the deceased patients had arrived from other Viennese hospitals for dissection, the histories were often sketchy. In two of the four patients, de Haen found haemorrhagic lesions – in one, subpial and intracerebral; in the other, it seemed limited to one ventricle. Another patient was a six-year-old girl, who will be discussed fully in the chapter on venous thrombosis. The story of the fourth patient is also complete:

> A tailor of 55 years had been overcome by anxiety, sadness and a strong rage on August 9, 1757, but went to bed in good health. On waking up on August 10, he noted that his entire right side felt swollen and paralytic; this [paralysis was] not only in his arm and leg, but also in his cheek and tongue, so that he could not be understood when he spoke. [*Treatment*] The effect was that the [feeling of] swelling of his limbs decreased and some movement returned in his leg, but the paralysis persisted in the other [body] parts.
>
> I first saw him on June 9, 1758; from then on, I started to treat him with the electrical machine. His voice became clearer, and the movement of the foot was already sufficient to let him walk alone around a large room, without a stick. However, on his way to the second afternoon at the machine, he had told the servant of the hospital that he did not feel well, but to me [he said] only at the tenth hour that he had a strong attack. He was immediately led to his bed, to let him calm down a bit, and so that I could see what was wrong with him. There he complained of a great cramp in the chest, and within half an hour he was no longer mentally sound. [*Treatment*] Since swallowing was eliminated, the use of medicines was barred. He expired within four hours.[25]

The role of emotions in causing apoplexy, already mentioned by van Foreest, who, in turn, cited earlier sources,[26] became a recurring subject in the eighteenth century, as will be more fully explained in Chapter 4. Electrical treatment for paralysis also emerged in the course of the eighteenth century and became standard procedure in the nineteenth century,[27] marking de Haen as very advanced in this respect. What he found on dissection was equally novel:

---

[23] Sigerist (1933), *The Great Doctors*, 205–18; Lindeboom (1984a), *Dutch Medical Biography*, 763–4.

[24] de Haen (1759), *Ratio medendi*, vol. IV, 163–78.

[25] de Haen (1759), *Ratio medendi*, vol. IV, 168–70.

[26] Forestus (1653 [1590]), *Observationes et Curationes*, vol. X, 509.

[27] Shorvon and Compston (2019), *Queen Square*, 123–6.

Under the arachnoid in the left and foremost part of the posterior lobe, much glittering lymph was visible, in some places reddish. [. . .] The left anterior ventricle, also called the superior one, was very wide everywhere, and full of very copious reddish serum as well as of clotted blood; the corresponding [ventricle] on the right had its natural width and lymph. The fourth ventricle was wide and distended with copious and coagulated blood, down to the large foramen of the occipital bone.

The abnormalities noted in the left hemisphere of the brain are a sufficient explanation for the paralysis of the right side. The abnormalities of the fourth ventricle appear also sufficient to understand the apoplexy and the rapidity of the fatal outcome.[28]

Apart from the 'serous' abnormalities in the left hemisphere, this seems to have been the first description of what today would probably be called a pontine or cerebellar haemorrhage. De Haen based the dynamics of apoplexy on the common premise that the capacity of the skull is limited, whereas the quantity of blood or fluids in general is variable and dependent on lifestyle or disease; even a small extra load in overfilled vessels, with consequent stretching or rupturing, might disturb the functions of the brain.[29]

Finally, de Haen reminds us of the vagueness in categorization of brain disease in his mind, as well as in the mind of many contemporaries. Overfilling of the head might have not only different causes, but also different effects:

Why does apoplexy so often follow paralysis, or generate it? The answer is that the same causes are found for paralysis, epilepsy, apoplexy, lethargy, cataphora, convulsion and other brain diseases.[30]

Interlude: Mistichelli's Novelties

Mention must be made of Domenico Mistichelli (1675–1715), though not for his contributions to the understanding of apoplexy.[31] Mistichelli was a young physician, born in Pisa. Having studied and subsequently taught in his home town, he moved to Rome and was active in several of its hospitals. In 1709, the same year in which Boerhaave first published his aphorisms, Mistichelli authored a monograph on apoplexy. It is probably the first book on apoplexy written in the vernacular, rather than in Latin, apart from William Cole's epidemiological musings in 1689. With respect to causes, Mistichelli offers a typical eighteenth-century repertoire of morbid processes implicating lymph, serum or viscous catarrh, blood, swelling in general, poisonous vapours,

---

[28] de Haen (1759), *Ratio medendi*, vol. IV, 170–1.
[29] de Haen (1759), *Ratio medendi*, vol. IV, 164–7.
[30] de Haen (1759), *Ratio medendi*, vol. IV, 180.
[31] Capparoni (1939), *Domenico Mistichelli e la sua scoperta*.

polyps, strangulations of vessels, and even convulsions.[32] His own experience was very limited – of the 12 patients he listed at the very end of the book, seven survived. Of the five with a fatal outcome, followed by dissection, three had resulted from head injuries, and the other two from 'malignant fever' (possibly malaria). But again, this is not the basis for Mistichelli's posthumous reputation.

Importantly, he began to understand the anatomical basis of 'crossed paralysis', also noted – but not quite explained – by de Haen.[33] This was despite Mistichelli's peculiar conception of brain anatomy by his assumption, following Erasistratus in ancient times,[34] that the meninges contained nerve fibres and conveyed animated spirits. Therefore, Mistichelli located apoplexy as much in the membranes as in the brain itself;[35] six years later, he elaborated on this view in a separately published addendum.[36] It is in this light that one has to interpret his novel description of a configuration on the ventral side of the transition between the medulla oblongata and the spinal medulla (Figure 3.1):

> The feature that has received most [of my] attention is the interlacement (*intrecciamento*) of the fibres of the membranes that surround it. If a part of the Medulla oblongata and the spinal [medulla] is kept in vinegar for the duration of eight or ten days, and after this has expanded to the thickness of a medium-sized knife, first of all a delicate removal takes place of the blood vessels wound around it (these run along the length of the spinal cord in the form of a net-like covering) and subsequently of the outer layer of fibres, which form the said membranes. Once the inside and the next layer has been reached, one observes that the entire brain stem on the outside resembles the plait of a lady, because many groups of straight fibres are superimposed on many transverse fibres, many oblique ones on transverse ones and other straight ones; according to this interlacement every kind in turn covers or is covered, until the said fibres leave the plait sideways to form the spinal nerves, which are at the side.[37]

The significance of this arrangement was not lost on Mistichelli; it helped to explain what Hippocrates had written about unilateral brain lesions causing paralysis or convulsion on the opposite side:

> To explain these [Hippocratic] texts it is necessary to recall what we have observed as a novelty: the medulla oblongata is on its outside covered by fibres that are mutually interwoven and represent a lady's braid; hence it

[32] Mistichelli (1709), *Trattato dell' Apoplessia*, 51–2.
[33] de Haen (1759), *Ratio medendi*, vol. IV, 194–200.
[34] Clarke and O'Malley (1996), *The Human Brain and Spinal Cord*, 12, 282.
[35] Mistichelli (1709), *Trattato dell' Apoplessia*, 46.
[36] Mistichelli (1715), *Aggiunta al Trattato dell' Apoplessia*.
[37] Mistichelli (1709), *Trattato dell' Apoplessia*, 13.

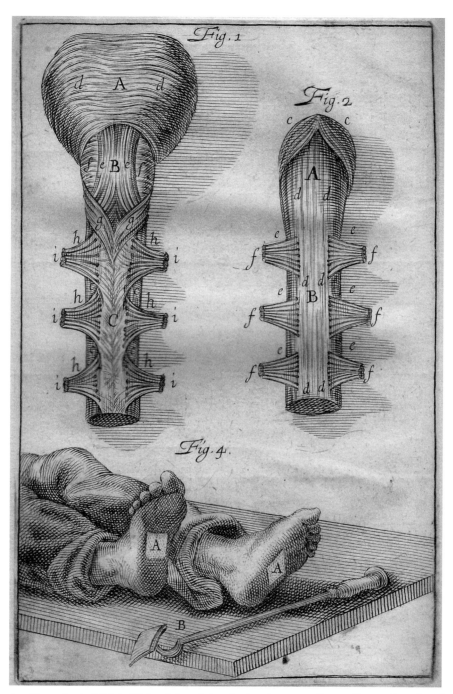

3.1 Engraving in Mistichelli's book (1790) showing interlacement of nerve fibres at the point of transition between the brainstem and the spinal cord. Mistichelli's 'Fig. 3' is not included; it shows the extracranial vessels, more or less schematically. Only the most relevant captions have been translated: 'Fig. 1' shows the front part of the medulla oblongata: dd, circular fibres of the membrane covering the part called 'protuberantia annularis'; ee, straight fibres of the same [membrane]; ff, transverse fibres; gg, oblique fibres, which, [coursing] above and below each occurs that many nerves branching out to one side contain the roots of another side. For example, the [nerves] extending to the right arm can easily contain, by this interlacement, roots from the fibres on the left side of the meninges; the same applies to the left ones, proceeding from the right side.[38]

The other remarkable feature in Mistichelli's book is his preferred treatment of apoplexy: the application of heat. His argumentation was holistic: despite some new chemical terms, he felt supported by Hippocratic writings that 'fire particles' are beneficial in all illnesses. He cited other physicians who had followed this lead by putting heated saucepans, a warm helmet, or burning cloth on the patient's head. Mistichelli himself preferred a branding iron, applied to the soles of the foot ('Fig. 4' in Figure 3.1; Figure 3.2), because he supposed that these parts were richly supplied with nerves and blood vessels.[39] He reported a cure in a patient with fever and, through hearsay, in two cases of his uncle.[40]

MORGAGNI: FROM FLUIDISM TO SOLIDISM

As the practice of dissecting human bodies slowly increased, there was place for a new book in which recent experiences were summarized, to supplant Bonet's rather haphazard and incompletely indexed *Sepulchretum*. This want was more than satisfied by Giovanni Batista Morgagni (1682–1771) (Box 3.2),[41] a towering figure in the history of medicine. His long career as Professor of Medicine in Padua marks a fundamental transition in the understanding of disease. Morgagni provided a wealth of evidence to counter the pervasive notion of disease as a disturbance of the balance between bodily humours. Gradually, disease became associated with changes in organs of the body – changes that could be located, seen, and felt.

Morgagni published his monumental work on clinico-pathological correlations in 1761, at the age of 79. Its title was telling: *De Sedibus et Causis Morborum*, or *About the Sites and Causes of Diseases*. Indeed, diseases could be

---

3.1 (*cont.*) other, form a kind of plait, as of lady's hair; hhhh, oblique fibres, which exit below each other to join in constituting the spinal nerves; iiiiii, site where the spinal nerves are tightly bound by a tendinous ring around these fibres. 'Fig. 2' shows the hind part of the medulla oblongata. 'Fig. 4' shows the soles of the feet and the sites (AA) where the red-hot branding iron (B) should be applied. (*Later readers have interpreted the drawing of the feet as showing the outward rotation of a paralysed left leg. Mistichelli himself is silent about this aspect.*)

[38] Mistichelli (1709), *Trattato dell' Apoplessia*, 58.
[39] Mistichelli (1709), *Trattato dell' Apoplessia*, 121–4.
[40] Mistichelli (1709), *Trattato dell' Apoplessia*, 169–71.
[41] Ongaro (2007b), Giovanni Batista Morgagni.

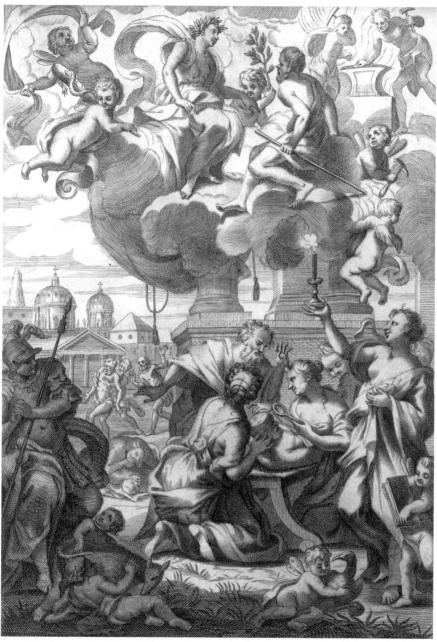

3.2 Frontispiece of Mistichelli's '*Trattato dell' Apoplessia*' (1709). The central object of the
engraving is the corpse of a patient; he has supposedly died from apoplexy. The top part of
the skull has been removed; part of his face, right shoulder, and trunk are visible. Three persons
surround his body: two women, one of whom is applying what looks like a magnifying glass,
and a man in Greek garments, perhaps Hippocrates. The woman to the right of this scene,
holding a candle, probably represents wisdom; the soldier to the left may signify courage. The
three running figures in the background symbolize attempts to escape the disease. Above, two
deities reside on a cloud. The person on the left, wearing a laurel wreath, is presumably Apollo.
The celestial being on the right, with a forge depicted behind him, must be Vulcan; the
branding iron he is holding has a role in the treatment Mistichelli proposes. Putti surround
the scenes.

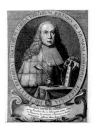

Box 3.2 Giovanni Battista Morgagni (1682–1771).

Morgagni was born in Forli, the central city of Romagna; his parents Fabrizio Morgagni and Maria Tornielli probably belonged to the upper middle class. Giovanni was their only child; his father died when he was seven years old. At the age of 16, he enrolled at the University of Bologna. Three years later, he obtained his degree in philosophy and medicine. His medical teachers had all been educated by Marcello Malpighi (1628–1694). The young Morgagni was especially close to Antonio Maria Valsalva (1666–1723), his senior by some 15 years. It was probably Valsalva's example that induced Morgagni to adopt the habit of keeping daily records of clinical and anatomical observations, post-mortem dissections, lectures, conversations, or anything else of interest. In 1706, Morgagni published his first anatomical work *Adversaria anatomica prima*. Soon afterwards he became involved in polemics with an influential faction of 'empirical' teachers who attacked Malpighi's anatomical approach to disease; he therefore moved away, first to Venice, where he became acquainted with chemistry, then to his native Forli as a practical physician. In this period, he married Paola Vergieri; they were to have 15 children, eight of whom would survive him.

Morgagni's ambition of obtaining a teaching post at the University of Padua, directed by the Venetian senate (*La Serenissima*), became reality in 1711; initially Second Professor of Medicine, he was promoted to the first position in 1714. Having reported several original observations about anatomical structures, he gradually shifted the centre of his attention to pathological anatomy. Eventually he realized the ambitious project of publishing hundreds of case histories, from his own records and those of his teacher Valsalva. Distinguishing features of this great work *De Sedibus et Causis Morborum* are the single authorship and the correlation between clinical features and anatomical changes.

Morgagni also wrote on history, geography, geology, and archaeology. His medico-scientific diary covered the entire period from 1699 to 1767.

Source: Portrait courtesy of Wellcome Foundation.

located. Incidentally, in the same year, the Viennese physician Leopold Auenbrugger (1722–1809) published a small book describing how one could detect diseases of the chest by means of percussion, a method he had seen applied to the wine casks in his father's hotel.[42] Morgagni's *magnum opus* filled two densely printed folio volumes, altogether counting some 750 pages, with each formatted in two text columns in small type. It represents the experience of two lifetimes, since Morgagni also included the records of his teacher Antonio Maria Valsalva (1666–1723). The text lacked illustrations, apart from a frontispiece with the author's stately portrait. Four parts, or 'books', dealt with affections of the head, chest, and abdomen and finally with surgical and

---

[42] Auenbrugger (1761), *Inventum novum ex Percussione Thoracis humani.*

general diseases. A supplementary fifth part contained later cases, encountered during the time of writing. Since the extra examples of diseases of the head, the first subject, date from the late 1740s, Morgagni must have been at it for the best part of 20 years.

He fully attained his aim of emulating the *Sepulchretum*: it represented his personal conviction, adopted from Valsalva, that changes in organ systems could and should be correlated with the patient's symptoms and signs. Overall, the tone of his book is informal, sometimes even conversational, since Morgagni styled the text as 'letters' (*epistulae*), directed to a – probably imaginary – young colleague. Each 'letter' contained observations about a distinct subgroup of diseases, for example tumours of the abdomen.

With regard to apoplexy, Morgagni adhered to the traditional view that its ultimate cause was a lack of animated spirits or obstruction of their pathways, or, in his own words, 'a sudden impairment of the internal motions performed in the brain, that is, when we move, think, or perceive'.[43] But his true ambition was to investigate the underlying changes in the body; some escape the senses, he thought, but many are observable.

Haemorrhages

The sheer number of Morgagni's observations is staggering. On 'sanguineous apoplexy' alone, collected in three *epistulae*, he reported 22 examples with extravasated blood in the brain (eight from Valsalva's records). In one stroke, he dwarfed everything previously written on the subject; the same applied to affections elsewhere in the body. But also, and true to what one might call 'the doctrine of fullness', he assigned to the category of 'sanguineous apoplexy' three patients who had suddenly collapsed and in whom the blood vessels in the brain and meninges looked strikingly engorged – fullness of the head by congestion, even without rupture.[44] Likewise, a patient who had been found dead was included, because much blood came out when the skull was opened, whereas the brain was intact.[45]

In five cases with true extravasation, blood seemed limited to the lateral ventricles; three of these dissections had been by Valsalva, probably long ago. In five other patients, the haemorrhage had occurred at the surface of the brain – a category discussed more fully in Chapter 11 on saccular aneurysms. Two other patients showed collections of blood under the *dura mater*; in one of these patients, with sudden hemiplegia, blood extended to the surface of the

---

[43] Morgagni (1761), *De Sedibus et Causis Morborum*, vol. I, 10 (epist. II, paragr. 5).

[44] Morgagni (1761), *De Sedibus et Causis Morborum*, vol. II, 403–4 (epist. LX, paragr. 8–12).

[45] Morgagni (1761), *De Sedibus et Causis Morborum*, vol. I, 24–5 (epist. III, paragr. 26–7).

brain;[46] in the other, the mode of onset was unknown and there was 'half a pound of blood between the dura and some other membrane, called arachnoid'.[47]

The remaining 10 patients had intraparenchymal haemorrhages. Two of these were in the cerebellum; Morgagni supposed, as Wepfer and Willis had done, that the cerebellum was important for maintaining respiration.[48] In several accounts of the other eight patients, with haemorrhage in a cerebral hemisphere, Morgagni repeatedly emphasized how Valsalva had taught him that with unilateral paralysis, the lesion was always in the cerebral hemisphere on the opposite side; he called this rule 'Valsalva's law'. Though he recognized Wepfer's earlier insight in the matter, Morgagni felt his assessment was somewhat tentative and claimed most credit for his teacher.[49] It also struck him how often these haemorrhages involved the deep medullary regions; he accentuated this aspect by putting a question about the location of haemorrhages in the mouth of his – fictional – correspondent:

> And you will perhaps want to know more things. First of all, why it is that in almost all the examples Valsalva, myself or others described or indicated in this or in earlier letters, [...] that in virtually all these examples, especially those where abnormal cavities were reported in which blood, as concluded from plain evidence, was either contained or poured out, these [cavities] were found in the Thalamus Opticus or the Corpus Striatum, in or near one or the other or both of them, often with perforation and laceration? Moreover, why [was the location] only once, with Wepfer, in the anterior lobe up to the front, and never in the posterior lobe up to the back? [...]
>
> The causes should be sought in the structure of the brain or in the distribution of its deepest vessels. For example, whether the small vessels dispersed over the areas I mentioned are either more numerous or have a greater diameter. Sometimes, when I cut the Corpora Striata horizontally in small slices, I recall having noted, on the anterior and outer side of each, a kind of small pit, through which unmistakably a blood vessel passed. Some other time, by cutting obliquely and slowly, I have shown on the same side several reddish threads, that is, blood vessels, parallel to each other and thicker than elsewhere.[50]

Apoplexies Neither Sanguineous Nor Serous

Apart from patients with haemorrhagic apoplexy, Morgagni classified other abnormalities as 'serous' – we return to these in Chapter 4 – or as 'neither'.

---

[46] Morgagni (1761), *De Sedibus et Causis Morborum*, vol. i, 14 (epist. ii, paragr. 17).

[47] Morgagni (1761), *De Sedibus et Causis Morborum*, vol. i, 23 (epist. iii, paragr. 20).

[48] Morgagni (1761), *De Sedibus et Causis Morborum*, vol. i, 15 (epist. ii, paragr. 24–5); vol. ii, 403 (epist. lx, paragr. 6–7).

[49] Morgagni (1761), *De Sedibus et Causis Morborum*, vol. i, 83–4 (epist. xi, paragr. 10).

[50] Morgagni (1761), *De Sedibus et Causis Morborum*, vol. i, 22 (epist. iii, paragr. 18).

This third category, to which he dedicated a separate letter,[51] was a mixed collection, seven case histories in all. Three showed purulent lesions or an abscess in one hemisphere (including two patients from Valsalva's notes). In a fourth patient, Morgagni had been asked to dissect the body of a tailor in Venice who had become speechless and died two days later; he found whitish fluid over the anterior lobes of the brain and polypous concretions in the sinuses. The fifth was an old man struck first by sudden headache, then 20 hours later by paralysis of the right limbs; he died a few days later. At autopsy, by Morgagni's assistant Nicolas Mediavia, the most striking abnormality in the brain was the brown colour of the entire right hemisphere.

In the two remaining patients, Morgagni put the blame on air – a new culprit. Both individuals had suddenly died. A Venetian fisherman of more than 40 years, liable to intestinal flatulence, had a bout of this malady at sea and died on the spot. The gastro-epiploic vessels were swollen; when these were cut, air escaped, with some blood. Frothy blood filled all veins in the body, the ventricles of the heart, and the sinuses of the brain. The other patient, a 30-year-old Ethiopian, had stood up with his trumpet and, while playing, collapsed and died instantly. In his brain, no lesions were apparent, except the presence of air in the artery running along the *corpus callosum* (current nomenclature: pericallosal artery) and in the artery in which both vertebral arteries are joined (now basilar artery).

Diagnostic Criteria Again Modified by Morphological Findings

One may wonder why some cases of sudden death were included as a form of apoplexy in Morgagni's series: three with either 'engorged' arteries or a profusion of blood on opening the skull, and two in whom cerebral and other vessels contained much air. What was left of the ancient triad that defined the diagnosis of apoplexy? Once more, the diagnostic criteria for apoplexy were stretched, this time to include patients who died within seconds, without a period of at least minutes during which respiration and heart action continued. In other words, the criteria for diagnosis were adapted by force of findings on dissection – a process called 'reverse logic' in Chapter 2.

Wepfer and other seventeenth-century physicians had sometimes relaxed the criterion of sudden onset if the brain of patients showed an excess of fluids other than blood, even if the 'apoplectic state' had developed in the course of an illness. Now Morgagni, also regarding unresponsiveness as the key feature of the disease, made the diagnosis even if heart action and respiration stopped at the very time of the collapse, as long as the cause could be attributed to the brain. This reflects the thinking of a pathologist, not that of a clinician, such as

[51] Morgagni (1761), *De Sedibus et Causis Morborum*, vol. I, 37–45 (epist. v, paragr. 1–27).

Pieter van Foreest, two centuries before; he had firmly excluded the diagnosis of apoplexy when a patient had stopped breathing at the moment he collapsed.[52]

THE GROWING DOMINANCE OF PATHOLOGICAL ANATOMY

Morgagni cast a long shadow. Once his morphological approach had been widely accepted, the body of medical knowledge remained rather stable until the second decade of the nineteenth century. From then on, momentous changes would again occur, at any rate in the understanding of apoplexy. The same timing applies to discoveries in neurophysiology; for this reason, some historians of neuroscience have used the term 'long eighteenth century'.[53] In keeping with this model, the paragraphs below will also cover developments up to the end of the Napoleonic era.

Not every physician writing after Morgagni was equally receptive to the morphological approach. For example, a treatise on apoplexy by G. B. Ponsart (n.d.), published in Liège 14 years after *De Sedibus et Causis Morborum*, cited only earlier works, apart from the opinions of a Parisian professor called Antoine Petit (1722–1794);[54] the book was completely silent about the Paduan experience.[55] In Montpellier, a thesis on apoplexy as late as 1804 barely mentioned Morgagni.[56] At around that same time, another Parisian of the old school was a productive writer himself: Antoine Portal (1742–1832) (Box 3.3).[57] An intriguing figure, he remained influential in medicine until the end of his long lifespan.

Remote Causes: The Last Gasps of External Causality

Portal is the embodiment of the alternative doctrine on causes of disease in eighteenth-century medicine. As touched upon above, reasoning of physicians in that era could be as much concerned with the question 'why did Mrs X have an apoplexy on that particular day and under those particular circumstances'? as with the question 'what happened in the brain of Mrs X when she had her apoplexy'?. Portal makes no bones about it in his book on apoplexy (1811), in his characteristic, insistent style:

> One has seen that physicians generally allowed two kinds: sanguineous and serous, or humoural. But since these can be recognised only by

[52] Forestus (1653 [1590]), *Observationes et Curationes*, vol. x, 513–14.
[53] Whitaker, *et al.* (2007), Introduction.
[54] Hirsch (1884–8), *Biographisches Lexikon*, vol. IV, 543–4.
[55] Ponsart (1775), *Traité de l'Apoplexie.*   [56] Bourée (1804), *Essai sur l'apoplexie*, 55, 60, 65.
[57] Hirsch (1884–8), *Biographisches Lexikon*, vol. IV, 618–19; Ramsey (2007), Antoine Portal.

Box 3.3 Antoine Portal (1742–1832).

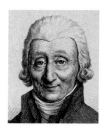

Portal, the eldest son of an apothecary in Gaillac on the river Tarn in southern France, studied medicine in Montpellier, where he developed a special interest in anatomy and surgery. Having defended a thesis on the treatment of dislocations in 1765, he went to Paris and, through family connections, obtained an appointment as a teacher of anatomy to the Dauphin, the future Louis XVI. His closeness to the royal family earned him the right to practise in Paris without a local doctorate and also, in 1785, the title of *chevalier*.

In 1769, he joined the section of anatomy of the *Académie des sciences* and was appointed to the chair of Medicine at the *Collège de France*. In 1778, he became Professor of Anatomy at the *Jardin du Roy*, after the revolution renamed as the 'Museum of Natural History'. He weathered not only the French Revolution and the Napoleonic era, as *citoyen Portal*, but also the restoration of the monarchy, becoming physician to Louis XVIII, as well as to his successor Charles X, who made him a baron and commander of the Legion of Honour. He was instrumental in the creation of the Royal Academy of Medicine in 1820, which replaced the Royal Society of Medicine, founded in 1778 and abolished in 1793.

Portal was a prolific writer. He published a seven-volume book on the history of anatomy and surgery since the earliest times (1770–1773), a five-volume textbook on medical anatomy (1805), and monographs on pulmonary phthisis (1792), apoplexy (1811), and epilepsy (1818), and on a variety of subjects related to public health.

---

dissection, [...] we have in no way thought it wise to adopt this or other distinctions authors have made. [...] We have preferred, following methodical pathologists and De Sauvages in particular,[58] in order to prescribe better treatment, to distinguish apoplexies according to well-recognised *external* causes rather than according to the result of the anatomical autopsy of the brain.[59]

Indeed, Portal arranged his large case series in 20 categories of 'external causes' (Table 3.2); today these would be called 'circumstances', perhaps 'contributing causes' or, at best, 'remote causes'. He illustrated each of the 20 categories with examples of patients, subdivided into 'cases with dissection' (few personal, most others culled from the literature) and 'cases with favourable treatment'; a comment concluded each section. Names of patients were mostly given in full and must have represented the Parisian *haute volée* of aristocracy, commerce, and army. Characteristically, the clinical details that led Portal to the diagnosis of apoplexy are as brief as his particulars about treatment are extensive.

As a sagacious society physician, Portal was keen on finding clues that might explain the occurrence of apoplexy, with a view to treatment. Insofar as he

---

[58] François Boissier de Sauvages de Lacroix (1706–1767), botanist and physician.
[59] Portal (1811), *Observations sur la Nature et le Traitement de l'Apoplexie*, 323–4.

TABLE 3.2 *'External causes' of apoplexy, distinguished by Portal (1811)*

1. During or soon after a meal	11. By convulsions or epilepsy
2. Plethoric	12. By pain, colic, worms, stones, or wounds
3. Inflammatory	13. During pregnancy or around confinement
4. Catarrhal	14. By compression, falls, blows, or straining
5. Arthritic and rheumatic	15. Through cold
6. In persons with emphysema or hydrops	16. By sexual intercourse or masturbation
7. With excess of fat	17. By suppressed evacuations or eruptions
8. Steatomatous congestion, or hereditary	18. With fever
9. Spasmodic or from emotions	19. By poisonous gases or narcotic drugs
10. In melancholic men or hysterical women	20. By strangulation

included findings at autopsy, sanguineous apoplexy was mostly synonymous with blood in the lateral ventricles. He also mentioned rupture onto the surface of the brain, but regarded a patient in whom a large clot was found in the brain tissue itself as so exceptional that he came back to the case in his summary.[60]

In 1826, a late follower of Portal, Jean-Étienne Granier (n.d.) from Marseille, elevated the classification of external causes to dizzying heights by copying the structure of a botanical album, with 'orders' subdivided into *genera* and again into *species*.[61]

Proximal Causes: Pathological Anatomy

Joseph Lieutaud (1703–1780) was also more of a compiler than a dissector. Born in Aix-en-Provence, he studied and worked in Montpellier, where he published a popular textbook of anatomy.[62] In 1750, he settled in Paris as a court physician, serving Louis XV and Louis XVI.[63] There, assisted by the young Antoine Portal, and perhaps trying to emulate Morgagni's 'bible' of 1761, he published six years later a book with summaries of all available post-mortem dissections, from Fernel and Platter up to his own time. His compilation had few clinical and pathological details and listed broad categories, despite a separate index of symptoms. In the section 'Effusions in the brain', subdivided as 'sanguineous', 'serous', 'viscid and gelatinous', and 'sordid',[64] there are many instances of head trauma and fever. Among the effusions that occurred spontaneously, one finds abridged versions of earlier case histories, including many

[60] Portal (1811), *Observations sur la Nature et le Traitement de l'Apoplexie*, 29, 335.
[61] Granier (1826), *Traité de l'apoplexie.*   [62] Lieutaud (1742), *Essais anatomiques.*
[63] Hirsch (1884–8), *Biographisches Lexikon*, vol. III, 708–9.
[64] Lieutaud (1767), *Historia anatomico-medica*, vol. II, 201–71.

by Valsalva and Morgagni. New additions were also brief, each time attributed to a particular physician or institution.

Portal's later approach to apoplexy, by classifying it according to circumstances, drew stiff criticisms from the brothers Montain in Lyon: Jean-François-Frédérik (1778–1851), physician, and Gilbert-Alphonse-Claudius (1780–1853), surgeon.[65] Their own main category was sanguineous apoplexy, subdivided as venous and arterial. The former they characterized as engorgement of the veins and right half of the heart, and the latter as overfilling of the arteries and left ventricle.[66]

Much more influential was the work of Matthew Baillie (1761–1823),[67] a physician at St George's Hospital in London, whose career was not a little helped by his uncles, the famous anatomists John and William Hunter.[68] Baillie published an inventory of his extensive pathological–anatomical observations, not in Morgagni's style with case histories, but in the form of general comments about the different types of morbid change in the organs of the body. The first edition appeared in 1793; in the second edition, in 1797, Baillie also included the most frequent symptoms, at the end of each section about a particular organ. The third edition (1799–1802) was accompanied by *A Series of Engravings* and contained the first illustration of apoplexy caused by extravasation of blood (Figure 3.3).[69] In the fourth edition, Baillie commented that changes in large arteries might predispose to rupture:

> It is very common in examining the brains of persons who are considerably advanced in life, to find the trunks of the internal carotid arteries upon the side of the sella turcica very much diseased, and this disease extends frequently more or less into the small branches. The disease consists in a bony or earthy matter being deposited in the coats of the arteries, by which they lose a part of their contractile and distensile powers, as well as of their tenacity. The same sort of diseased structure is likewise found in the basilar artery and its branches. The vessels of the brain under such circumstances of disease, are much more likely to be ruptured than in a healthy state.[70]

He also found serous effusions in brain tissue, but attributed these to previous haemorrhage, an interpretation we also encountered when Wepfer, Brunner, and Morgagni found old lesions of this kind:

> Cavities containing a serous fluid are sometimes observed in the substance of the brain. They almost constantly occur in the medullary part of the hemispheres, and the substance of the brain immediately surrounding

[65] Hirsch (1884–8), *Biographisches Lexikon*, vol. IV, 270–1.
[66] Montain and Montain (1811), *Traité de l'Apoplexie*, 39–54.
[67] Nicolson (2007), Matthew Baillie.   [68] Moore (2005), *The Knife Man*.
[69] Baillie (1803), *A Series of Engravings*, 226–7.   [70] Baillie (1812), *The Morbid Anatomy*, 453–4.

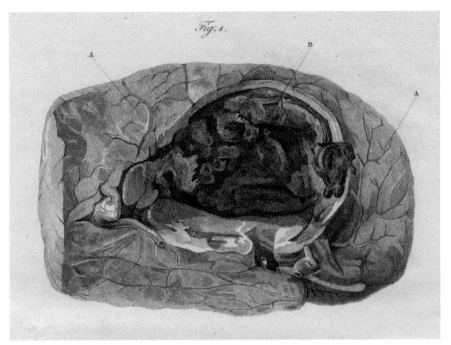

3.3 Apoplexy. Engraving after a drawing by William Clift (1775–1849), in a book by Ballie (1803, p. 226); he provided the following legend:
'Represents the greater part of the half of the cerebrum upon the right side, its anterior extremity being cut off. The flattened side of the hemisphere is presented to view, viz. that which lies in contact with the falciform process of the dura mater.
A. The flattened surface of the right hemisphere of the cerebrum.
B. A large mass of extravasated and coagulated blood. The blood during its extravasation had broke down a considerable part of the medullary substance of the hemisphere, and had burst into the right ventricle.
(This drawing was taken from a very fine preparation presented to the author by Dr Hooper.)'

these cavities is tough and smooth, so as to resemble a membrane. They would appear to be the remains of the cavities formed by extravasated blood, in cases of apoplexy, where the patients have not been carried off immediately, but have lived afterwards for some months or years. The extravasated blood would seem to have been dissolved in such cases, and taken up by absorption; but the injury is not repaired, and a cavity remains afterwards, filled with a serous fluid.[71]

The Site of Vessel Rupture

More specific were the writings of John Cheyne (1777–1836) (Box 3.4),[72] a Scot, about a decade younger than Baillie. Cheyne differed from Lieutaud, Baillie, and Portal in that he documented clinical, as well as anatomical,

[71] Baillie (1812), *The Morbid Anatomy*, 455.
[72] Hirsch (1884–8), *Biographisches Lexikon*, vol. II, 8; Cheyne (1843), Autobiographical sketch.

Box 3.4 John Cheyne (1777–1836).

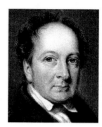

Cheyne was born in Leith, near Edinburgh. From the age of 13, he accompanied his father John in attending to poor patients. Not even 16, he became a medical student in Edinburgh. Having graduated two years later, Cheyne became a military surgeon. Some four years later, in 1799, he returned, joined his father's practice, and was appointed to the hospital in Leith. During this period, he befriended Charles Bell (1774–1845), only a few years older, who instructed him in the techniques for performing dissections. Acute and epidemic diseases of children were Cheyne's special interest; on these conditions, he published selected cases and dissections, and also works on croup, bronchial and bowel disease, and hydrocephalus.

In 1809, he moved to Dublin, where he saw professional opportunities because most Irish physicians had been groomed by Cullen and paid more attention to symptoms than to pathology. Eventually he was appointed to Meath Hospital and soon also as Professor of Military Medicine at the Royal College of Surgeons of Ireland. In 1812, he published his famous *Cases of Apoplexy and Lethargy, with Observations on the comatose Diseases*. In 1815, he relinquished his official medical duties on his appointment to the House of Industry, established by the government 'for the employment and maintaining the poor thereof', but maintained his prolific practice. He continued to publish on a variety of subjects, such as epidemic fevers. Around 1820, he left the House and became Physician-General to the army in Ireland. As his health declined, he at first limited the bounds of his practice, then in 1831 retired to Sherington, Buckinghamshire. Even there, he continued for some time to give medical advice, if requested.

Cheyne had married in Scotland and had at least two sons. He is eponymously remembered by the phenomenon of periodic (Cheyne–Stokes) breathing.

Source: Portrait courtesy of Wellcome Foundation.

---

features. He published on several subjects other than the 'comatose diseases' that concern us here and deserves to be called a true representative of the tradition established by Morgagni.

Cheyne performed more than ten dissections of the brain in patients with apoplexy or 'lethargy'; he found intracerebral haemorrhage in seven of them.[73] Most extravasations involved the ventricular system, but clots also occurred near the centre of the hemisphere, especially in the corpus striatum or the pons, or they involved the surface of the brain. His opinion about the role of the 'bony or earthy matter' in the coats of arteries differed from that of Baillie, who had regarded these lesions as potential sites of rupture:

> In reality, I believe, it generally proceeds not from one considerable vessel, but from a number of the smaller vessels; and, consequently, the

---

[73] Cheyne (1812), *Cases of Apoplexy and Lethargy*, 88–128.

more the larger arteries, by communicating a great impulse to the blood which they are propelling, can add to the increased irritability of their ramifications, the more, one would expect, they would promote that action of the minute vessels which ends in extravasation. [...] Rupture is not necessarily the consequence of the deposition of the gritty matter, even when it exists along the whole course of an artery. For example, the coronary artery, which must feel the effects of occasional distension as much as any vessel in the body, and which I have seen ossified, trunk and branch, is not ruptured in angina pectoris.[74]

The book contained a few illustrations of brain lesions in patients with apoplexy. These were not drawn after Cheyne's own dissections, but from preparations in the museum of Sir Charles Bell (1774–1842),[75] a famous anatomist and surgeon in London; Cheyne and Bell had collaborated as young men in Scotland. One of Bell's specimens showed an intracerebral haemorrhage from which the patient had soon died (Figure 3.4); in another case, the patient 'survived for some time' (Figure 3.5).

Proximal Causes: Other Possibilities than Haemorrhage

When eighteenth-century authors described the pathological anatomy of apoplexy, they rarely distinguished more than two categories: sanguineous and serous. Yet we saw that Boerhaave's list from 1709 (Table 3.1) was much longer; it included any fluid that might lead to overfilling of the head and a variety of space-occupying lesions. He was not alone – van Swieten did the same in his extensive comments on Boerhaave,[76] and also Borsieri (see below);[77] even Portal included 'gelatinous, albuminous and mucous materials'.[78] Yet very few well-documented case reports linked such uncommon anatomical changes with the traditional clinical features of apoplexy; Morgagni was exceptional with his reports of pus, air, and polyps. Most items on such lists had never been observed but were included for the sake of completeness.

The same applies to Wepfer's theoretical suggestion that occlusion of the arterial supply of the brain might lead to apoplexy. Willis had rejected this possibility, given the number and the interconnections of the cerebral arteries, but Boerhaave had kept the idea somewhat alive.[79] Morgagni did the same, despite the experiments of Valsalva who had failed to produce apoplexy after

---

[74] Cheyne (1812), *Cases of Apoplexy and Lethargy*, 37–9.
[75] Gordon-Taylor and Walls (1958), *Sir Charles Bell*; Kaufman (2007), Charles Bell.
[76] van Swieten (1755), *Commentaria*, vol. III, 258–77.
[77] Burserius (1781), *Institutiones Medicinae practicae*, vol. III, 50.
[78] Portal (1811), *Observations sur la Nature et le Traitement de l'Apoplexie*, 346–91.
[79] Boerhaave and van Eems (1761), *Praelectiones academicae*, vol. II, 672.

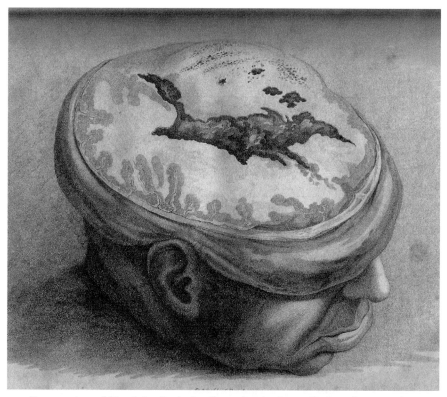

3.4 Extravasation of blood in the brain. Engraving by James Stewart (1791–1863). From Cheyne (1812), who was permitted to have drawings made from specimens of morbid anatomy in the museum of Charles Bell. Cheyne's legend reads as follows:
'This plate represents the section of the brain of a watchman who was found dead in his box. There were no marks of injury in the head, nor was there any suspicion of violence. He had taken several glasses of gin early in the night.
It was remarkable, that, on laying open the surface of the brain, no blood was to be seen in the vessels. On cutting into the substance of the brain it was of a cheesy firmness, and no spot of blood was any where to be observed: but, on opening the ventricles, they were found distended with dark coloured blood, and the coagulum was traced into all the cavities of the brain. From the left ventricle it was traced through the torn substance of the brain, to the corpus striatum, and central part of the hemisphere.'

tying the carotid arteries of three different dogs.[80] Cheyne disagreed; such occlusions, he thought, would cause fainting ('lipothymia').[81]

Hemiplegia

Given that unresponsiveness was the hallmark of apoplexy, isolated paralysis of the arm and leg on one side was mostly labelled as a separate disorder.

[80] Morgagni (1761), *De Sedibus et Causis Morborum*, vol. I, 180 (epist. XIX, paragr. 25–7).
[81] Cheyne (1812), *Cases of Apoplexy and Lethargy*, 27.

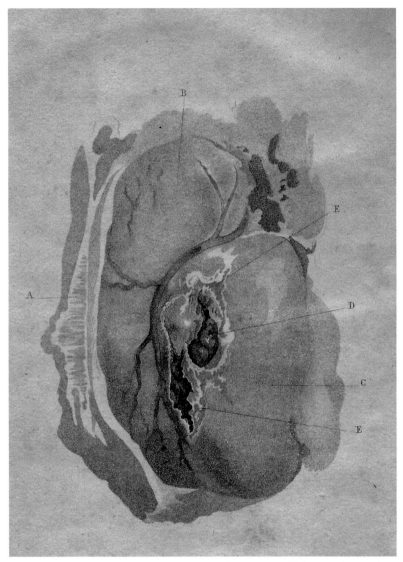

3.5 Same provenance and artist as Figure 3.4. The legend of Dr Cheyne is as follows: 'Represents the effect of an extravasation of blood between the corpus striatum and the thalamus nervi optici. [...]

A. Corpus callosum

B. Corpus striatum

C. Thalamus nervi optici

D. Coagulum of blood contracted and in part absorbed

E. The extent of the irregular cavity formed by the extravasation, now chiefly containing serum.'

However, Giovanni Battista Borsieri de Kanilfeld (1725–1885),[82] Professor of Practical Medicine in Padua and later in Pavia, distinguished apoplexy into a

[82] Hirsch (1884–8), *Biographisches Lexikon*, vol. I, 532.

'true, exquisite' and a 'spurious, mild' form;[83] in the mild form, hemiplegia was not accompanied by a disorder of consciousness. In this way, Borsieri formalized the relationship between unilateral paralysis and apoplexy, explicitly mentioned by Morgagni ('What convulsion is to epilepsy, is paralysis to apoplexy').[84] In Nancy, François-Nicolas Marquet (1683–1759) had expressed himself in the same way,[85] as did Thomas Kirkland (1721–1798) in Edinburgh:

> The moderns agree [. . .] in there being a great affinity betwixt apoplexy and palsy, because they seize in a similar manner, and because they change vice versa from one in the other.[86]

That patients might become apoplectic during sleep was a novel experience, reported by François-Emmanuel Foderé (1764–1835).[87] Born in a poor family in the Savoy region, he studied in Turin, settled as a physician in Martigues, at the Provence coast, and became an expert in a diversity of medical subjects.[88] In a treatise on apoplexy, Foderé recounted how he accidentally detected a mild form of hemiplegia:

> One of the surgeons in the community of Martigues, an old man of nearly eighty years, a slender and honest man, met me last summer when I was visiting patients, in order to carry out a venesection I had ordered. I perceived that he was stammering; when I had noticed his distorted mouth I had also a look at his right hand, of which two fingers were immobile. Unaware of it, he had recently sustained a mild apoplectic attack – not for the first time in his long life. Step by step the movement and sensation returned to the right hand, so that by now the good man can still devote himself to his craft; also, he stammers less.[89]

A THIRD MAIN GROUP OF CAUSES

'Serous apoplexy' is not the only form of apoplexy that faded into oblivion after the medical minds of the late seventeenth and long eighteenth century had paid serious attention to it. Another example is 'nervous apoplexy'.

Near the end of the seventeenth century, Thomas Willis' idea that apoplexy might occur by chemical or other subtle factors inspired a younger colleague in Brandenburg to hypothesize that apoplexy might occur without obvious changes in the brain on dissection. His name was Michael Ettmüller (1644–1683), Professor of Botany and later of Surgery at the University of

[83] Burserius (1781), *Institutiones Medicinae practicae*, vol. III, 57.
[84] Morgagni (1761), *De Sedibus et Causis Morborum*, vol. I, 82 (epistula XI, paragr. I).
[85] Marquet (1770), *Traité de l'Apoplexie*, 142–7.
[86] Kirkland (1792), *Apoplectic and Paralytic Affections*, 81.   [87] Foderé (1808), *De Apoplexia*, 6.
[88] Hirsch (1884–8), *Biographisches Lexikon*, vol. II, 391–2.   [89] Foderé (1808), *De Apoplexia*, 7.

Leipzig.[90] He died of lung disease before he was 40, according to some as a consequence of chemical experiments. In a posthumous edition of his works, prepared by his son and later successor at the university, Ettmüller explained:

> For this same reason *Willis* does not agree with the exclusive [role of] abnormal collection of serous or other humours in the centre of the brain, but he also incriminates a virulent force chasing as well as inactivating the animated spirits. [...] And let me be silent about the quite commodious and almost common fallacy of *a cause for the sake of a cause* in the *interpretation of Anatomical Observations*, so that an abnormality found by chance is held for the cause of disease or death, or that a consequence of the disease is regarded as its origin.[91]

The notion of functional varieties of apoplexy slowly took root in the first half of the eighteenth century; it even broadened to include 'spasm' of nervous structures. The most common names for this category of disease were 'nervous apoplexy' or 'spasmodic apoplexy'. As might be expected, this belief was not generally shared. But since a man like Borsieri, an authoritative and well-referenced textbook writer, had in 1781 listed the three main categories of apoplexy as sanguineous, serous, and convulsive,[92] and since we shall see that even the great Morgagni took recourse to functional mechanisms in explaining some of his findings, 'nervous apoplexy' cannot be written off as just one of countless idiosyncrasies in the history of medicine. Instead, it has truly belonged to the mainstream of medical practice. Therefore, not only 'serous apoplexy', but also a 'nervous' variant, merits separate discussion in Chapter 4 on ephemeral forms of apoplexy.

---

[90] Hirsch (1884–8), *Biographisches Lexikon*, vol. II, 310–11.
[91] Ettmüller (1685), *Opera omnia theoretica et practica*, part II, 302–3.
[92] Burserius (1781), *Institutiones Medicinae practicae*, vol. III, 67.

FOUR

FORGOTTEN FORMS OF APOPLEXY

SUMMARY

In one of the four patients with apoplexy, Wepfer described in 1658 the excess of fluid in the brain was not blood, but 'serum' – a gelatinous form of it covered the entire surface. Wepfer therefore distinguished 'serous apoplexy' from the sanguineous form, even though the apoplectic state had occurred as part of a protracted illness. Later he reported similar cases. In retrospect, thanks to Wepfer's meticulous recording, a retrospective diagnosis of chronic infectious disease seems inescapable. In the eighteenth century, Boerhaave and van Swieten implicated the accumulation of brain lymph as a cause of apoplexy, but without providing anatomical proof. In Morgagni's large series of dissections, patients classified as having 'serous apoplexy' showed a variety of lesions; in a patient with 'paralysis', he found unilateral 'erosion' of the striate body, like Willis before him. In the decades around 1800, once it had become fashionable to diagnose apoplexy in a variety of attacks, the 'serous' form was considered less often.

The term 'nervous apoplexy' emerged towards the end of the seventeenth century (Ettmüller, Friedrich Hoffmann). It was often diagnosed when the brain showed no abnormalities despite a fatal apoplectic disorder or if a patient recovered from an unresponsive state. The explanation was sometimes sought in the brain itself (emotions, mental exhaustion, tightness, or convulsions of the meninges), sometimes in the chest or abdomen. In the latter case, the 'sympathic action' was attributed to toxic particles, retained menstrual blood, 'vapours', dregs of gout, or intense pain, with or without increased blood flow to the brain. In clinical terms, the diagnosis of 'apoplexy' became so much stretched in the eighteenth century that it was applied to almost any form of unconsciousness.

SEROUS APOPLEXY

Wepfer was the source of the notion 'serous apoplexy'. He distinguished it from sanguineous apoplexy, apart from impaired arterial flow towards the brain, which remained a theoretical possibility – for him, at least. 'Serous apoplexy' was to remain prominent in the thoughts of later generations of physicians, up to the early nineteenth century. Wepfer regarded serum as a possible cause since he found, in one of the four patients with apoplexy he dissected, not blood but a large collection of clear fluid. Importantly, the patient had lapsed into an apoplectic state only in the final stage of his illness. Wepfer found this observation so compelling that he overlooked the incongruity that the onset of the patient's disease had been progressive and not instantaneous, as the ancient definition of apoplexy had it. In other words, morphological changes no longer merely served to explain a given set of symptoms; they were conspicuous enough to overrule an atypical onset – reasoning backwards. Here are the details.

Chest Pain and Gelatinous Serum

Jacob Reutinger, some 50 years of age, had always been employed in the vineyards. Red blotches disfigured his face; some people attributed it to wine drinking. A few months before the current illness, he had consulted Wepfer on account of excruciating chest pain; at first, his treatment seemed successful, but when the pain persisted, the patient sought help from a hangman, who apparently moonlighted as a healer. 'A couple of weeks' before his death, Jakob developed a vicious headache; at times, the pain drove him out of his mind; yet he refused all treatment. Three weeks before his death, he became blind; examination of the eyes showed no cataract or other abnormality. Soon afterwards, he became bed-bound; he tossed around with pain, eventually wetting his bed; his feet became paralysed. Four days before his death, he was found 'apoplectic': he could not be roused and did not speak or move. No fever had occurred at any time. After his death, in February 1656, the widow allowed dissection of the head, but not of the chest and abdomen.[1]

> After the dural membrane had been incised, pale, corn-coloured serum flowed out with some force, in the same way as blood gushes from the median vein of the arm when it is cut; here even in such large quantity,

---

[1] Wepfer (1658), *Observationes anatomicae*, 15–17.

that it could have filled more than one cup with a few ounces. For the most part this serum was collected in the space between the dura and pia mater, which [space] seemed to me larger and more capacious than normal. By its excessive volume the serum everywhere stretched the dural membrane, unless an obstacle was in the way, and it depressed the brain and the cerebellum. Indeed, even more serum was contained between the pia mater and the cerebrum and cerebellum. Furthermore, the entire surface of the cerebrum and cerebellum, gyri as well as sulci – where the gyri had been forced apart – were covered far and wide with something like gelatine. When it was cut with a knife it oozed clear serum, almost similar to that between the dura and pia mater. I could very clearly recognise that the actual substance of the brain and cerebellum was drenched in serum, for both were extraordinary flabby and soft. [...] In all ventricles there was also an excess of serum.[2]

At this time, the arachnoid membrane had not yet been identified (see below). Serum was a well-known constituent of blood; if blood was collected after venesection in a receptacle and was left standing, sedimentation of particles occurred, with a supernatant layer of serum. For the notion of 'serum overload', Wepfer had found support in the writings of Carolus Piso, or Charles Le Pois (1563–1633) (Box 4.1). In a monograph published in 1618, Le Pois highlighted the role of serum in the pathogenesis of several diseases, including apoplexy. If the changes were so rapid, Piso argued, for example in 'mild' apoplexy, in which sudden prostration was followed by paralysis on one side, how could phlegm be displaced so quickly?[3] Wepfer not only praised Piso for having drawn attention to the role of serum in apoplexy, but he also exculpated him for some mistakes, since at the time when his book appeared, the circulation of blood was not yet known.[4] Wepfer reasoned as follows:

Serum [...] is an inseparable companion of blood; because they are transported together through the entire brain within the capillary arteries, and [because] it is fine-spun and almost free of viscosity, it can pass through the smallest openings and make its way into the narrowest channels, in the same way as water gets into the little cavities of sponges, or into substances even tighter than sponges. In addition, it is not difficult to separate it from blood; this is testified not only by urine, tears and sweat, but also by certain diseases, as proved by catarrh, serous diarrhoea, arthritis, etc.[5]

Thus, Wepfer imagined, this separation of serum from the rest of the blood was driven by the same pulsatile force that could also cause haemorrhage into

[2] Wepfer (1658), *Observationes anatomicae*, 17–19.
[3] Piso (1618), *De praetervisis hactenus Morbis*, 89–90.
[4] Wepfer (1658), *Observationes anatomicae*, 271.
[5] Wepfer (1658), *Observationes anatomicae*, 246.

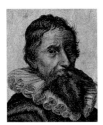

Box 4.1 Charles Le Pois (1563–1633).

Charles Le Pois was born in Nancy where his father was a physician to the count of Lorraine. Having studied medicine in Paris and Padua, Charles started a practice in his home town, until he also became physician to the count – first Charles III, then Henri II. In 1598, he became Professor and Dean of Medicine at the University of Pont-à-Mousson (Lorraine), newly founded as a Jesuit bulwark against the dominant Protestantism beyond the eastern border of France.

Source: Portrait courtesy of Wellcome Foundation.

the brain. But here, the explanation went, it is not whole blood, but only serum that is squeezed through tiny openings in the terminal ramifications. Next, serum was thought to obstruct the entry of animated spirits by blocking minute openings in nerve tissue. It was rather commonly supposed at the time that brain tissue and nerves contained tiny, invisible channels, at least for physicians who no longer believed in transport of spirits via ventricular fluid.[6] It was an inescapable hypothesis, in Wepfer's eyes:

> The first thing that must be mentioned before everything else with regard to the obstruction is that the brain and the cerebellum are porous, not only because of the relationship with arteries, of which [both] receive very many – pores of this type are visible in great number – but also because of the animated spirits that have to be transported from both these [bodies] into nerves. That these spirits must consist of some kind of material is clear from the diverse paralyses of body parts and ligatures of nerves. For if these spirits had to be allocated to the category of spiritual qualities, they might easily overcome these obstacles (in the same way as light goes through the thickest window panes and smells of bait are perceived by fishes swimming in the deepest pools).[7]

Obstruction of nervous pathways by serum was not an all-or-nothing phenomenon, according to Wepfer; patients might suffer hemiplegia or other partial defects and subsequently recover or at least survive. In this way, he explained a gradual course of the disease. He also recalled patients in his practice who had experienced premonitory symptoms, even repeatedly, before ending up with a true apoplexy. In one patient, who went through an episode of being unable to read what he had written himself, Wepfer described these symptoms in such admirable detail that a modern neurologist can exactly

---

[6] Smith (2007), Brain and mind in the 'long' eighteenth century, 17–18.
[7] Wepfer (1658), *Observationes anatomicae,* 244.

localize the site of the lesion.[8] Wepfer could not actually prove that serum caused these episodes in his patient, but he based his conclusions on circumstantial evidence.[9]

A 'Postscript' in 1675

Seventeen years after the publication of his first treatise, when Wepfer's fame had spread throughout Europe, he had the book reprinted – at the request of his friends, as he wrote in the introduction. In addition, he added 17 new cases of apoplexy, seven of which were from colleagues. At the end of each case report, Wepfer added a section with commentaries (*scholia*) to explain the course of events, often in great detail, especially if autopsy of the brain had been performed (ten patients). In these 10 cases, the cause of death had been head injury in four and disease outside the head in two; a seventh patient, a boy of 19, admitted to hospital with fever and delirium, showed purulent changes in the brain. In the remaining three new case reports, Wepfer's diagnosis was 'serous apoplexy'; one of these, to whom he had only briefly alluded in his earlier book,[10] shared some characteristics with Jacob Reutinger, above:

Jacobus Spoerlin, a basket-maker in his 70s, had an eventful life before ending up in the municipal hospital of Schaffhausen. He was in a miserable state of health but eventually recovered and became an expert in his craft. In later years, he had several ailments, which Wepfer successfully treated and dutifully recorded. In the final year of his life, Spoerlin started to cough, especially in the morning; the phlegm was 'greenish, opaque, thick, viscid, smooth, certainly not smelling, sometimes tinged with blood'. The coughing gradually worsened, until it troubled him day and night. A few weeks before his death, he felt suffocated, started to run a fever, lost weight, became bed-bound and died. What follows are relevant details of the dissection; Wepfer performed it with a colleague:

> When the chest was opened, we found that the upper lobes of both lungs were increased in size, especially on the left; they were both rather hard and solid, yet they had not reached the degree of hardness that I had observed elsewhere in patients with phthisis. Cut open, they were ulcerated in the top part and had formed holes with the size of walnuts, yet not completely round nor equally hollow, but torn as it were, as if the

---

[8] Wepfer (1658), *Observationes anatomicae*, 264–9; van Gijn (2015), A patient with word blindness in the seventeenth century.

[9] Wepfer (1658), *Observationes anatomicae*, 263–70.

[10] Wepfer (1658), *Observationes anatomicae*, 360.

lungs had been eaten by a weasel or a dormouse. [...] After the top of the skull had been removed, much pale serum flowed out from the space between the two membranes, but not in such mass as I had seen in the case of Jacob Reutinger, for the intervening space was narrower. The entire surface of the convolutions was covered with a kind of gelatine, from which water emerged if it was pierced with a knife. We also found much of this serum in all ventricles.[11]

A Modern Reinterpretation

The interpretation of the preceding two case histories by a modern neurologist must be different from that of Wepfer. Retrograde diagnosis of diseases in the past is notoriously difficult and deservedly suspicious, but especially in the case of the first patient, Jacob Reutinger, the temptation is impossible to resist. In the final phase of his illness, probably a fortnight at most, Wepfer recorded the sequential occurrence of excruciating headache, blindness, unresponsiveness, and death; with this order of events and a gelatinous layer covering the surface of the brain, few neurologists can suppress the suggestion of tuberculous meningitis.[12] In addition, Reutinger's initial chest pain may well have indicated the source of the brain disease, even though the lungs could not be examined after death; after all, phthisis was rampant at the time.[13] The 'gelatine-like' (*seu gelatina*) substance corresponds to illustrations of tuberculous meningitis in the early nineteenth century in atlases of pathological anatomy by Bright and Cruveilhier,[14] and later by photography.[15] In the case of Jacobus Spoerlin, the diagnosis of pulmonary tuberculosis is also inescapable; involvement of the brain was less obvious from the nervous symptoms, but more so from the anatomical changes.

In all his comments, Wepfer did his utmost to reconstruct the course of events; some examples will follow. With hindsight, his reasoning may seem long-winded and forced, but fortunately he kept his observations and his interpretations strictly apart. Modern interpretations of his findings, tricky as they are, would not have been possible without Wepfer's meticulous inspection and reporting.

[11] Wepfer (1675), *Observationes anatomicae, cum Auctuario*, 370–6.
[12] Marais, *et al.* (2010), Tuberculous meningitis.
[13] Barberis, *et al.* (2017), The history of tuberculosis.
[14] Bright (1827–31), *Reports of Medical Cases*, vol. II, part 2, plates XXIX and XX; Cruveilhier (1829–42), *Anatomie pathologique du Corps humain*, vol. I, livraison VI, planche I.
[15] www.flickr.com/photos/pulmonary_pathology/6541111989/in/set-72157628488912495. [Accessed 20 October 2021]

Young Women with Hemiplegia and, Much Later, Serous Apoplexy

Wepfer's new case reports of 1675 included two more examples of what he regarded as serous apoplexy, but with a more complicated course.

Ursula Aberlin, an unmarried girl of 23, employed as servant at a village inn, twice felt something snap in her head while she was hauling a heavy load of cattle food, in summer of 1667. From that time onwards, she had some difficulty holding her water. In December of that same year, after she had sought shelter against the cold in a church, she suddenly lost all sensation and movement in the left arm and leg, within a few minutes; her mouth was also awry and she spoke with difficulty. Taken home, she stayed in bed for two weeks, was sometimes delirious, and complained of headache. When Wepfer saw her, eight weeks after the event, the paralysis of the arm and leg was unchanged; she spoke well and had a good colour. The countess of the region supplied the drugs Wepfer prescribed. The patient learnt to walk again with a stick, but in the following summer (of 1668), the weakness of the left side worsened; the headache returned and became steadily worse. In January of the next year, she suffered from 'catarrh of the chest'; she coughed not only phlegm, but also blood clots. Her abdomen and left arm became swollen; she developed dropsy and painful gangrene of the right foot, became delirious, and died on 24 March 1669.

By persistent entreaties, Wepfer was permitted to perform a dissection. On opening the *dura mater* of the brain, yellowish serum flowed out; a gelatinous, transparent, yellow membrane covered the entire surface of the brain. The right half of the brain, near the ventricle, contained two abscesses, about the size of a hen's egg; one of these was inadvertently cut. The chest was not opened, because Wepfer was called away and the patient had not voiced complaints about that region of the body.[16]

In his comments, Wepfer related the two abscesses (or tumours – he used both terms) to the episode in which the patient had carried a heavy load, almost two years before. This is but one example of his attempts to fit all recorded observations into a logical framework. He attributed the left-sided hemiplegia that occurred six months later to an excess of serum, perhaps with some contribution from the two 'tumours' (he was by now well aware that body parts often corresponded to areas of the brain on the opposite side). He blamed dietary factors for the recurrence of the headaches that initially accompanied the hemiplegia, and the two tumours for the dizziness, after an extensive discourse about his experience with brain cysts in mules. With regard to the cause of death, he remained somewhat evasive – after all, he had not examined the lungs and the heart.[17]

---

[16] Wepfer (1675), *Observationes anatomicae, cum Auctuario,* 392–400.
[17] Wepfer (1675), *Observationes anatomicae, cum Auctuario,* 400–10.

Ursula Pulen Frisen, 37 years old, had given birth to several children and was again four months pregnant. For a long time, she had complained of headache and dizziness, when, one morning in May 1661, crouching because of violent headache, she suddenly lost her voice, fell down like a log and was deprived of all sensation and motion, except breathing. Transferred to bed, she was motionless for three days; then it became clear that she could no longer move her right arm and leg. Within a month, she was again able to walk when supported, dragging her foot, while the arm remained useless. In October, she was delivered of a healthy baby but showed no concern for this infant or the other children. She was often 'delirious' or afraid of harmless noises, and made several attempts to hang, or otherwise harm, herself. Gradually she became quieter, but she lost weight and became pale in the face. She became pregnant once more and bore another child, which she breast-fed until her death. On 21 February 1664, she was woken up by a severe pain in the right part of her chest, which became even worse in the next few days. She coughed continuously, with blood-tinged sputum, became delirious, and died on 26.

Wepfer had not been involved in her treatment but received permission for autopsy, thanks to the abbot of a nearby monastery. In the head, the dural membrane was swollen and tense, as if inflated by vapours; its vessels were full of blood. The pia mater seemed to squeeze and flatten the convolutions. The surface of the brain looked swollen on both sides – everywhere copious serum flowed out when it was damaged. Both ventricles contained blood-tinged serum; the same fluid was found at the base of the brain. The walls of the ventricles 'looked orange-yellow, as if covered by rust; for it was lined with yellow slime, similar to what is seen around iron-containing waters and often incrusts the surface of stones and the soil'. The right lung was firmly attached to the pleura; when this had been torn loose, almost two pounds of pale serum stagnated in the back of the chest. The lobes of the right lung were all large, hard, tense, and red, or rather spotted with red, and their outer membranes solid and thickened. On incision, both lungs were full of blood-tinged grime, watery, foamy, and in the deeper parts purulent.

Wepfer's reconstruction of this sad tale was, in brief, that swollen blood vessels of the *dura mater* had caused the headache, which, in turn, had caused a temporary surge of serum that caused apoplexy but was no longer found at the time of the patient's death, caused by inflammation of the lungs and its membranes.[18]

The symptoms and findings in the two women, incidentally both named Ursula, have a few things in common with those in the two men called Jacob. No doubt all aspects of the disease of the servant girl, in the brain as well as in the

---

[18] Wepfer (1675), *Observationes anatomicae, cum Auctuario*, 410–16.

lungs, are explained by some form of chronic inflammation, while the gelatinous layer covering the brain is again suggestive of tuberculosis. The farmer's wife died of a pulmonary infection. Her history of progressive headache and the 'yellow slime' in the brain are equally consistent with chronic infection. Less obvious is the explanation of the sudden hemiplegia both had experienced before.

SEROUS APOPLEXY: AN ESTABLISHED NOTION IN THE EIGHTEENTH CENTURY

Why did the notion of serous apoplexy catch on and have such a relatively long life, up to the early 1900s? One of the reasons is Wepfer's growing reputation. After all, he had been the first to explore the inside of the brain in patients with intracerebral haemorrhage and to describe the resulting anatomical changes. Later generations also followed his example in extending the diagnosis of apoplexy to patients who had become unresponsive only in the course of an illness.

Furthermore, the remembrance of Galen's 'thick phlegm' has undoubtedly facilitated the acceptance of more fluid counterparts, variously described as serum, water, or 'lymph'. As the battles over Harvey's theory of circulation illustrate, acceptance of new knowledge is extremely difficult unless there is some relationship with existing knowledge.[19]

Wide Acceptance

The idea that excess of serum was a potential cause of apoplexy did not remain restricted to isolated researchers or centres of learning. The notion soon percolated to less prominent medical centres. In 1709, Domenico Mistichelli (1675–1715), a physician in Rome, mentioned effusions of serum or lymph in his book on apoplexy.[20] Another example is an inaugural dissertation at the University of Halle, Brandenburg in 1728:

> From what I have so far reviewed, it seems sufficiently clear there are two kinds of apoplexy, sanguineous and serous; the former is due to overly abundant and copious blood, excessively distending the vessels of the brain, the latter to phlegm and relaxation of tissues.[21]

The supervisor of the thesis, Friedrich Hoffmann the younger (1660–1742), reproduced in his popular textbook Wepfer's explanation of exudation via small pores.[22] Also influential was Boerhaave's interpretation of serous

---

[19] Fleck (1980 [1935]), *Entstehung einer Tatsache*, 53–5.
[20] Mistichelli (1709), *Trattato dell' Apoplessia*, 51–2.   [21] Adam (1728), De Apoplexia, 15–16.
[22] Hoffmann (1732), *Medicina rationalis*, vol. IV, part II, 172.

apoplexy (see Table 3.1, p. 90). It shows how physicians could implicate different colourless fluids in the pathogenesis of apoplexy, from Wepfer's 'gelatinous layer' to Boerhaave's 'normal humour' surrounding the brain.

Boerhaave's Brain Fluid and Its Obstruction

Given his lack of personal experience with apoplectic brains, Boerhaave's approach was necessarily theoretical. He emphasized, even more than Wepfer did,[23] the limited capacity of the skull, so that the addition of any extra fluid should lead to compression of nervous structures.[24] In his list of fluids that could act as potential causes of apoplexy, by rupture or distension of vessels, he rarely applied the term 'serum', at least not in the sense of a filtrate of blood, as Wepfer had done. Boerhaave designated the normal content of brain cavities as 'fluid', 'humour', or 'water', because he was uncertain about its origin. By this time, the subarachnoid space had been identified (Figure 4.1);[25] Boerhaave therefore noted in his lectures:

> Since the entire brain with all its appendages is surrounded by this arachnoid layer and it does not merge with the dura mater, the pool can overflow all these parts. It can thus occur over its entire circumference, for the four lobes of the brain are quite freely accessible.[26]

Boerhaave assumed the fluid was somehow secreted from blood and located the problem at its exits. He was critical, as Wepfer and Willis had been,[27] of the ancient belief that fluid, having passed from the infundibulum to the pituitary gland, somehow dripped across the skull base to the palate and the nose. In fact, Conrad Schneider, Professor of Medicine at the University of Wittenberg, had experimentally proved in the middle of the seventeenth century that fluids could not pass out along this route, neither below the pituitary gland nor more anteriorly, through the cribriform (sieve-like) plate.[28] Willis had been aware of these studies.[29] Boerhaave exhorted anatomists to find the tiny hidden pathways,[30] which, he thought, allowed an exit to brain fluid but disappeared soon after death.[31]

[23] Wepfer (1658), *Observationes anatomicae*, 290–1.
[24] Boerhaave and van Eems (1761), *Praelectiones academicae*, 659–60.
[25] Ruysch (1743 [1697]), Responsio ad Goelicke; Ridley (1695), *The Anatomy of the Brain*, 15–16.
[26] Boerhaave and van Eems (1761), *Praelectiones academicae*, 666.
[27] Wepfer (1658), *Observationes anatomicae*, 153; Willis (1664), *Cerebri Anatome*, 144–8.
[28] Schneider (1655), *Liber de Osse cribriformi*; Schneider (1660), *De Catarrhis*.
[29] Willis (1664), *Cerebri Anatome*, 56.
[30] In 1875, the 'exits' were definitively located in Pacchioni's granulations (Key and Retzius (1873), *Studien in der Anatomie des Nervensystems*, vol. I, 168–87).
[31] Boerhaave and van Eems (1761), *Praelectiones academicae*, 671.

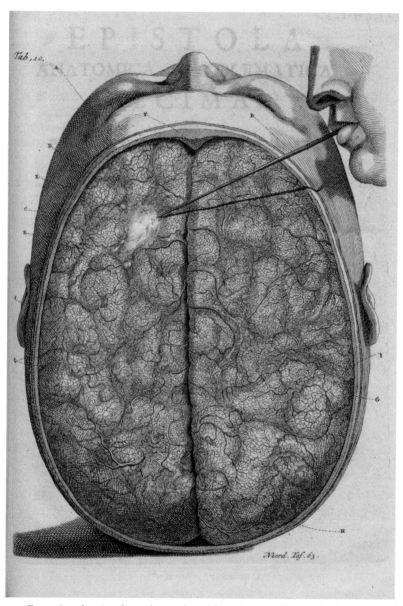

4.1 Engraving showing how the arachnoid layer bulges when air is blown through a straw inserted between the arachnoid and pial membranes (from Ruysch, 1697).

Gerard van Swieten broadly followed Boerhaave's reasoning on the many possible ways in which 'fullness of the skull' could result in apoplexy, including excess of serum – or lymph, as he often called it. And, like Boerhaave, van Swieten could not cite post-mortem observations, but he alluded to two other reports;[32] one of these was a case of sudden death,[33] and in the other, the

[32] van Swieten (1755–72), *Commentaria*, vol. III, 262.
[33] Mangetus (1700), *Theophili Boneti Sepulchretum*, vol. I, 138–9.

disease onset had been gradual.[34] Given van Swieten's authority – even Morgagni was to cite him – the following passage is illustrative:

> But because that accumulation of lymph occurs gradually, the symptoms worsen slowly, as the disturbed functions of the brain show; patients suffer from these for months and sometimes even years before apoplexy ensues. Sometimes they even perish from other diseases, before lymph had accumulated in such excess that it abolished all functions of the brain, by pressing on it. In contrast, when vessels have ruptured and blood flows out, apoplexy occurs mostly immediately.[35]

How Serous Apoplexy Could Be Cured But Not Seen

In 1770, serous apoplexy was mentioned in a posthumous booklet on diseases of the brain by François-Nicolas Marquet (1683–1759).[36] Born in Nancy, Marquet studied in Pont-à-Mousson and Montpellier before settling as a physician in his home town.[37] Marquet's 33 case histories of apoplexy contain few clinical details, in contrast to his treatments – combinations of shaking the patient, venesection, enemas, emetics, scarifications or blistering plasters, simple or composite drugs (with recipe), and *bouillon*. Not a single post-mortem dissection was included. In fact, Marquet was hugely successful with his treatment, since only 3 of the 33 patients failed to recover completely within a few days or weeks; the only fatality occurred when Marquet was away. Nevertheless, it is useful to reproduce his reasoning about the distinction between sanguineous and serous apoplexy:

> On December 26, 1734, I was called to see Mr Saint-Jean, carpenter in Nancy, who had been seized with apoplexy, without sensation or move-ment. Of the natural functions only the pulse was preserved, as well as the respiration, which was irregular and difficult. The paleness of the face and also the weakness and contraction of the pulse allowed the conclu-sion that this apoplexy was caused by an effusion of a serous fluid on the brain, which compressed the cortical substance and at the same time impeded the outflow of spirits to the body parts and so suppressed their functions. [*treatment*] When the patient had regained complete conscious-ness, I ordered him to take [...] every fortnight, to prevent a recurrence.[38]

---

[34] Schwencke (1733), *Rari Casus Explicatio anatomico-medica.*
[35] van Swieten (1755–72), *Commentaria*, vol. III, 263.
[36] Marquet (1770), *Traité de l'Apopléxie*; presumably published by his son-in-law Pierre-Joseph Buc'hoz.
[37] Hirsch (1884–8), *Biographisches Lexikon*, vol. IV, 138; Dos Santos (2008), François-Nicolas Marquet.
[38] Marquet (1770), *Traité de l'Apopléxie*, 33–5.

MORGAGNI: SERUM AS A CAUSE OF APOPLEXY, SUDDEN DEATH, OR PARALYSIS

Even Morgagni primarily distinguished between sanguineous and serous apoplexy ('a celebrated division') in his monumental *De Sedibus et Causis Morborum*. 'Some oppose the notion of serous apoplexy,' Morgagni wrote, 'either because they think serum is an effect rather than a cause, or because they want to stamp out ancient notions to do with phlegm and ventricles, but they went too far in their modernism.'[39]

Serous Apoplexy in Padua: A Mixed Lot

After the many examples of sanguineous apoplexy listed in Chapter 3, Morgagni presented 15 instances of what he classified as serous apoplexy, in a separate 'letter'.[40] He gleaned some dissection findings from Valsalva's notes made in Bologna, but Morgagni had not always seen the patients himself and depended on secondary information. The common feature in these 15 patients was the presence of serum in the ventricles of the brain or between its membranes. Its quantity was not always abnormal; Morgagni insisted that even a small volume of serum might precipitate apoplexy if combined with other factors, such as engorgement of blood vessels or an acrid, erosive quality of serum.[41] In most cases, the aspect of serum was translucent, but sometimes 'gelatinous', 'thick', or 'ash-coloured'. In one case, Valsalva had tested its coagulability by heating, but it completely evaporated.[42]

The symptoms of patients in this category were diverse. Only three of them fitted the classical definition of apoplexy: the disease onset had been gradual in three patients, unknown in two, four had died on the spot, and three had been found dead. In other words, in 7 of the 15 patients, there was no proof for continued breathing and heart action in the apoplectic state. As Chapter 3 showed, Morgagni had been similarly inclusive in patients with sanguineous apoplexy, reasoning more as a pathologist than as a clinician.

Only three 'typical' patients remained in Morgagni's series of serous apoplexy, with sudden onset of deficits and death some days or weeks later. In two of them, both culled from Valsalva's notes (numbers 2 and 4 in Morgagni's narrative), there is almost no information on clinical features, except that one patient suddenly lost his speech. The history of the last patient allows the modern reader a better impression:

---

[39] Morgagni (1761), *De Sedibus et Causis Morborum*, vol. I, 11 (epistola II, paragr. 6).

[40] Morgagni (1761), *De Sedibus et Causis Morborum*, vol. I, 26–37 (epistola IV).

[41] Morgagni (1761), *De Sedibus et Causis Morborum*, vol. I, 26–7 (epistola IV, paragr. 1 and 3) and 35 (epistola IV, paragr. 32).

[42] Morgagni (1761), *De Sedibus et Causis Morborum*, vol. I, 27 (epistola IV, paragr. 3).

Joh. Baptista Anguissola, that most honourable priest [...] in 1707, in his
61st year, [...] initially had a fainting-fit while travelling in a gondola in
Venice, where he was on a mission for the pope. At home, he fell down
in his room, without any cause; finally, he was seized by apoplexy, so that
the physicians predicted a speedy death. All this happened in the middle
of July; however, he did not die until the middle of August. They gave
him [...]; yet they never achieved the goal: the patient failed to regain
command of his speech or his right limbs, which were paralytic. [...] At
last the grunting, which had been often present before, increased, and he
ended his life. [...]

On cutting through the cranium, water flowed out [...] When the
dura mater was removed, a kind of ash-coloured gelatine shone through
here and there, lying upon the convolutions of the brain. The vessels on
the surface of the brain and the cerebellum were a little more swollen
with blood than usual. In the substance of the brain no abnormality
appeared, except perhaps some laxity. For the rest, I saw water in all
ventricles, but not much.[43]

Whatever the true explanation of the priest's illness, and despite the scarcity of
fully documented reports of serous apoplexy, Morgagni's role was important
from a historical point of view, in that his authority confirmed the existence of
serous apoplexy as a separate category.

Paralysis as a Mild Form of Apoplexy, by Blood or Serum

'Paralysis is to apoplexy, what convulsion is to epilepsy,' Morgagni wrote in
the first sentence of his 'letter' on 'palsy'.[44] This should no longer be a surprise,
since many physicians struggled with the distinction between apoplexy and
paralysis, mostly in the form of hemiplegia. Wepfer was lenient, whereas Willis
was more strict: the latter had described a brain haemorrhage under the
heading of 'paralysis', while he also had seen 'a lack of firmness' in the striate
body of patients who had previously suffered from sudden paralysis (see
Chapter 2). Morgagni further obscured the distinction in his (supplementary)
Book V, by classifying some additional cases of patients with intracerebral
haemorrhage, all of whom had been in an 'apoplectic state', as 'paralysis',[45] but
most as sanguineous apoplexy.[46]

As a matter of course, all seven patients Morgagni listed under the heading
'paralysis' had shown hemiplegia, shortly before they died (two cases) or at least
months before (five). In none of them, the brain contained extravasated blood.

[43] Morgagni (1761), *De Sedibus et Causis Morborum*, vol. I, 28–9 (epistola IV, paragr. 13).
[44] Morgagni (1761), *De Sedibus et Causis Morborum*, vol. I, 82 (epistola XI, paragr. 1).
[45] Morgagni (1761), *De Sedibus et Causis Morborum*, vol. II, 411–12 (epistola LXII, paragr. 7–13).
[46] Morgagni (1761), *De Sedibus et Causis Morborum*, vol. II, 401–5 (epistola LX, paragr. 1–14).

The reports about the two patients who survived for days only (both were dissections by Valsalva) allow most insight, especially the first:

> A man, some sixty years of age, troubled by colics and diarrhoea as well as by persistent sleeplessness, had rubbed his abdomen with oil from quinces. While the diarrhoea continued up to his death, he was seized by hemiplegia the following night, without any warning symptom of the head; the entire right side of his body was motionless. On the first day he could somewhat move his hand and foot, when he felt the venesection or stimulation of the sole of the foot, but not at all on the next day. For the rest, his right eye was half closed, his cheeks were red, and he hardly spoke but only stammered. Yet, by nodding he responded in such a manner to those who questioned him that he gave the impression his internal senses were intact. Respiration was easy in the beginning, but more difficult as the days went on – until his death at day four.
>
> When the brain was lifted from the skull and especially when the infundibulum was cut free from the pituitary gland, clear serum and bright blood came out. On the left, next to the meningeal vessels, some gelatine-like material was detected. Similarly, below the tender membrane on the left, the substance of the brain itself was somewhat eroded. For it was found that, owing to the erosion, the corpus striatum was completely separated from the rest of the brain, perhaps by serum that had stagnated in the ventricles.
>
> Whatever the cause of this separation of the corpus striatum, in a previous letter I have sufficiently shown you how often hemiplegia seems to result from a lesion of this [structure] or of a neighbouring region.[47] I add what I have read in the Sepulchretum, that also Willis 'on examining people who had passed away after long-standing paralysis and severe inactivity of nerves, had always found these bodies less firm than the other regions, and discoloured, like the dregs of olive oil'.[48]

Thus, Morgagni compared Valsalva's report with Willis' finding of soft tissue in the corpus striatum of patients with paralysis. Alternatively, the term 'gelatine' may suggest a similarity with some of Wepfer's patients, but there are no other symptoms suggesting an infectious disorder of the brain. Whatever the truth may be, the salient point is that invasion by serum could cause not only apoplexy, but also paralysis, in the sense of hemiplegia. Whether such disease was classified under 'apoplexy' or 'paralysis' depended sometimes on the presence of 'internal senses' – in other words, on the degree of responsiveness before death, but on other occasions, on the physician's preference.

---

[47] Morgagni (1761), *De Sedibus et Causis Morborum*, vol. I, 22 (epistola III, paragr. 18).
[48] Morgagni (1761), *De Sedibus et Causis Morborum*, vol. I, 82 (epistola XI, paragr. 2–3).

THE DIFFICULTY OF DIAGNOSING SEROUS APOPLEXY DURING LIFE

That apoplexy was generally caused by extravasation of either blood or serum became firmly accepted in the course of the eighteenth century. Examples abound. Samuel-Auguste André-David Tissot (1728–1797),[49] a Protestant physician in Lausanne and one of the most popular writers of his time about health issues,[50] clearly distinguished the two categories not only in a book for lay persons, written in the vernacular,[51] but also in a text for physicians.[52]

One finds similar descriptions of serous apoplexy in later books of the 1770s and 1780s, for example in Borsieri's medical textbook[53] and in the monographs on apoplexy by Ponsart and Cerulli.[54]

A Pale Face and a Weak Pulse?

It was often taught that serous apoplexy could be distinguished from the sanguineous form during life. Signs believed to be most indicative of the serous variant were paleness of the face and a feeble pulse, as the above citation from Marquet's text testifies, while Tissot added that respiration was less impeded than with extravasation of blood.[55] Morgagni was rather critical of these criteria,[56] but the most vociferous dissent came from Antoine Portal, the physician with a chameleonic career in the eventful years around 1800. In 1781, he attacked the relevance of physical signs in the *Académie royale des sciences*, by presenting brief case histories of patients who had been dissected after a fatal apoplexy in the period of 1767–80:

> I might report other examples with the same result; they would prove that a pale face, a weak pulse and the presence of foam around the mouth are by no means certain signs of a serous apoplexy and that one errs, when these are present, by prescribing a treatment which is different from what had been necessary in case of a sanguineous apoplexy.[57]

Portal's necessary treatment was bloodletting. He recounted instances of patients with signs of 'serosity' in whom, on dissection, the vessels of the brain and meninges were nevertheless swollen with blood. Therefore, he did no

---

[49] Hirsch (1884–8), *Biographisches Lexikon*, vol. v, 687–8; Emch-Dériaz (2007), Samuel-Auguste Tissot.
[50] He is now mainly remembered by his diatribes against onanism.
[51] Tissot (1764), *Avis au Peuple*, vol. i, 192.
[52] Tissot (1761), *De Variolis, Apoplexia, et Hydrope*, 124.
[53] Burserius (1781), *Institutiones Medicinae practicae*, vol. iii, 69.
[54] Ponsart (1775), *Traité de l'Apoplexie*, 9–11, 34–5; Cerulli (1806), *Riflessioni intorno ai Mali apopletici*, 123.
[55] Tissot (1764), *Avis au Peuple*, vol. i, 197.
[56] Morgagni (1761), *De Sedibus et Causis Morborum*, vol. i, 13 (epistula ii, paragr. 14).
[57] Portal (1781), *Observations sur l'Apoplexie*, 626.

longer abstain from venesection in patients with a weak pulse and a pale face, as he used to do before; as a result, he claimed, the Marquess of Brida, 55 years of age, had been completely cured from his apoplexy by repeated bloodletting.[58] In a later communication, as *citoyen Portal*, he repeated his conviction that 'serous apoplexy' was diagnosed too often and repeated venesection was far more effective than emetics, even in aged patients.[59]

Unavoidably, there were dissenters. Portal's most ardent opponent was Jean-Antoine Gay (n.d.); he had moved from Montpellier to Paris and was a crusader against bloodletting.[60] Gay's polemical treatise on apoplexy, published in 1807 and translated into English in 1843,[61] is purely theoretical, with a rather eclectic and tortuous interpretation of ancient and modern literature. The root of apoplexy lies in the digestive system, Gay argued; irritation and convulsive activity lead to rarefaction of blood, and secondarily to dilatation of blood vessels. In the end, sanguineous and serous apoplexy were essentially one and the same thing. In his view, bloodletting was the worst possible treatment under these circumstances, and emetics the best.[62]

Again, Serum Excreted by the Force of Blood?

Maximilian Stoll (1742–1787) (Box 4.2) was an outstanding representative of the 'old Viennese school' of medicine,[63] established by van Swieten and de Haen. He questioned the theoretical validity of the distinction between sanguineous and serous apoplexy, by arguing that blood flow formed the primary impetus through which serum was expelled, thus reverting to Wepfer's original theory and Boerhaave's later variant, though without citing them. Stoll's attention to details was already noticeable from his description, in Chapter 3, of the circumstances preceding the apoplexy of a 74-year-old widow found speechless and with right-sided hemiplegia, the morning after a sumptuous meal; she died two days later. Here follows Stoll's report of the dissection:

> The cadaver, opened a few hours after death, showed on either side much serum between the meninges. The pial membrane, harder and thicker than usual, resembled a tendinous membrane. The vessels of this same membrane were much wider on the left than on the other side and had a swollen aspect, distended by too much blood. The substance of the brain appeared softer than usual. The carotid arteries, where they entered

---

[58] Portal (1781), *Observations sur l'Apoplexie*, 627.
[59] Portal (1800), *Mémoires sur la Nature et le Traitement de plusieurs Maladies*, vol. II, 216–28.
[60] Gay (1808), *Traité contre la Saignée*.
[61] Gay (1843), *An Essay on the Nature and Treatment of Apoplexy*.
[62] Gay (1807), *Vues sur l'Apoplexie*, 29–33 and 48–68.
[63] Eyerel (1790), *De vita et scriptis Maximiliani Stollii*.

Box 4.2 Maximilian Stoll (1742–1787).

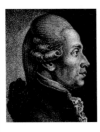 Stoll was born in the village of Erzingen, in southern Bavaria, where his father practised as a surgeon. After two years' tuition by a local priest, he assisted his father. Almost two years later, having been very much affected by a patient who had accidentally amputated his own hand, he was allowed to attend the village school instead. His zeal for study earned him a place at the distant gymnasium of Rottweil, led by Jesuits. On finishing school in 1761, his teachers persuaded him to enter the Society of Jesus, to the disappointment of his father. After three years as a novice, he became a teacher of classical languages in Hall (Tirol). His method of being brief on grammar to make room for adventurous texts earned him the popularity of pupils, but the censure of superiors, who transferred him to two other schools, in quick succession. Stoll had had enough and left the order in 1767.

After a brief period at home, he decided to study medicine. He started in Strasburg but continued in Vienna, attracted by Anton de Haen, famous for his bedside teaching. In 1772, he graduated with honours. It was not easy to establish oneself as a physician; Stoll tried his luck in Hungary, where he became inspired by Sydenham's work and made a systematic study of fevers. Because of illness, he had to return to Vienna. After his recovery, he replaced de Haen, who had become ill, at the medical school. After de Haen's death, Stoll was appointed Professor of Medicine in 1777; he continued the practice of bedside teaching. Stoll kept notes about his patients and, if possible, performed dissections at the Hospital of Holy Trinity. He published these experiences in annual instalments, *Rationis Medendi*, continuing de Haen's tradition; by the time of Stoll's death, three volumes had appeared (1777–9). His colleagues published four more volumes; the entire series was reprinted several times, in different countries. Stoll had married not long after his return from Hungary; the couple had a son and a daughter.

Source: Portrait courtesy of U.S. National Library of Medicine.

the skull, were found entirely bone-like and were in a similar state, as far as time allowed me to follow them within the bony canal. The branches of the carotid artery were for a large part bone-like, in the sense that the normal and bone-like parts alternated. On the left side the arteries were bone-like over a greater distance than those on the opposite side. Some smaller branches showed only bone-like walls.[64]

The words 'softer than usual' (*mollior solito*) applied to brain tissue will probably prompt readers to think of a modern diagnosis; Stoll mentioned the softness even twice, but he did not limit it to a single hemisphere. Although Stoll continued to believe that serous apoplexy truly existed, in this case, he regarded the impetus of blood as the primary cause:

[64] Stoll (1786), *Ratio medendi*, vol. I, 135–6.

> I did not believe that the present case belongs to the serous apoplexies, although much serum was contained between the meninges on either side. Given that blood was being retained and congested in the skull, the more subtle part, that is, serum, had been forcefully expressed from the more lateral small vessels and it was necessary for it to percolate. Though produced by *blood*, the apoplexy was worsened by *extravasated serum*.
>
> In the dissected brain of apoplectics, one often reads, the *vessels of the brain are swollen and much serum has flowed out*. Apoplexies of this type often have the name '*serous*', but should be properly called sanguineous.[65]

In the ensuing paragraph, Stoll acknowledged, with due respect, that Morgagni would probably have classified the apoplexy as 'serous', but he was happy to find that they at least agreed on the need for venesection in patients with swollen blood vessels.

SEROUS APOPLEXY BECOMES A NEBULOUS NOTION

Thus, by the end of the eighteenth century, several dissections in which excess of serum was regarded as the cause of apoplexy concerned patients with a long-standing, or at least complex, history or instances of sudden death. Only a few of the proposed cases had been seized by sudden hemiplegia and died after a few days or weeks. The issue was further compounded by physicians who, like Stoll, doubted, or at least qualified, the original distinction from sanguineous apoplexy.

The Early Nineteenth Century: Serous Apoplexy as a Controversial Diagnosis

As time went on, autopsy reports of serous apoplexy became increasingly sparse, even though a spate of no fewer than seven monographs about apoplexy appeared in the first 12 years of the nineteenth century. One cannot escape the feeling that several writers felt uncomfortable with the issue. Gay, cited above, was first on this list in 1807, but he was more concerned about the benefits of emetics and the dangers of bloodletting than about the existence of serous apoplexy.[66]

A more traditional treatise was that by François-Emmanuel Foderé (1764–1835). He presented a case of serous apoplexy, with dissection, of a feverish soldier who had died suddenly. Foderé leant heavily on Morgagni's opinion that serum, though a normal finding in the brain, could lead to sudden brain dysfunction and collapse by the suddenness of its appearance or by its acrid properties. He also dissected two patients with sanguineous apoplexy.[67]

---

[65] Stoll (1786), *Ratio medendi*, vol. i, 137–8.   [66] Gay (1807), *Vues sur l'Apoplexie*.
[67] Foderé (1808), *De Apoplexia*, 39–46.

Foderé's colleague Pierre Richelmi (1769–1841), who practised in Marseille and Nice, where a street has been named after him, admitted in his book on apoplexy that the 'pituitous' form, as he named it, was much rarer than the sanguineous form; yet he remained convinced it did exist. Of the five case histories he cited, three were taken from authors cited above. In the two personal – and fatal – cases he contributed, the onset had been gradual and there was no anatomical proof. Richelmi based his diagnosis on circumstantial evidence such as freezing weather, cold food, preceding catarrh, or dropsy.[68]

A 'Catarrhal' Form of Serous Apoplexy

Portal, cited above as a fierce opponent of the idea that serous apoplexy could be diagnosed during life, later extended his views on apoplexy in a separate book. He did not go as far as denying that serous apoplexy existed, but he doubted whether his colleagues had searched closely enough for distended vessels in the brain, including those of the choroid plexus.[69] In catarrhal disease, he reasoned, no doubt with Galen in mind, the membranes of the brain might indeed secrete too much fluid: watery, mucous, or albuminous. After all, why suppose that membranes of the brain reacted otherwise than membranes of the nose, throat, intestines, bladder, and joints?[70] Also, Portal found it conceivable that the serous part of blood was sometimes not properly mixed with the red part, or that it was too fluid, or – echoes of Boerhaave – that the absorption of brain fluid was somehow impeded.[71] Portal gave an example of 'catarrhal apoplexy' that stands out because, a colleague having passed it on, there are more clinical details than in the terse reports of Portal himself:

> A bookbinder [. . .], aged about fifty, stout and obese, usually with red cheeks and a drowsy disposition, complained during a rainy winter of severe headache; this was regarded as accompaniment of the catarrh of the nose and eyes from which he suffered, together with hoarseness. He then experienced weakness of the muscles of the trunk and the extremities, in that he could not sufficiently move the limbs to straighten them normally; as a result, he walked with great difficulty and often stumbled. Also, the patient's mouth remained half open, the lower lip being turned down towards the chin. The tactile sense was diminished; he said it seemed as if there was fine muslin between his fingers and fabric or a small mattress under his feet. However, he lapsed into extreme drowsiness and remained in this state for some days. The patient lost all sensation

[68] Richelmi (1811), *Essai sur l'Apoplexie*, 68–78.
[69] Portal (1811), *Observations sur l'Apoplexie*, 346–7.
[70] Portal (1811), *Observations sur l'Apoplexie*, 99–100 and 351–3.
[71] Portal (1811), *Observations sur l'Apoplexie*, 350 and 354–8.

and movement of the limbs, respiration became laboured and he died apoplectic.

   The opening of the body was performed by an assistant, who noted that the vessels of the brain were filled with black blood, that the ventricles contained much water and that there were rather large cysts in the choroid plexus.[72]

Today's physicians will interpret this story as a neuromuscular disorder adorned with many eponyms, rather than as apoplexy; in this case it was – once more – the final phase of unresponsiveness that must have prompted a diagnosis of apoplexy.

   The brothers Jean Montain (1778–1851) and Gilbert Montain (1780–1853), physicians in Lyon,[73] were not at all convinced by the catarrhal origin of the above case, in the treatise they published somewhat later than Portal in 1811.[74] They altogether dispensed with the notion of serous apoplexy, regarding superfluous serum as an effect rather than a cause. They also reclassified the case of Wepfer's 50-year-old vine-dresser as a form of 'nervous apoplexy',[75] another forgotten form of apoplexy (see below).

'One of the Most Complete Specimens'

In Chapter 3, we already encountered the monograph *On Cases of Apoplexy and Lethargy* by John Cheyne (1777–1836). It appeared in 1812, the year of Napoleon's failed Russian campaign. With regard to serous apoplexy, Cheyne steers a middle course, by acknowledging that its existence is a contentious issue and its causes 'involved in great obscurity'.[76] He summarily disqualified Morgagni's 15 examples, save two or three, but admitted that in two patients from his own practice, the diagnosis of serous apoplexy might have been applicable. He could retrieve his case notes on one of these.

   A meticulous historian and observer, Cheyne relates in great detail how, one night, the spouse of a 72-year-old man, a dyer by trade, discovered he had 'lost the power of articulating' and also 'the use of the whole left side of his body'. He had been in a declining state of health for two years and had complained of intermittent headache for the last three weeks, after a long journey by mail coach. Cheyne saw the patient on the following day:

   He sometimes breathes with stertor, but in general, calmly and regularly. His right hand, in constant motion, is very often directed to his forehead, the skin of which is red, from the pressure of his hand. His eyes are shut,

[72] Portal (1811), *Observations sur l'Apoplexie*, 91–2.
[73] Hirsch (1884–8), *Biographisches Lexikon*, vol. IV, 270–1.
[74] Montain and Montain (1811), *Traité de l'Apoplexie*, 24–31.
[75] Montain and Montain (1811), *Traité de l'Apoplexie*, 59–62.
[76] Cheyne (1812), *Cases of Apoplexy and Lethargy*, 41–9.

as if the light were irksome; his pupils are generally contracted. He cannot articulate, and seems very imperfectly to understand what is said: he attempted, after having been repeatedly importuned, to show me his tongue. There is some moisture on his tongue. His pulse is 60, full and regular. There is some moistening on his skin.

One day later, Cheyne paid another visit. The patient was 'unable to expectorate the loose mucus', became extremely restless as the day advanced, and died at seven o'clock.

Dissection. In denuding the skull, not a drop of blood was effused. There was no mark of the increase of red vessels in the dura mater. On the pia mater there prevailed signs of inflammation. There was a slight effusion of clear serous fluid between the tunica arachnoides and pia mater. The minute blood vessels were in increased number, but there was no extravasation in the form of red striae: the veins in the pia mater were full of blood. The substance of the brain was unusually soft. In the right ventricle there was a small quantity of limpid fluid: the ventricle was of a natural size. The other lateral ventricle was very much dilated, and full of clear serous fluid. One part of the ventricle was particularly distended, viz. the anterior horn. From the first descending part to the bottom, it was so large as to give passage to the little finger, without is touching the sides of the ventricle. [...] The quantity of fluid in the ventricle was about an ounce and a half. We were not permitted to open the thorax or abdomen.[77]

In the ensuing discussion, Cheyne presented this case as 'one of the most complete specimens' of serous apoplexy.[78] Modern neurologists and pathologists will wonder how to reconcile the left hemiplegia with the abnormalities found in the left hemisphere and they may well disagree with Cheyne's idea of an inflammatory process; there is no mention of pyrexia, but he had few alternatives from which to choose.

Cheyne also mentioned cases he could not classify as apoplexy, either sanguineous or serous, and went on to explain the nosological specifics of other states of disturbed consciousness, such as 'catalepsis, extasis, carus, cataphora and lethargus'; the famous Professor William Cullen (1710–1790) in Edinburgh had regarded these states as 'mere modes of apoplexy'. Cheyne, however, argued that 'lethargy' nevertheless deserved to be distinguished as a separate disorder of the brain.[79]

The last treatise to be discussed in the context of serous apoplexy appeared in 1817; its author was Johann Karl Friedrich Leune (1757–1825),[80] Professor of Medicine at the University of Leipzig. In the introduction, he promised to deal

---

[77] Cheyne (1812), *Cases of Apoplexy and Lethargy*, 125–8.
[78] Cheyne (1812), *Cases of Apoplexy and Lethargy*, 182.
[79] Cheyne (1812), *Cases of Apoplexy and Lethargy*, 184–213.
[80] Hirsch (1884–8), *Biographisches Lexikon*, vol. ii, 686–7.

with what he called 'The doctrine of serous apoplexy' in Chapters 2 and 3,[81] but unfortunately the book ends with Chapter 1, on p. 130. So the reader is left with only a portent of possible criticism.

Not so with James Abercrombie (1780–1844) from Edinburgh, who will appear more prominently in the following chapters. One year after Leune's book, he wrote in an article on apoplexy:

> I object to the term 'Serous Apoplexy' entirely, and I think it extremely doubtful whether there really exists such a disease.[82]

His arguments were, in condensed form, that serous effusion in other organs always occurred as a sequel of other diseases, that it always developed slowly and that the small quantity of effused fluid was disproportionate to the massive symptoms. With this conclusion, almost an obituary notice, the story of serous apoplexy comes to an end. In the course of the nineteenth century, only faint echoes of this 'entity' could still be heard.[83]

NERVOUS APOPLEXY

Now follows the other forgotten form of apoplexy. Chapter 3 ended with the story of how, at the close of the seventeenth century, Michael Ettmüller (1644–1683) from Leipzig grumbled that explanations of apoplexy were exclusively based on anatomical changes. Sometimes, he intimated, post-mortem dissection had failed to explain the supposed dysfunction of the brain.

APOPLEXY AND INTACT BRAINS

Ettmüller had not buttressed his opinion with descriptions of actual patients and their symptoms. A few decades later, Antonio Vallisneri (1661–1730),[84] Professor of Theoretical Medicine in Padua and a contemporary of Bologna's Antonio Valsalva, voiced a similar postulate:

> Why have I dissected many Cadavers of persons succumbed by Apoplexy, as the medical histories recounted, and how has it happened that I failed to observe any lesion whatsoever (to the amazement of the physicians, who had never thought this possible), not in the meninges, not in the cortical substance or the medulla of the brain, not in the ventricles, not even in the vessels for blood or lymph, nor anywhere else in the head?[85]

[81] Leune (1817), *De Apoplexia*, 16.   [82] Abercrombie (1818), On apoplexy, 584–6.
[83] Trousseau (1882), *Clinique médicale de l'Hôtel-Dieu de Paris*, vol. II, 53.
[84] Hirsch (1884–1888), *Biographisches Lexikon*, vol. VI, 62–3.
[85] Vallisneri (1727), *Bevande e Bagnature calde o freddo*, 35.

Also, at around the same time, the great Boerhaave had lectured:

> Thus, you see that all nervous diseases, down to apoplexy, can arise
> without any material [cause] or change of humours.[86]

But none of these general comments were accompanied by the patients' stories.

The Ultimate Inclusiveness of Diagnostic Criteria for Apoplexy

Before considering the miscellaneous forms of 'apoplexy without pathology'
proposed especially in the eighteenth century, it is fitting to contemplate briefly
for what reason this new nosological entity gained a firm foothold in medicine.
First of all, it provided a link with ancient 'fluidism' and its effects at a distance.
Also, a diagnosis of 'nervous apoplexy' provided a convenient way out in patients
without abnormalities on brain dissection (negative evidence), and especially in
patients who survived or even recovered (no evidence at all). If the clinical features
of such 'nervous' attacks were mentioned at all, they were brief. It seems,
admittedly with hindsight, that, as the diagnosis of 'spasmodic' or 'nervous'
apoplexy caught on, the diagnosis came to be applied to episodes of fainting or
swooning that only faintly resembled the classical Galenic triad of a sudden
collapse with complete loss of sensation and movement.

If symptoms were mentioned at all, they were not uniform, as one might
expect. Of course, given the hypothetical nature of the entire category, a
diagnosis of 'nervous apoplexy' was attached to a wide range of phenomena.

Intrinsic and Extrinsic Causes

The variety of explanations can be distinguished into two groups, depending
on whether the supposed disturbances are primarily taking place in the brain or
in other organs, through a kind of 'consensual action' on the brain. Borsieri
and some others called the former kind *idiopathic* and the latter *sympathic*.[87] The
two categories are not strictly separated, since sometimes a combination of
factors is implied, within, as well as between, these two main categories.

CAUSES IN THE BRAIN

Mental Effort and Emotions

In the course of time, the relationship between body and mind has troubled
physicians and philosophers alike. Friedrich Hoffmann the younger (1660–1742)

---

[86] Boerhaave and van Eems (1761), *Praelectiones academicae*, vol. II, 549.
[87] Burserius (1781), *Institutiones Medicinae practicae*, vol. III, 64.

Box 4.3 Friedrich Hoffmann (1660–1742).

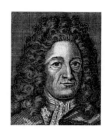

Hoffmann was born in Halle, Saxony. His father, a respected physician, died when he was 15 years old. Despite modest means, he managed to study medicine – mostly in Jena where he graduated in 1681, and for a short time in Erfurt. After a brief period of teaching in Jena, he started a practice in Minden, Westphalia. In 1683, he made an educational journey to the Low Countries and England, where he met Robert Boyle. Back in Minden, he exchanged his private practice for a position as a physician at the local garrison; somewhat later, he became a district physician in Halberstadt, again in Saxony. In 1793, the Elector Frederick III, later King Frederick I of Prussia, appointed him to the chair of Medicine at the newly established University of Halle. He was to stay there for the rest of his life, apart from a brief stint as a court physician in Berlin. Together with Georg Ernst Stahl, he made Halle a leading academic centre for medicine in German-speaking countries. Saddened by the death of his wife in 1737, he followed her five years later.

Hoffmann was a proponent of a mechanistic conception of living organisms and rejected iatrochemical principles. Influenced by Descartes, he included mental activities in his modelling and attributed the function of signalling to nervous fluids, closely related to the *spiritus animales* of antiquity. He published extensively; best known is his collected *Medicina rationalis*, in many volumes. He is said to have been not only didactic and impressive, but also kind and helpful. His prescriptions were few and simple; the 'Hoffmann drops' were to become proverbial.

Source: Portrait courtesy of Wellcome Foundation.

(Box 4.3), briefly mentioned above in relation to 'serous apoplexy',[88] and Professor at the University of Halle in Saxony, reiterated that the interaction of mind and body should not be neglected in the understanding of any disease. Some later writers saw him as the father of 'nervous apoplexy', together with Ettmüller.[89] Hoffmann wrote:

> Not only the state of the body must be studied, but also one should inquire about the nature of its mind and consider disorders from which this may suffer. For there is a very intimate and intense harmony and communion between the actions of both body and mind.[90]

In keeping with his conviction that all physiological processes are material events, Hoffmann regarded animated spirits of the brain as an expendable

---

[88] Hirsch (1884–8), *Biographisches Lexikon*, vol. III, 238–1; Helm and Stukenbrock (2007), Friedrich Hoffmann.
[89] Ullersperger (1864), *Der Hirnnervenschlag*, 12 and 19.
[90] Hoffmann (1732), *Medicina rationalis systematica*, vol. III, 10.

commodity, so that excessive mental activity might cause apoplexy by exhaustion:

> One must also ask whether – a vice especially of literate persons – excessive study, burning midnight oil during deep and exhausting meditations, common in abstract disciplines such as metaphysics and mathematics, might perhaps impose great weakness on the brain and nervous system, when the so-called animated spirits have been drained? After all, such weakness paves the way for most serious diseases of the head, to wit, apoplexy, melancholy, mania and loss of memory.[91]

The belief that strong emotions, such as excessive joy, grief, rage, or terror, can cause apoplexy is as old as humanity. Earlier physicians recounted examples, for example Forestus and Georg Nymmann in the sixteenth and seventeenth century.[92] Later generations duly transmitted these tales; van Swieten recounts a contemporaneous story about a Frenchman who stayed unconscious for two months after a fright.[93] Samuel-Auguste André David Tissot, a physician in Lausanne and a popular author of medical works for the laity, stretched the facts even further, writing to his learned compatriot Albrecht von Haller (1708–1777):

> Repressed rage or repressed, intense grief that no one knows about cause apoplexies every day. When a generous man puts on a happy face and congratulates his victorious rival with having obtained the position they were both competing for, he may collapse during the kiss.[94]

In the early nineteenth century, social upheaval and political turmoil in urbanized society were again blamed for a perceived increase in the incidence of apoplexy.[95]

Tight or Convulsing Meninges

Membranes of the brain can be seen to move, in rhythmic fashion, in live animals with head wounds and in the fontanelle of newborns. Whether the movement is a passive reflection of the pulsatile blood flow or an intrinsic activity of the meninges, the dura mater in particular, is a question that has long divided medical opinion.[96] In the seventeenth century, the consensus veered towards assigning a contractile property to the dural membrane; Thomas Willis and Humphrey Ridley (1653–1708), both of whom had found fibres in it,

---

[91] Hoffmann (1732), *Medicina rationalis systematica*, vol. III, 11.
[92] Forestus (1653 [1590]), *Observationes et Curationes*, vol. X, 509; Nymmanus (1629), *Tractatus de Apoplexia*, 156–7.
[93] van Swieten (1755–72), *Commentaria*, vol. III, 271; Imbert (1717), Assoupissement extraordinaire.
[94] Tissot (1761), *De Variolis, Apoplexia, et Hydrope*, 89.
[95] Foderé (1808), *De Apoplexia*, 63–7.
[96] Neuburger (1897), *Entwicklung der Gehirn-und Rückenmarksphysiologie*, 69–86.

agreed with this view but limited the capacity for movement to special circumstances.[97] In 1703, Ridley showed in a crucial experiment that the regular, pulsatile movements entirely depended on the inflow of blood into the brain,[98] but nevertheless the idea of contractility stuck. In the course of the eighteenth century, it was reinforced by the notion of 'irritability': a supposedly intrinsic property of some types of fibres to shorten when touched,[99] disseminated especially by Albrecht von Haller.[100]

Since overfilling or compression of the brain was the final common pathway in all instances of apoplexy where structural changes were found or supposed, some thought constriction or spasm of the meninges might squeeze the brain and cause apoplexy by interfering with transport of blood and spirits. Giovanni Francisco Scardona (1708–1800),[101] who wrote a three-volume textbook of medicine and practised in his native Rovigo (Veneto), alluded to meningeal spasm in order to explain the negative findings in the dissections of Vallisnieri he had watched in Padua.[102]

Even the great Morgagni sometimes had to invoke a role for compression by the meninges, on at least two occasions. As early as in 1719, he took recourse to an earlier experiment by Valsalva when faced with the problem of explaining hemiplegia if dissection of the brain had failed to show a relevant cause:

> For if in hemiplegics one finds nothing, or only serum, in either half of the brain, at least [serum] of the kind one observes in a perceptible and material lesion of the brain, then it is surely permitted to argue that in some part of the brain a defect is hidden, especially since an experiment recorded by a most experienced Author [*i.e. Valsalva*] sufficiently shows how easily very serious but invisible damage can be inflicted on the brain itself.
>
> 'For if the nerves to the heart of a dog are tightly bound by a string and immediately released, they are so much disturbed in their invisible structure, that the dog dies within a few days in the same way as if the nerves had been amputated. If [the nerves] are inspected once more, they fail to show a single trace of a lesion.'
>
> When I considered this experiment at the time, I saw that it could also be understood how easily an overall paralysis can result from an overall convulsion, that is, of the dura mater, and how easily a local paralysis can result from a similar but local cause. I conclude this from the nervous or

[97] Willis (1664), *Cerebri Anatome*, 85; Ridley (1695), *The Anatomy of the Brain*, 5.
[98] Ridley (1703), Experimentum anatomicum; Neuburger inadvertently omitted this reference.
[99] von Haller (1758), *Primae Lineae physiologiae*, 151; Frixione (2007), Irritable glue.
[100] Steinke (2007), Albrecht von Haller.
[101] Hirsch (1884–8), *Biographisches Lexikon*, vol. v, 197.
[102] Scardona (1746), *Aphorismi de cognoscendis et curandis Morbis*, 11. Scardona admired Boerhaave and copied the title of his aphorisms.

membranous filaments, which, if stretched, can tightly compress one or more nerves.[103]

Many years later, when writing his main work *De Sedibus et Causis Morborum*, Morgagni recalled this passage when again confronted with an anatomically unexplained hemiplegia.[104]

CAUSES ELSEWHERE IN THE BODY

'The Vapours'

Disturbances elsewhere in the body could, some thought, also interfere with animated spirits in the brain, acting at a distance. Ettmüller, the godfather of nervous apoplexy, had been influenced by Willis' iatrochemical approach and regarded the intestines as a possible source of 'poisonous particles':

> With regard to *apoplexy evoked by internal causes*, damaging the animated spirits and rendering them numb and slack (to explain the matter in common language), they operate in a *positive* way, being located or sticking at the region of the stomach or at its uppermost orifice; in other words, a *positive apoplexy* is evoked from the entrails. [...] I cured a woman who had become apoplectic by an internal cause that had arisen spontaneously. She had been excited and had an attack in which she complained exclusively of oppression and anxiety in the region of the chest, of great cardiac distress, together with a marked propensity to fall asleep.[105]

But Friedrich Hoffmann, a few decades later, envisaged a mechanical, rather than chemical, explanation, by assuming that this 'sympathic' apoplexy was mediated by the meninges:

> But if the course of the blood is halted by rigid spasm of the dura mater, and the vessels are overfilled with blood and compress the origin of the nerves, a mild form of apoplexy arises. I call this a spasmodic form; it is often seen in severe hysterical passion and is sometimes immediately relieved by timely venesection.[106]

Hoffmann and subsequent authors on the subject did not usually explain how they envisaged the supposed 'spasm' of the dura mater – only as a reaction to an increase in blood flow to the brain, or as mediated by the nervous system, or both. At any rate, Hoffmann regarded the spasmodic form as less life-

[103] Morgagni (1719), *Adversaria anatomica VI*, 110.
[104] Morgagni (1761), *De Sedibus et Causis Morborum*, vol. I, 85 (epistula XI, paragr. 17).
[105] Ettmüller (1685), *Opera omnia theoretica et practica*, 301.
[106] Hoffmann (1732), *Medicina rationalis systematica*, vol. III, 73.

threatening than the sanguineous or serous form. In his time, the term 'hysterical' did not have today's Freudian ring, but of course, it referred to the womb and menstrual bleeding:

> It is very often a symptom of hysterical women and results from violent spasm in the abdomen, by which blood, redundant through stagnation of periods, is transported with great force to the brain and, by halting in its vessels, interrupts all sensation and motion, except the pulse and breathing.[107]

Here at least, Hoffmann used the term 'spasm' for events in the abdominal cavity. Of course, venesection was the preferred treatment for 'stagnation of periods'. His notion of apoplexy had much in common with attacks in women that, in earlier times, had been named 'suffocation from the uterus', and later 'hysteria'. The subject deserves its own history; at any rate, at least in the early seventeenth century, some physicians clearly distinguished these attacks from apoplexy.[108]

In males, indigestion and other intestinal troubles could cause similar attacks; Thomas Sydenham called them 'hypochondriac'.[109] His writings, and those of Hoffmann, were well known to Pierre Pomme (1735–1812), who practised at first in his native Arles, later in Paris (with royal patronage), and finally in Montpellier.[110] He assembled all hysterical and hypochondriac attacks under the term 'vapours' (*affections vaporeuses*), without specification. According to Pomme, the central problem was the effect on nervous tissue, especially on the meninges: dryness and shrivelling (*racornissement*).[111] In the case of hemiplegia or apoplexy:

> [The brain] is permanently exposed to the repeated pressure of the meninges, which squeeze it from all sides and, in case of shrivelling, bear down on it with some force and impede the movement of fluids, which presents even more obstacles to the circulation of blood in this organ and enhances the stuffing that is the ultimate cause. [. . .] Each time the blood enters, too fiery and impetuous, it is unavoidable that this leads to dilatation of the different sinuses and arterial and venous vessels. These will imperceptibly increase their calibre and form varicose swellings, which interferes with the circulation of blood and spirits, and gives rise to apoplexy, epilepsy, paralysis and all other diseases such compression produces.[112]

[107] Hoffmann (1732), *Medicina rationalis systematica*, vol. III, 53.
[108] Nymmanus (1629), *Tractatus de Apoplexia*, 18–19.
[109] Sydenham (1684b), *Dissertatio epistolaris ad Guilelmum Cole*, 82.
[110] Hirsch (1884–8), *Biographisches Lexikon*, vol. IV, 605.
[111] Pomme (1765), *Traité des Affections vaporeuses des deux Sexes*, xxviii.
[112] Pomme (1765), *Traité des Affections vaporeuses des deux Sexes*, 259–60.

Fullness of the head, once more, but in a different guise. Pomme's recommended treatment for this variety of apoplexy is completely different from that for the sanguineous or serous form. In a later edition of his book, he recites an occasion where he arrived just in time to forestall venesection in a patient with hemiplegia, subsequently cured with tepid baths.[113]

Gout

Painful swelling of joints, or gout, was a common disease, at least in the affluent part of society. The morbid material, though at great distance from the brain, could also contribute to apoplexy, according to Thomas Sydenham (1624–1689):

> If the quantity of harmful material is too large, so that the affected part cannot harbour it, it soon diverts [the material] to other joints, followed by swelling and bubbling up or fermentation of blood as well as other fluids. If the body abounds with serous dregs capable of generating Gout, one has to fear an attack of Apoplexy.[114]

The story was perpetuated in the eighteenth century, for example by van Swieten, elaborating on Boerhaave's list,[115] and later by Kirkland.[116] In 1811, Pierre Richelmi, after stating 'everybody knows that gout can have an outburst in the brain', illustrated this dictum by the history of a 60-year-old citizen of Marseille with *apoplexie goutteuse* who first became hemiplegic and one year later died of a second 'metastatic attack'.[117]

Pain in the Abdomen or Elsewhere

Once 'nervous apoplexy' had earned its place in the nosological system, it was not a far cry to suppose that severe pain, especially in the abdomen, but sometimes also in the chest, might disturb the nervous system and even cause apoplexy, especially in combination with other factors, such as emotional upsets, toxic particles, or vapours. Hoffmann asserted the role of intestinal spasm as a cause of increased blood flow to the brain, with overfilling or even rupture of brain vessels:

> The more, and the more certainly, the excess of blood is able to inflict the damage I mentioned, if it results from the accession of another cause, that is, spasm in other parts, outside and even remote from the head. [...]

[113] Pomme (1782), *Traité des Affections vaporeuses des deux Sexes*, 268–9.
[114] Sydenham (1684a), *De Podagra et Hydrope*, 23.
[115] van Swieten (1755–72), *Commentaria*, vol. III, 276.
[116] Kirkland (1792), *Apoplectic and Paralytic Affections*, 75.
[117] Richelmi (1811), *Essai sur l'Apoplexie*, 106–8.

And one has to conclude it occurs through this cause that, as experience testifies, people are often victim of this haemorrhage when they have for some time been in the grip of spasm, mostly of the abdomen: people who have suffered from intestinal colics, chiefly the spastic form, from hypochondriac illness, pain from a stone in the bladder or the gall bladder, but from also daily cramps in the rectum.[118]

The next decades saw a rapid increase in the number of disorders associated with apoplexy by some sort of distant effect, especially in the abdominal cavity. Theses were written on the subject, for example in Göttingen, supervised by Professor Philipp Georg Schroeder (1729–1772)[119] or by August Gottlob Richter (1742–1812).[120]

A rather radical proponent of the 'violent irritation' of the intestines as a cause of apoplexy was Thomas Kirkland (1721–1798), a remarkable figure in Ashby, Leicestershire; he graduated first as a surgeon in Edinburgh and only later as doctor of medicine.[121] In his opinion, the abdominal form was the only true form of apoplexy, mostly with fatal outcome. Vertigo he considered as an early warning symptom of intestinal trouble; progression could be averted by proper remedies, but susceptible persons were less fortunate:

To account for this kind of apoplexy therefore, it is only necessary to suppose the nerves of the stomach to be more violently affected under an apoplectic diathesis, and that this affection is communicated as quick as lightning along the medullary part of the nerve to the same substance in the head, and hence an apoplexy, or sudden stroke, is produced.[122]

Kirkland even questioned whether apoplexy at all occurred by extravasation of blood or serum. He relied on two arguments. The first was absence of brain abnormalities in some dissections, for which he cited Ettmüller, Morgagni, and a local colleague.[123] The second argument was his own experience – in patients with penetrating head injuries, described in hair-raising detail, he had found blood clots and other effusions at the surface or even within the substance of the brain, but without the well-known symptoms of apoplexy.[124] Nevertheless, Kirkland recognized a mild form of apoplexy, 'of the kind which so often leaves a hemiplegia behind', but he was silent about its pathogenesis.[125]

[118] Hoffmann (1732), *Medicina Rationalis Systematica*, vol. IV, part 2, 167–8.
[119] Koch (1779 [1767]), De apoplexiae ex praecordiorum origine.
[120] Moll (1780), *De Apoplexia biliosa*.
[121] Hirsch (1884–8), *Biographisches Lexikon*, vol. III, 481.
[122] Kirkland (1792), *Apoplectic and Paralytic Affections*, 33.
[123] Kirkland (1792), *Apoplectic and Paralytic Affections*, 27–9.
[124] Kirkland (1792), *Apoplectic and Paralytic Affections*, 18–26.
[125] Kirkland (1792), *Apoplectic and Paralytic Affections*, 40–1.

Another unconventional approach to apoplexy was that of Giuseppe Cerulli (n.d.) from the University of Naples. In his book *Reflections on Apoplexy*, he proposed an interaction between, on the one hand, particulate, purulent debris from solid organs and, on the other hand, fever and intense heart action, resulting in transudation or vessel erosion.[126]

How complex the subject of apoplexy had become, not least by the emergence of a nervous variant, is illustrated by the table (Figure 4.2) in the book by Pierre Richelmi (1764–1841),[127] who made a few brief appearances above. He subdivided both the idiopathic and the sympathic form of nervous apoplexy into cases with a material cause and those without – the 'spastic' or 'convulsive' forms. His table not only reflects the passion for 'botanical' system-building in eighteenth-century medicine, but also the sub-sub-subdivisions of nervous apoplexy showing the variety of internal organs that, by 1811, were considered potential sources of apoplexy.

Two Books on 'Nervous Apoplexy'

Francesco Zuliani (1743–1806) undertook the task of describing all the ins and outs of apoplexy without visible brain changes; he had studied in Venice and practised in Brescia.[128] In his first few chapters he briefly dealt with sanguineous and serous (or 'lymphatic') apoplexy, which he attributed to agitation, expansion, and inflammation of humours,[129] and to mucous clogging, respectively.[130] However, the nervous variant was his main subject. Certain premonitory symptoms, he wrote, should alert physicians that a nervous (or 'spastic', or 'convulsive') apoplexy might be in the offing:

> Apoplexies of this kind are often preceded for several days by shady dizziness, mild shivering and muscle tremors, as well as by some sensation as if a trickle of water runs over a limb; also dryness of the skin anticipates it, or shaking of the knees, severe weakness of the entire body, perturbation in the lower belly, and some difficulty in thinking as well as in making decisions. Now, when apoplexy is imminent, the pulses of the arteries are increased, especially of the carotids, and they become harder; sometimes monstrous headaches supervene, or horrible convulsions of the limbs; the extremities of the body, especially the limbs, become stiff with cold, and something like heat rages through the head. At times feelings of oppression are felt in the chest or the lower abdomen.[131]

---

[126] Cerulli (1806), *Riflessioni intorno ai Mali apopletici*, 81–5 and 118–24.
[127] Richelmi (1811), *Essai sur l'Apoplexie*, 7.
[128] Hirsch (1884–8), *Biographisches Lexikon*, vol. VI, 381–2.
[129] Zulianius (1789), *De Apoplexia, praesertim nervea*, 12–41.
[130] Zulianius (1789), *De Apoplexia, praesertim nervea*, 41–5.
[131] Zulianius (1789), *De Apoplexia, praesertim nervea*, 50–1.

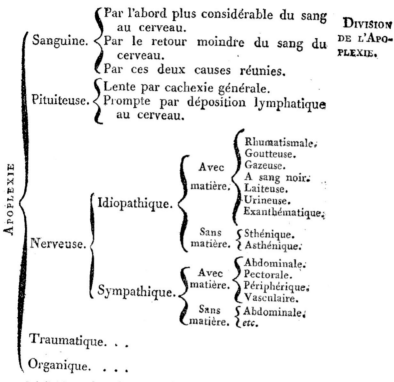

4.2 Subdivisions of apoplexy, according to Pierre Richelmi (1811).

Of the four personal case histories Zuliani presented, one concerned a monk who had studied too much and was struck by hemiplegia from which he only partially recovered; the other three were young women, all restored to good health by appropriate medical assistance.[132] Zuliani distinguished nervous apoplexy from 'hysterical suffocation', in which he found the pulse 'thin and depressed' and the eyes closed.[133] He duly explained the subcategories of the idiopathic and sympatic form; as an example of the former, he referred to the sudden death of the famous mathematician von Euler, when he was applying calculus to astronomical problems.[134] For aficionados of the genre, Zuliani's

[132] Zulianius (1789), *De Apoplexia, praesertim nervea*, 66–71.
[133] Zulianius (1789), *De Apoplexia, praesertim nervea*, 72–3.
[134] Zulianius (1789), *De Apoplexia, praesertim nervea*, 82–3.

book is a treasure trove of tales in which victims were suddenly carried away by strong emotions or unusual circumstances, from antiquity to his own time.[135]

Despite a German translation of Zuliani's treatise,[136] the belief in nervous apoplexy slowly fizzled out in the early nineteenth century. Cerulli (1806) and Gay (1807) paid merely some lip service to it.[137] But Portal, who was not very precise in defining the symptoms of apoplexy, even in patients who had died and in whom he had found corresponding brain lesions on dissection, went along with all emotional, convulsive, and painful afflictions (Table 3.2, p. 104, items 10–13) as possible causes.[138] He confesses to ignorance about their explanation, but – of course – he is ready to treat them.[139] Also the brothers Montain believed in this purely functional entity; they even distinguished a 'sthenic' and an 'asthenic' form, representing hyperactivity and languor of the brain, respectively.[140] But as far ahead as in 1840, in a doctoral dissertation on apoplexy in Vienna, for which the candidate had read up on the work of all relevant authors in Europe, the reader can almost feel his distaste when he perfunctorily closed with two brief and wholly theoretical sections on serous and nervous apoplexy.[141]

As a last gasp, a booklet on nervous apoplexy appeared in 1864,[142] by Johann Baptist Ullersperger (1798–1878), a ducal physician and later a private practitioner in Bavaria; after 1835, he devoted himself entirely to literary work. A firm believer in 'nervous stroke', Ullersperger attempted to present both a historical overview and an explanation. Though he failed to achieve either aim, the book can serve as a fitting farewell to the subject.

APOPLEXY: UNCONSCIOUSNESS OF ANY KIND

At the beginning of his book on 'nervous apoplexy', Francesco Zuliani lamented that a definition of apoplexy was hard to give because there were so many symptoms and so many causes.[143] He hit the nail on the head.

To begin with, the Galenic triad, already somewhat diluted by the inclusion of hemiplegia, or an incomplete loss of sensation and movement, had been further broadened by Wepfer. He, and then others, included case histories in

[135] Zulianius (1789), *De Apoplexia, praesertim nervea*, 84–96.
[136] Zulian (1791), *Ueber den Schlagfluss*.
[137] Cerulli (1806), *Riflessioni intorno ai Mali apopletici*, 92; Gay (1807), *Vues sur le Caractère et le Traitement de l'Apoplexie*, 29–36.
[138] Portal (1811), *Observations sur la Nature et le Traitement de l'Apoplexie*, 150–209.
[139] Portal (1811), *Observations sur la Nature et le Traitement de l'Apoplexie*, 162–7.
[140] Montain and Montain (1811), *Traité de l'Apoplexie*, 55–68.
[141] Melicher (1840), *Tractatus de Apoplexia*.   [142] Ullersperger (1864), *Der Hirnnervenschlag*.
[143] Zulianius (1789), *De Apoplexia, praesertim nervea*, 1–2.

which the apoplectic state had not been a bolt from the blue, but developed in the course of a progressive illness.

This inclusiveness went on in the eighteenth century. Morgagni not only confirmed previous anatomical findings with a mass of new observations and added air as a new cause, but he further expanded the clinical spectrum of apoplexy by including episodes of sudden death.

And finally, when the idea took hold that in some fatal cases of apoplexy, the aspect of the brain was normal, a variety of functional explanations found their way into medicine and provided a free-for-all of possible symptoms. The only more or less constant symptom that remained was a decrease in the level of consciousness. See what Anne-Charles Lorry (1726–1783),[144] a fashionable and royal physician in Paris, wrote in his book on melancholical diseases:

> Stagnation, or merely slowing of the circulation in the brain implies the threat of not only Melancholy, but also Apoplexy. [...] A woman of about twenty-five years old was always very active but prone to some sadness when her periods were about to come on. Instead of the usual evacuation she was seized by distortion of the mouth, paralysis of one side of the body and deep sleep. The uterus was also tense, and she experienced manifest pain from the hand that touched her. Jerks were present in tendons, also in the paralysed parts. Her abnormally livid face betrayed an impeded return of blood via the jugular veins. She was unchanged when woken from her sad and anxious slumber. This state lasted a few days, but ended unexpectedly. For with a shock in all body parts she suddenly came to herself and was able to move all her limbs, once the menstruations had started to flow copiously.[145]

The clinical definition of apoplexy was not only expanded by pathologists, but also watered down by physicians, who made the diagnosis in a wide range of episodes of altered consciousness, from swooning to sudden death. Something had to change.

---

[144] Hirsch (1884–8), *Biographisches Lexikon*, vol. IV, 43.
[145] Lorry (1765), *De Melancholia*, vol. I, 115 and 298.

FIVE

HAEMORRHAGE

SUMMARY

The French Revolution accelerated the increase of medical knowledge. Rochoux, a typical exponent, dissected several patients who had died of apoplexy. In his view, sudden hemiplegia always signified a haemorrhage in the brain. He regarded other brain lesions, particularly serous effusion and softening, found always after an interval of at least one month, as secondary complications. However, Riobé, Cruveilhier, and Moulin soon elucidated the usual course of tissue changes following intracerebral haemorrhage. Elsewhere, Abercrombie distinguished forms of apoplexy according to the initial symptoms: loss of consciousness, headache, or paralysis. Serres categorized brain haemorrhage without paralysis as 'meningeal apoplexy'.

With regard to causation, Rochoux assumed that local softening of brain tissue preceded and prompted haemorrhage, but others increasingly recognized an association with hypertrophy of the heart. Gradually, ideas about the source of cerebral haemorrhage converged on arterioles in the deep regions of the brain. Charcot and Bouchard proposed 'miliary aneurysms' of arterioles as the site of extravasation, preceded by 'peri-arteritis'. After an avalanche of morphological studies and theories, most opinions revolved on degenerative change of arterioles, without an inflammatory origin. In the twentieth century, the relationship between hypertension and fatty degeneration of arterioles emerged, as quantification of blood pressure became possible (Riva Rocci). Fisher identified a few types of damage in arteriolar walls other than miliary aneurysms, but the exact source of bleeding remained somewhat conjectural.

In the first decades of the nineteenth century, the notion 'apoplexy' had become a quagmire. Many fresh ideas emanated from Paris, in the aftermath of the French Revolution. Paris has therefore been often designated the cradle of modern medicine, at least for the first half of the century.[1] Other historians have, however, contested this view as mythical rhetoric.[2] Indeed, science did not come to a halt everywhere else, yet it is useful to begin with a sketch of the Parisian milieu in which many of the transitions occurred.

MEDICINE AND THE FRENCH REVOLUTION

The French Revolution ousted not only royalty and aristocracy, at least for some time, but also the power of the Catholic Church. As a consequence, health care was no longer a matter of religious benevolence, but a responsibility of the state. In the course of the three decades after the storming of the Bastille on 14 July 1789, Paris hospitals came to provide not only patient care, but also bedside teaching and research: *peu lire, beaucoup voir, beaucoup faire* (read little, see much, do much).[3] In two important institutions, this hospital function was joined with that of an old people's home, intended for Parisians no longer able to live at home because they were handicapped by palsy, dementia, incontinence, or mental disturbance. For women, this institution was the Salpêtrière, a name recalling the building's past as a gunpowder house;[4] needy men went to the Bicêtre. The number of inmates in these institutions ran into the thousands.[5] The revolutionary authorities replaced the medical faculty of the university by *Écoles de Santé,* in Paris, but also in Montpellier and Strasbourg; the revised medical curriculum abolished the traditional division between medicine and surgery. Academic staff were salaried, so their income no longer entirely depended on private practice.

The innovations produced luminaries such as Jean-Nicolas Corvisart (1755–1821), who introduced Auenbrugger's percussion method, René Laennec (1781–1826), the inventor of auscultation, Xavier Bichat (1771–1802), champion of pathological anatomy and father of the tissue doctrine, and Pierre Charles Alexandre Louis (1787–1872), who used a 'numerical method' to compare groups of patients. The meeting of doctor and patient lost the previous aloofness in which physical contact was limited to feeling of the pulse; internal organs were not only talked about, but actually probed and sounded out.

---

[1] Foucault (1963), *Naissance de la Clinique.*
[2] Hannaway and La Berge (1998), Paris medicine: perspectives past and present.
[3] Ackerknecht (1967), *Medicine at the Paris Hospital 1794–1848*, 15–44.
[4] Vessier (1999), *La Pitié-Salpêtrière.*   [5] Guillain and Mathieu (1925), *La Salpêtrière*, 35–51.

The teaching facilities stood out in comparison with universities elsewhere. It is no wonder that medical students and physicians from other European countries and the United States of America flocked to Paris in droves, as in the past they had gone to Northern Italy, Leiden, or Edinburgh.[6] An example was the young Englishman Thomas Hodgkin (1798–1866); he spent a full year in Paris before becoming one of the stars of London's Guy's Hospital.[7]

Admittedly, the success of Parisian medicine tended to overshadow developments elsewhere. Pathological anatomy had already been established at other European universities, notably in Vienna and Edinburgh. Although the public hospital system in Paris ensured that the number of post-mortem examinations far outstripped that in other European centres, physicians elsewhere addressed the same problems, and with some success. Another qualification is the uneven, and sometimes erratic, fashion in which new experience found its way across the medical world. The story in this book cannot but follow its vanguard.

Advances in knowledge were, of course, not limited to medicine. Antoine Lavoisier (1743–1794), a nobleman dedicated to chemistry who tragically lost his head in the Terror,[8] had discovered that combustion depended on a single element in the air; he baptised it 'oxygen'. Until that time, most people had believed the key element was some intrinsic principle in the burning object, called 'phlogiston'.[9] The link between oxygen and respiration was obvious, and as early as in 1819, a physician used the term 'oxygenated blood' as if it were a household term.[10] Also, 'animated spirits' were giving way to 'animal electricity'.[11]

APOPLEXY SYNONYMOUS WITH INTRACEREBRAL HAEMORRHAGE?

A Bold District Physician

Jean-André Rochoux (1787–1852) (Box 5.1),[12] described as 'one of the most original figures of our time',[13] studied the clinical and pathological aspects of apoplexy during his time as physician at the *Maison de la Santé* in the Parisian district of Saint Martin. Having submitted a thesis on the subject in 1812, he

---

[6] Ackerknecht (1967), *Medicine at the Paris Hospital 1794–1848*, 191–4.
[7] Kass and Kass (1988), *The Life and Times of Dr. Thomas Hodgkin*, 85–104.
[8] Poirier (1993), *Lavoisier*, 371–414.
[9] Gregory (2008), *Natural Science in Western History*, 211–14.
[10] Bricheteau (1819), La circulation et les fonctions cérébrales, 17.
[11] Galvani (1791), *De Viribus Electricitatis in Motu musculari*.
[12] Walusinski (2017a), Jean-André Rochoux.
[13] Raige-Delorme (1852), Notice nécrologique sur le Dr. Rochoux.

Box 5.1 Jean-André Rochoux (1787–1852).

Rochoux was born as the son of a postmaster in Argenton-sur-Creuse (Centre-Val de Loire). He studied medicine in Paris and became *interne des hôpitaux* at the age of 20. He was employed in a hospital for venereal diseases and in a children's hospital before being appointed around 1810 as a physician at the *Maison de Santé* in the district of St Martin and, one year later, as an assistant for anatomy at the Faculty of Medicine. It is in this period that he wrote his book on apoplexy. The prospects of establishing a private practice in Paris must have been bleak, for in 1814 he became a military physician in Guadeloupe, a group of islands under French control in the Caribbean area, where he stayed until 1819. On his return, he published a book with his observations on yellow fever, concluding that the condition was not contagious. In 1824, he passed the *agrégation*, an examination required for access to academic positions, but he failed in subsequent competitions for a professorial chair. After a period at the central office of the Paris hospitals, he was in 1830 appointed as physician to the Bicêtre, a hospital, nursing home, and mental institution for male patients. Rochoux became a member of the Royal Society of Medicine and was an active discussant at its meetings; otherwise, he led a reclusive life.

In his outlook on life, Rochoux was a convinced materialist, mentioning Epicurus whenever he could; he also wrote on microscopy of the central nervous system, on psychology, and against phrenology. He remained single all his life, retired in 1848, and died four years later of septicaemia. He was known as stubborn and satirical in his opinions, but never unfair.

published a full book two years later. Rochoux exemplified his simple approach to the chaos surrounding apoplexy by beginning his book with eleven case histories of patients with sudden hemiplegia, often accompanied by loss of consciousness – all showed extravasated blood in the brain, almost always in a deep region of one hemisphere.[14] He also made sure he was on firm ground with the clinical features:

> There is only one way to characterise the disease: paralysis of one or more voluntary organs of movement, and a more or less similar trouble of sensation, both of which appear suddenly and persist for a certain time, and are usually not preceded by any warning event.

He then went on to deliver a final blow to the diversity of notions with regard to apoplexy:

> Since all patients who died after suffering from these two symptoms have *invariably* shown an effusion of blood with tearing of brain tissue, one cannot but assume the same cause in those who survive such attacks, and these [two symptoms] become the pathognomonic sign through which one can be infallibly certain that there exists an effusion of blood in the

[14] Rochoux (1814), *Recherches sur l'Apoplexie*, 9–62.

brain. *Nobody*, as far as I know, has up to now demonstrated the co-existence of these two categories of phenomena, the haemorrhage and the symptoms mentioned above. To me it seems an incontestable truth of fact.[15]

Rochoux's Two Premises

So this bold district health officer, about to seek temporary employment in Guadeloupe, to be followed by an equally erratic career, postulated two facts:

1. 'Apoplexy is sudden loss of power and sensation in several body parts';
2. 'The cause is always haemorrhage in the substance of the brain.'

The first premise meant that, in defining apoplexy, Rochoux moved away from the issue of consciousness and declared sudden paralysis and numbness as the key symptoms. He might have added 'on one side of the body', but that was implicit from his cases. This view eliminated three categories of patients that had, in the course of time, diluted the diagnostic criteria: sudden deaths, patients in whom the course of the disease was progressive, and patients with short-lived faints or fits.

The second premise, however, immediately prompts a question, at any rate from modern readers: how is it possible that Rochoux had in his dissections *always* found extravasated blood and never something else? The answer is that indeed he did find other abnormalities, in no fewer than ten patients, but that in all of these, there had been a considerable interval between the attack and death. As a result, Rochoux interpreted these different lesions as complications of a haemorrhage that, he supposed, had occurred initially.

CHANGES IN THE BRAIN AFTER HAEMORRHAGE

'Complications' after Intracerebral Haemorrhage?

It was difficult for Rochoux to arrive at any other conclusion. All patients with an acute apoplectic event in whom he performed an autopsy and failed to find a recent haemorrhage, 10 in number, had died fairly long after the apoplectic event. The interval had always been more than one month, in six even between 3 months and 20 years.[16] At the time, there was very little knowledge about the manner and the velocity in which blood was cleared from the brain, or about other later changes. Thus, whether or not Rochoux's interpretation

---

[15] Rochoux (1814), *Recherches sur l'Apoplexie*, 237. Page numbers are cited as printed, despite some misnumbering (192 is followed by 189).

[16] Rochoux (1814), *Recherches sur l'Apoplexie*, 92–129.

of previous haemorrhages was correct, it was not at odds with existing knowledge. The time interval had been much shorter in the 11 patients in whom Rochoux had indeed found extravasated blood: a week or less in nine, and 11 and 21 days in the remaining two.

The abnormalities Rochoux found in patients with a longer interval between apoplexy and death often consisted in softening or in 'serous effusion'. The haemorrhages had not been lethal, he reasoned, but the complications had caught up with them after all. In 5 of the 10 patients, Rochoux found mainly serous effusion (*épanchement séreux consécutif*); in the other five, the main abnormality was softening and disintegration of brain tissue (*ramollissement consécutif*), accompanied by serosity.

Rochoux explained the relationship between the – supposed – initial haemorrhage and the complications as follows:

> 1° Softening always manifests itself at a time quite remote from the initial apoplexy, usually after one or two years, sometimes six or even eight [years]. 2° The serous effusion, in contrast, mostly takes place in the first months after the illness, and it is exceptional that an apoplectic person, if he does not completely regain his health, survives for a year without being attacked by it. 3° Finally, each time softening of the brain occurs, there is always secondary effusion of serum, while one often sees serous effusion without softening.[17]

What happened in the brain of patients who survived an intracerebral haemorrhage was a question that had so far not received much attention; scarce observations of later changes had been made by Brunner and de Haen, as mentioned in previous chapters, and also by Valsalva.[18] This gap in medical knowledge was soon to be filled.

Resorption of Extravasated Blood

In August 1814, a certain Dr Mathurin Riobé (1788–?), employed at the *Hôpital de la Charité* and unaware of Rochoux's work, defended a thesis in Paris on the question of whether recovery after apoplexy was possible. He presented a series of six patients who had died at different intervals after apoplexy, between one day and five years. In all of them, he found a cystic lesion in the central area of one hemisphere, filled with blood and surrounded by serous fluid, with the relative proportions depending on the interval. The borders of the cyst consisted of a pale, semi-transparent membrane, with a yellow-brown colour, often containing small blood vessels. This membrane,

---

[17] Rochoux (1814), *Recherches sur l'Apoplexie*, 130.

[18] Morgagni (1761), *De Sedibus et Causis Morborum*, vol. I, 14 (epistula II, paragr. 15–16) and 83 (epistula XI, paragr. 6).

Riobé concluded, secreted a fluid that dissolved blood and gradually absorbed it, in parallel with recovery of paralysis.[19] After two years, as confirmed by two personal observations and supported by those of Valsalva and Brunner, the walls of the cyst are almost joined and form a narrow scar.[20]

Riobé's thesis was well reviewed in a journal article by the young Isidore Bricheteau (1789–1861),[21] attached to the *Hôtel-Dieu* in Paris. Bricheteau added five brief case histories of his own to support Riobé's views.[22] Also he had consulted his colleague and contemporary Jean Cruveilhier (1791–1874), whose special interest was pathology, as will emerge again below. Cruveilhier's extensive response evokes almost cinematographic impressions:

> In the first two or three days after the attack of apoplexy one finds an irregular destruction of the substance of the brain, and [also] blood that is partly clotted, partly fluid. Towards the fourth or fifth day, the surrounding brain substance shows a yellowish colour, quite similar to that of skin or cellular tissue with external contusions. At the ninth, tenth, or fifteenth day, the clot is firmer and touches the walls, which are red and soft. If one divides these regions in very small layers, one finds, after the innermost one, other layers formed by the substance of the brain, sprinkled with red spots. There is no real membrane yet, but the superficial red coating seems to be its base. At a more advanced stage, the redness diminishes and the membranous aspect becomes more evident.
>
> Ultimately, if one dissects deceased persons after one, two, six, etc. years after an attack of apoplexy, one finds a cyst of variable size, formed by a very thin membrane, yellowish or reddish in colour, containing yellowish etc. serum. As the effused blood and the serous fluid diminish by absorption, the contents of the cysts are reduced, its walls thicken, form adhesions and its cavity gradually vanishes; the structure merges more and more with the substance of the brain and after a certain time its shows nothing but a yellowish scar, or layered tissue, sometimes infiltrated by equally yellowish fluid.[23]

Rochoux's speculations about later 'complications' of extravasation were not adopted by subsequent authors on the subject, neither with regard to its morphological aspects – softening or serous effusions – nor to explain clinical features. Five years later, a new book on apoplexy again described post-haemorrhagic changes in the brain. Its author Étienne Moulin (1795–1871)[24] was employed at the *Hospice des femmes incurables*, later in several other Parisian hospitals. Moulin had carefully read Riobé and Bricheteau; supported by his own dissections, he extensively described the gradual transformation of a

[19] Riobé (1814), Apoplexie et guérison, 10.   [20] Riobé (1814), Apoplexie et guérison, 10–14.

[21] Hirsch (1884–8), *Biographisches Lexikon*, vol. I, 571.

[22] Bricheteau (1818), Considérations et observations sur l'apoplexie, 146–9.

[23] Bricheteau (1818), Considérations et observations sur l'apoplexie, 151.

[24] Hirsch (1884–8), *Biographisches Lexikon*, vol. IV, 295–6.

haemorrhagic lesion into an 'apoplectic cyst' and exemplified it with new case histories; one of his patients had four attacks of apoplexy before she died.[25]

Rochoux's simple solution for the bewildering diversity of symptoms eighteenth-century physicians interpreted as apoplexy was to limit its definition to sudden hemiplegia, whether or not accompanied by some loss of consciousness. Others, however, still recognized other initial symptoms as a hallmark of apoplexy.

SUBDIVISIONS OF HAEMORRHAGIC APOPLEXY

John Abercrombie (1780–1844) (Box 6.3, p. 201), a leading physician in Edinburgh, published several case histories of patients with apoplexy in *The Edinburgh Medical and Surgical Journal*, of December 1818 and January 1819. Before an explanation of his views on the subject, it is proper to pay some attention to the medical journal as a new medium of communication.

Medical Journals Take Over

Previous sources of medical facts were mostly books, sometimes letters. Articles were at first limited to memoirs for closed organizations such as the Royal Society. Scientific journals open to all interested subscribers started to appear at around the beginning of the nineteenth century, for example the *Medical and Physical Journal* in London. Accordingly, this periodical published not only medical items, for example cases of cerebral haemorrhage,[26] but also about surgery, pharmacy, chemistry, or natural history. Instead, the Edinburgh journal covered merely medical subjects, as did the Parisian *Journal complémentaire du dictionnaire des sciences médicales*, in which Bricheteau wrote on the resorption of extravasated blood. In the course of the nineteenth century, medical journals were to become increasingly important in the diffusion of medical knowledge.[27] The inclusion of surgery in the title of the Edinburgh journal, founded in 1805 to replace the *Annals of Medicine* (1796), indicates that not only in Paris physicians and surgeons had ceased to live in separate spheres; their colleagues in northern Italy had been allied even earlier.

Three Possible Symptoms at Onset: Unconsciousness, Headache, and Paralysis

Back to John Abercrombie. Though a private practitioner without hospital facilities, he nevertheless performed post-mortem dissections. From this

---

[25] Moulin (1819), *Traité de l'Apoplexie*, 68–77.
[26] Howship (1810), Observations on diseases of the brain.
[27] Csiszar (2018), *The Scientific Journal*.

experience, he distinguished three types of apoplexy, depending on whether the first symptom had been loss of consciousness, headache, or paralysis.[28] Abercrombie recognized that, in the course of the disease, these three symptoms could combine, replace each other, or recur. Nevertheless, post-mortem dissection in fatal cases had revealed different 'morbid appearances', he wrote, in each of these three categories.

In the first group, with initial loss of consciousness ('simple apoplexy'), patients either quickly recovered or they died on the spot or at least soon afterwards, without headache or paralysis. Of his patients in this group, one had a cerebellar haemorrhage, but the other eight dissections showed no abnormalities in the brain or only some serous effusion, a feature Abercrombie regarded as a secondary phenomenon. In trying to explain these deaths without apparent cause, he supposed there had been some 'interruption of the circulation', either within the brain itself, particularly with regard to its venous channels, or by some disorder of the heart or the lungs. Abercrombie did not believe in the widespread notion of arterial overfilling as a cause of apoplexy:

> I know no principle on which we can suppose, that, in the natural state of the vessels, the blood can be sent with greater impetus, or in greater quantity into the carotid than into the subclavian, or any other great artery.[29]

This sounded rather heretical to John Cooke, a contemporary in London who compiled a book about nervous diseases, but without any personal experience of apoplexy; he bolstered his more traditional view with the judgement of others, from Aretaeus of Cappadocia to John Cheyne.[30]

Abercrombie's second group consisted of six patients with sudden and severe headache, sometimes preceded by a brief loss of consciousness. They all lapsed into a comatose state and died later on; all six showed brain haemorrhages on dissection. As a distinguishing feature of these extravasations, not only was blood found in brain tissue itself, but sometimes it had ruptured to the surface (two patients) or to the ventricles of the brain (four patients).[31] Abercrombie located the primary abnormality in the wall of blood vessels and dismissed not only congestion, but also an inflammatory disorder.[32]

In the third and last group, the onset had been sudden 'paralysis' – hemiplegia or loss of speech. At the time Abercrombie wrote his article, there were only two patients of this type and he still made some distinction between sudden hemiplegia and apoplexy.[33] This was no longer the case when, 10 years

[28] Abercrombie (1818a), On apoplexy, 553–5.   [29] Abercrombie (1818a), On apoplexy, 571.
[30] Cooke (1820), *A Treatise on Nervous Diseases*, 210–16.
[31] Abercrombie (1818a), On apoplexy, 560–5.
[32] Abercrombie (1818a), On apoplexy, 588–91.   [33] Abercrombie (1819), On paralysis, 1–22.

later, he revised the text for a book on diseases of the brain and could add 10 more cases. The other two categories also contained more patients, but this had no effect on his conclusions. In all patients with initial paralysis in the later and larger series, he found remnants of a previous haemorrhage, in agreement with the description of the Parisian physicians, except two patients in whom the interval between the attack and death had been 10 or more years.[34]

'Cerebral Apoplexy' and 'Meningeal Apoplexy'

Antoine (Étienne-Renaud-Augustin) Serres (1786–1868), a physician at the *Hôtel-Dieu* and the *Hôpital de la Pitié* in Paris, professed extensive experience, with more than 100 autopsies in patients with apoplexy. His journal article was planned in 1814 but, for some reason, did not appear until five years later.[35] He failed to refer to Rochoux's text of five years before; yet, after a historical review that cannot even be called superficial,[36] he announced the subject needed some fresh air.

Serres started by attacking the notion that apoplexy – defined as unresponsiveness – and effusion of blood or other fluids are virtually synonymous. First of all, he referred to his own experimental brain haemorrhages in a variety of species, from pigeons and dogs to cows and horses: some animals were paralysed, but none were unconscious.[37] The same dissociation occurred in several autopsies, published by others or representing personal observations. Conversely, Serres also claimed that apoplexy can occur without effusion of blood. With a strange twist of reasoning, he concluded that effusions of fluid are not the cause, but an effect of apoplexy.[38]

A 'new division of apoplexy', Serres proposed, was to distinguish two kinds, depending on whether or not the patient showed paralysis. Of his purported 100 Parisian patients, 79 had shown paralysis of one or more limbs – with or without concomitant loss of consciousness at onset, thus unlike Abercrombie's classification. Serres called these cases 'cerebral apoplexy'. He specified only eight of them, with different combinations of limb paralysis; in this small group, he found blood clots in the deep regions of one hemisphere, sometimes the brainstem.[39]

The remaining 21 patients, without paralysis, all showed signs of inflammation, irritation, or injection in the *pia mater*, the arachnoid membrane, or the walls of the ventricles. In view of these superficial changes and of the absence

---

[34] Abercrombie (1828), *Diseases of the Brain and the Spinal Cord*, 247–68.
[35] Serres (1819), Nouvelle division des apoplexies, 255.
[36] Serres (1819), Nouvelle division des apoplexies, 249–55.
[37] Serres (1819), Nouvelle division des apoplexies, 257–62.
[38] Serres (1819), Nouvelle division des apoplexies, 262–71.
[39] Serres (1819), Nouvelle division des apoplexies, 332–58.

of paralytic symptoms, Serres classified them as 'meningeal apoplexy'. Current readers will have associations with superficial haemorrhages or even ruptured aneurysms, but that is not what Serres had in mind. Of the 21 patients, as many as 16 had only 'serous effusion', between the membranes of the brain or in the ventricles. Of the five remaining patients, two had a sero-sanguineous effusion between the arachnoid and the pia, and one a similar sero-sanguineous effusion in one lateral ventricle, while two patients showed no effusions at all.[40]

Comments from Berlin

The publications from Paris and Edinburgh attracted the attention of Moritz Romberg (1795–1873).[41] He had recently graduated (1817) from the Friedrich-Wilhelm University of Berlin, founded just seven years before. This new institution and Prussian education in general owed much to Wilhelm von Humboldt (1767–1835), a diplomat, linguist, and champion of research and academic freedom; he wished universities to focus on research, as well as on teaching.[42] Romberg started his medical career as a physician for the poor in Spandau, a Berlin suburb. Through his ambition and talents, he received permission to perform autopsies at the university hospital, the *Charité*. At present, his name is eponymous; it will probably remain so, because 'Romberg's test' is a more convenient expression than 'asking patients to keep their balance while standing with the feet together, arms outstretched, and eyes closed'.

Romberg wrote a series of three articles about apoplexy in the journal *Archiv für medizinische Erfahrung &c.*, at the time the main vehicle for medical communication in Prussia. His doctoral thesis, a few years later, contained a summary.[43] Romberg cited foreign work, sometimes with a full translation, mixed with his own comments or experiences. With regard to the classification of apoplexy, he reserved his judgement about Serres' 'meningeal apoplexy', if only because Morgagni's findings only partly agreed with it.[44]

In a review of Abercrombie's journal articles of 1818–19, Romberg was critical on two counts. With regard to Abercrombie's classification according to presentation (collapse, headache, or paralysis), Romberg wrote that he understood the rationale, but he criticized the lack of an unequivocal common denominator. He was concerned about the possible confusion by

[40] Serres (1819), Nouvelle division des apoplexies, 274–5.
[41] Schiffter (2010), Moritz Heinrich Romberg; Hirsch (1884–8), *Biographisches Lexikon*, vol v, 73–4.
[42] Geier (2009), *Die Brüder Humboldt*, 233–314.
[43] Romberg (1830), De cerebri haemorrhagia.
[44] Romberg (1820), Ueber den Schlagfluss, 82–7.

combinations of the three symptoms, and by the inclusion of sudden deaths from disease of the heart or lungs.[45] Regrettably, Romberg struck a shrill false note in his critique.[46] Furthermore, Romberg opposed the Scot's dismissal of 'cerebral congestion' as a cause of apoplexy, with a variety of arguments.[47]

Still, vessel rupture was the most common cause, Romberg admitted in a new article, with his own findings; two of his three cases were associated with trauma and showed extravasations between the arachnoid and dural membranes. The third patient had a spontaneous haemorrhage in a cerebellar hemisphere; Romberg managed to find the site of rupture, in a branch of the superior cerebellar artery.[48]

COLOURED ILLUSTRATIONS

So far, almost every description of lesions in the brain consisted of words; the only exceptions were the black-and-white engravings of brain haemorrhages in the books of Matthew Baillie and John Cheyne.

Printing in Colour

In the early nineteenth century, hand-colouring was the preferred method for adding colour to prints made by classical *intaglio* techniques, where the lines of the images are below the surface. This is different from the older woodcut technique whereby the areas around the image are cut away. In engraving, linear grooves are cut in a copper plate by a kind of chisel (burin). Another *intaglio* technique is etching: the copper plate is covered with an acid-resistant coating; the design is drawn with a needle through the coating, followed by immersion of the plate in acid, which bites away the metal. Combinations of the two techniques are possible (for example, in 'stipple engraving').

Commonly the ink for printing plates was black, brown, or grey-brown. For detailed colour printing, different parts of the plate were inked with different colours (*à la poupée* inking) and printed in a single press run. In special cases, different colours were printed from different plates, with each plate containing part of the total design.[49] Such techniques, sometimes in combination with hand-colouring, were applied in the volumes of Richard Bright

---

[45] Romberg (1822), Kritische Prüfung von J. Abercrombie's Abhandlung, 459–61.

[46] Romberg (1822), Kritische Prüfung von J. Abercrombie's Abhandlung, 473–5. Romberg flubbed not only by misunderstanding the scientific issue, but also especially by accusing the Scot of 'excessive scepticism . . . to which English authors have a greater tendency anyway'.

[47] Romberg (1822), Kritische Prüfung von J. Abercrombie's Abhandlung, 461–73.

[48] Romberg (1823), *Hämorrhagieen*, 413–20.

[49] Goldschmid (1925), *Bibliographie der pathologisch-anatomischen Abbildung*, 126–7; Bertoloni Meli (2017), *Visualizing Disease*, 166–75.

Box 5.2 Richard Bright (1789–1858).

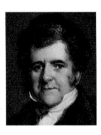 Bright was born as the fourth child of a prosperous merchant in Bristol. His mother was Sarah Heywood; four more children were to follow. Father Richard was an avid collector of minerals, plants, and insects. In 1808, the young Bright became a student of medicine in Edinburgh; his father had some initial doubts on this choice, given this son's tacit and slightly melancholic nature. After theoretical training and a five-month geological expedition to Iceland, Richard Jr. went to London for his clinical rotationships, in the united hospitals of Guy's and St Thomas'. His role model was the physician William Babington (1783–1833), excelling by his modesty and gentle manners with patients.

After graduation (Edinburgh in 1813), Bright made a grand tour of the continent, for which he prepared himself by learning some French, German, and Italian. Among the many cities he visited was Vienna, where the conference about the future of Europe was in progress. Fascinated by Hungary, he traversed the country, tried to master the gypsy language, and made notes, drawings, and watercolours, later condensed in a book. Returning via the Low Countries, he found the battle of Waterloo had just taken place and assisted for some time in the care for sick and wounded soldiers in Brussels.

After having settled in London, initially employed at the Caley Dispensary, the Lock Hospital, and the Fever Hospital, he made another long journey to the continent, now with special interest for post-mortem rooms. In 1820, he was appointed assistant physician at Guy's Hospital; he was to stay there for the rest of his professional life, collaborating with other luminaries such as Thomas Addison (1793–1860) and Thomas Hodgkin (1798–1866). Bright developed a special interest for diseases of the kidney and set up an exclusive ward for this category of patients. He detected that 'dropsy' was often related to albuminous (coagulable) urine, and associated with different morbid appearances of the kidneys. Between 1827 and 1837, he published his famous *Reports of medical Cases*. He retired from the hospital in 1844 but retained his practice well into the 1850s.

In 1822, he had married Babington's daughter Martha; Bright adored her and was devastated when she died a year later, a few days after the birth of their son William. In 1826, he married Eliza Follett; they had seven children, six of whom survived childhood.

(1789–1858) (Box 5.2),[50] a physician at Guy's Hospital in London, after extensive experiences on the continent. Bright, though an accomplished draughtsman himself, relied for his illustrations on professional artists; most often Frederick Richard Say (1804–1868) produced the initial watercolours, after which his father William Say (1768–1834) etched the printing plates.

Lithography, or printing from stone, was the first technique for printing in which the image was transferred to paper from the same plane as the background and not above or below it.[51] The technique was developed between

[50] Bright (1983), *Dr. Richard Bright*; Peitzman (2007), Richard Bright.
[51] Bouquin (2005), Lithographie.

1796 and 1798 by Alois Senefelder (1771–1834), a Bavarian student in chemistry and amateur actor. The essence of the method is to draw on stone, usually limestone, with oily crayon or ink, which forms a strong chemical bond with the surface. After the stone has been moistened with water, it is rolled up with an oil-based ink, usually black, which attaches itself to the drawing but is repelled by the damp part of the surface. When the stone is printed on paper, only the design is transferred. For colour printing, separate stones are prepared for each colour; the colours are printed over each other.

Two authors writing on apoplexy were early adopters of lithography: Jean Cruveilhier, mentioned above, and Robert Carswell (1793–1857). Cruveilhier commissioned the original drawings, mostly to the artist Antoine Chazal (1793–1854); at the printing shop, these would be copied on stone, again separately for each colour. Only Carswell was an artistic prodigy who made his own watercolours.

Images of Brain Haemorrhage

The illustrated atlases of the authors mentioned above all appeared around the 1830s. Richard Bright's text included case histories of all patients with cerebral haemorrhage who had been under his care up to the time of publication, with dissection in 22 of them.[52] Most were located in or near the striate body or thalamus, in keeping with the descriptions of Morgagni and Rochoux (Figure 5.1).[53] Bright commented, as Abercrombie had done, that the large arteries of patients with apoplectic haemorrhage were often diseased, with cartilaginous patches or even ossification (Figure 5.2).[54] Bright also noted that headache was especially prominent if the effused blood had reached the surface of the brain.[55] He did not cite Rochoux but followed him by attributing older, cystic lesions to previous bleeding episodes;[56] he regarded 'serous effusion' as a form of general brain congestion, unrelated to apoplexy.[57]

Jean Cruveilhier (1791–1874) (Box 6.4, p. 208) appeared earlier in this chapter, as an informant of Bricheteau about changes in the brain after haemorrhage. Later on, he held the first chair of Pathological Anatomy in Paris. In the course of 13 years, he published 40 fascicles with his findings in assorted organs, with texts and lithographies; the order of subjects was not systematic but depended on recent experiences. The serial instalments were sent to

[52] Bright (1827–31), *Reports of Medical Cases*, 266–332.
[53] Bright (1827–31), *Reports of Medical Cases*, vol. II, part 1, 290–2, and part 2, plate XXIII, figure 1.
[54] Bright (1827–31), *Reports of Medical Cases*, vol. II, part 1, plate IXX, figure 2.
[55] Bright (1827–31), *Reports of Medical Cases*, vol. II, part 1, 329.
[56] Bright (1827–31), *Reports of Medical Cases*, vol. II, part 2, 296–312.
[57] Bright (1827–31), *Reports of Medical Cases*, vol. II, part 1, 223–65.

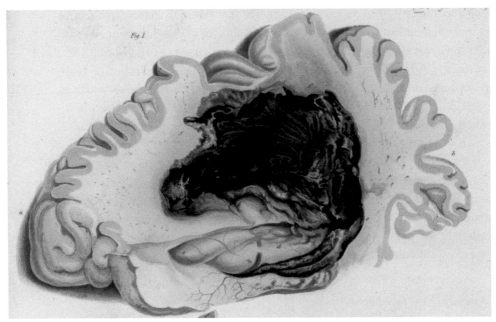

5.1 Coloured engraving of intracerebral haemorrhage (Bright, 1831). The patient, a man of 58, became suddenly paralysed on the left side, while driving a cart; he died 12 days later. Drawing by C. J. Canton (n.d.), engraving by W. T. Fry (n.d.). The legend by Bright reads, somewhat abbreviated: 'Horizontal section of the right hemisphere, a little below the level of the top of the ventricle, showing a large clot of blood which had found its way into the right lateral ventricle by a rupture of the cerebral substance, near the optic thalamus. a) The anterior and b) the posterior portion of the right hemisphere; c) corpus striatum; d) the optic thalamus; e) the posterior horn filled with the clot; f) the brain around the clot, discoloured and somewhat softened.'

subscribers and eventually grew into two hefty tomes, together weighing 42 English pounds. In the fifth fascicle, Cruveilhier described the histories of four patients in whom he had found extravasated blood in the deep regions of the brain, with illustrations (Figure 5.3).[58] In a later fascicle, he added four case histories of patients with haemorrhages in the pons, plus a rather lurid illustration of a fifth patient whose history he was unable to retrieve (Figure 5.4).[59]

Robert Carswell made more than 1000 watercolours in the dissection rooms of Paris and Lyon, also of brain haemorrhage (Figure 5.5).[60] The images are not linked to symptoms, since Carswell stayed as a guest and was not involved in patient care.

[58] Cruveilhier (1829–42), *Anatomie pathologique*, vol. I, livraison V, planche 6.
[59] Cruveilhier (1829–42), *Anatomie pathologique*, vol. II, livraison XXI, planche 5.
[60] Carswell (1838), *Pathological Anatomy*, section 'Haemorrhage' (there is no numbering of pages).

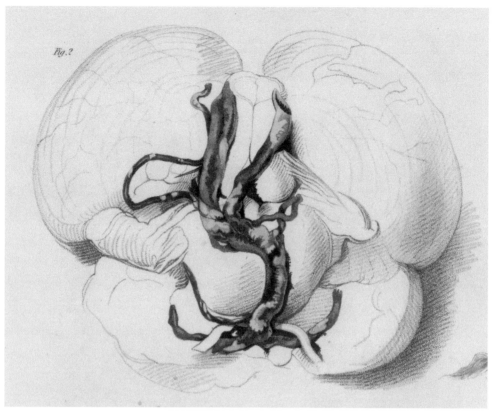

5.2 Coloured engraving of cerebral arteries at the base of the brain (Bright, 1831). The patient, a man of sixty-one, had been seized by hemiplegia on the left side, while aboard ship; he died three days later. Dissection showed that a haemorrhage had destroyed the right thalamus, with rupture into the ventricle. Drawing by C. J. Canton (n.d.), engraving by W. T. Fry (n.d.). The legend by Bright is as follows: 'The under part of the cerebellum, the pons Varolii, and the medulla oblongata are seen in outline, and the vertebral and basilar arteries, and several of the arteries proceeding from them, are in a highly diseased state, their coats having become studded with cartilaginous patches, which are gradually passing into bone: by this disease the diameter of the vessels is rendered irregular, and considerable contortion is produced in their course.'

The artistic representations also mark a shift of attention in this story of cerebral haemorrhage. Apart from its morphology, its clinical features, and its relation with other disorders, an aspect not yet fully explored was that of the causes of extravasation.

PRIMARY CHANGES IN THE BRAIN – OR ELSEWHERE?

When Rochoux postulated, in 1814, that all apoplexies with 'paralysis' were haemorrhagic in nature and that softening or serous effusions were secondary complications, he did not leave it at that. He also tried to understand the origin

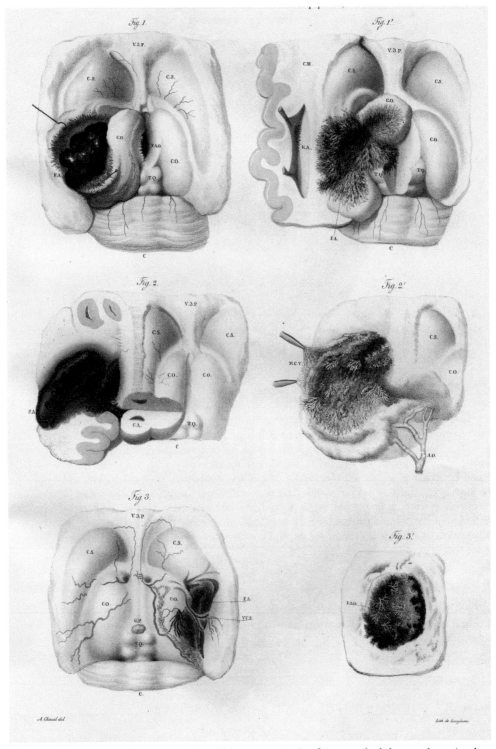

5.3 Lithographic images (Cruveilhier, 1829–1842) of intracerebral haemorrhage in three patients, from top to bottom. All sections are viewed from below. On the left side of the page, the clotted blood is still in place; on the right, it has been removed to show the wall of the abnormal cavity. Drawings by Antoine Chazal (1793–1854).

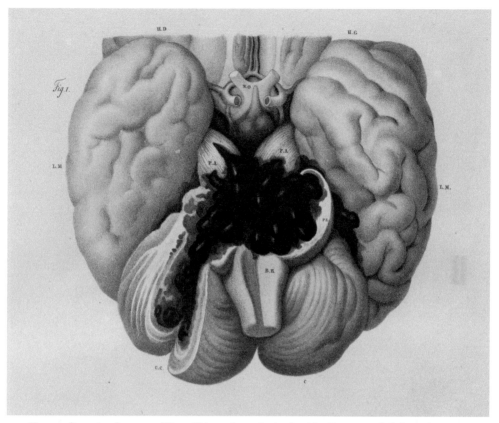

5.4 Haemorrhage in the pons (Cruveilhier, 1829–1842); the bleeding extended into the cerebral peduncles. The history of the patient could not be retrieved. Drawing by Antoine Chazal (1793–1854).

of the haemorrhage and wondered whether a local alteration of brain tissue might be at its root. Still unencumbered by the information that was to come from later studies of resorption, he described the area bordering the extravasated blood as follows:

5.3 (cont.) 'Fig. 1'. Man, 52 years, who suddenly lost consciousness; having come round, he was paralysed on the right side and could not speak. He died five days after the event. Dissection: haemorrhage in the left thalamus (CO), with rupture into the third ventricle (FAO). There is an old apoplectic cyst in the right centrum semiovale.
'Fig. 2'. Woman, 72 years, seized by paralysis of the left arm and leg. The weakness showed some improvement, but then she developed a fever from an infection in the right leg; she died 28 days after the attack. Dissection: brown coagulum of blood in the right centrum semiovale; the effusion had reached a part of the right ventricle.
'Fig. 3'. Man, 65 years. He was admitted in a comatose state and died after five days. He was said to have had an attack of apoplexy one month before. Dissection: brown clot in the posterior part of the left thalamus and the lateral part of the thalamus, with rupture into the left ventricle. An intact vein traverses the haemorrhage.

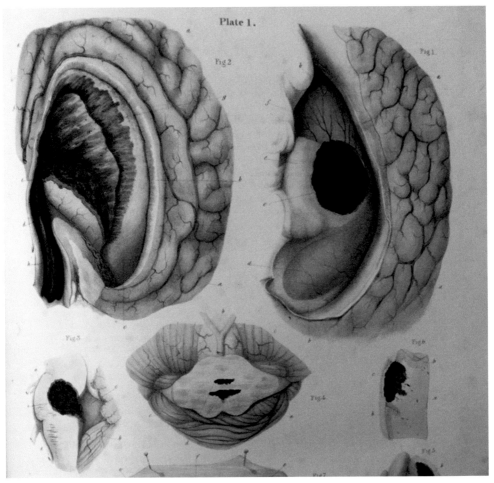

5.5 Cerebral apoplexy (Carswell, 1838; he is also the artist). The patients' histories are not available. His legend is as follows:

'Fig. 1. aa) external surface of the brain; bb) left lateral ventricle laid open; c) thalamus; d) corpus striatum; e) a large effusion consisting of fluid and coagulated blood, protruding into the ventricle through an extensive laceration of the thalamus; f) large congested vessels opening into the haemorrhagic excavation.

Fig. 2. Haemorrhage in the same situation; aa) external surface of the brain; b) corpus callosum divided longitudinally; c) corpus striatum; d) thalamus; e) the lacerated surface of this body; f) and g) layers of the fibrous structure of the brain separated by the effused blood, and presenting deep red points in the situation of the ruptured vessels; h) a quantity of coagulated blood in the fourth ventricle and commencement of the spinal canal.

Fig. 3. A longitudinal section of the pons Varolii and medulla oblongata, representing haemorrhage of the former, and rupture of the inferior wall of the fourth ventricle. a) the pons; b) portion of the cerebellum; c) fourth ventricle; d) vertebral and basilar arteries; e) the haemorrhage.

Fig. 4. The same part of the brain cut transversely, representing haemorrhage in the direction of its fibrous structure. a) the pons; b) medulla oblongata; d) cerebellum; d) the effused blood.'

> The walls of these artificial cavities are very soft, coloured bright red by the blood, one or two lines in thickness,[61] uneven, sinuous, visibly torn at its inner surface, and they show floating shreds when rinsed with water. They are surrounded by a layer of cerebral substance, a few millimetres in thickness, pale canary yellow, very soft, hardly firmer than certain creams, poorly soluble in water. The colour and the softness of this layer, most marked at the inside, gradually diminish outwards, so that it is impossible to determine precisely where the brain regains the integrity of its texture.[62]

These changes set him thinking about the order of events:

> Such an alteration of the brain has not been described by anybody, as far as I know. Is it simply the effect of the presence of blood? Does it precede the haemorrhage? The latter opinion seems the most probable to me, and it is not invalidated by the absence of preceding symptoms. Does one not know that certain organic lesions, for example tubercles of the lung, reach a great size before manifesting their presence by some derangement of function?[63]

Rochoux left it at this tentative speculation, at least in 1814.

Brain Softening as the Primary Event?

But in a second edition of his book, 19 years after the first, with twice as many pages, Rochoux adopted a much firmer stance. He drew an analogy with haemorrhages in other organs, but his key argument was that he had found softening around the blood clot, even in patients who had died only a few hours after the haemorrhage.[64] He had designed a Graeco-Latin name for this purported primary change in brain tissue: *ramollissement hémorrhagipare* or *apoplectipare*, in other words 'softening about to give rise to bleeding or apoplexy'. He distinguished this 'pre-haemorrhagic' type of softening from secondary areas of softening, which, Rochoux wrote, had a different texture and represented either inflammation or complications of the earlier haemorrhage.[65]

Others thought more or less along the same lines. Maxime Durand-Fardel (1815–1899), in a book on diseases of old age published two decades later, slightly adapted Rochoux's theory by incriminating a more generalized atrophic process in brain tissue of elderly people: 'interstitial atrophy'.[66] And Robert

---

[61] A *ligne* is one-twelfth of an inch, corresponding to 2.25 mm; revolutionary metrics (Alder (2002), *The Measure of All Things*) was not yet applied to small objects.
[62] Rochoux (1814), *Recherches sur l'Apoplexie*, 88.
[63] Rochoux (1814), *Recherches sur l'Apoplexie*, 89.
[64] Rochoux (1833), *Recherches sur l'Apoplexie*, 153–9.
[65] Rochoux (1833), *Recherches sur l'Apoplexie*, 180–96.
[66] Durand-Fardel (1854), *Maladies des Vieillards*, 293–8.

Bentley Todd (1809–1860), in his textbook on paralysis and other diseases of the brain, proposed a nutritional disorder of brain tissue and its minute nutrient blood vessels alike.[67]

Jaundice and Other Counterarguments

Rochoux's strongest argument, that a zone of softened brain tissue around the haematoma could be distinguished even if only a few hours had elapsed between the attack and death, came under attack in the 1860s. A Parisian thesis, discussed more fully below, also contained the story of a patient who, severely jaundiced by liver cancer, had finally died of multiple intracerebral haemorrhages; on dissection, each of these haemorrhages was surrounded by an intensely yellow zone.[68] This definitively proved that 'softening' of brain tissue around a fresh haematoma is nothing but secondary 'imbibition' of serum by brain tissue.

The common finding that haemorrhages had ruptured into the ventricular system was another objection against Rochoux's hypothesis of a primary change in brain tissue, Romberg argued.[69] He also adduced the frequent finding of cardiac hypertrophy in patients with apoplexy.[70] Romberg was not alone in noting this association.

Hypertrophy of the Heart

In 1658, Wepfer had attributed the occurrence of intracerebral haemorrhage to the propulsive force of the heartbeats. Early in the nineteenth century, the Parisian surgeon Anthelme Richerand (1779–1840)[71] found that 'hypersarcose' of the heart often accompanied haemorrhagic apoplexy;[72] the physician Isidore Bricheteau soon confirmed this.[73]

Rochoux, however, dismissed this association.[74] A few years later, in 1836, he came back on the subject in a meeting of the *Académie royale de médecine*. He reiterated his arguments for *ramollissement* as the primary event and ventured new arguments against a vascular cause. He also maintained that hypertrophy of the heart was almost equally common in patients who had

---

[67] Todd (1856), *Clinical Lectures on Paralysis*, 126–30.
[68] Bouchard (1866), La pathogénie des hémorrhagies cérébrales, 20–1 and 106–9.
[69] Romberg (1819), Ueber den Schlagfluss, 556–7.
[70] Romberg (1820), Ueber den Schlagfluss, 91–6; Romberg (1823), Hämorrhagieen, 420–4.
[71] Hirsch (1884–8), *Biographisches Lexikon*, vol. v, 14–15.
[72] Richerand (1806), *Nosographie chirurgicale*, vol. iii, 14–15.
[73] Bricheteau (1819), La circulation et les fonctions cérébrales.
[74] Rochoux (1833), *Recherches sur l'Apoplexie*, 424–9.

died of pneumonia.[75] Many opponents took the floor.[76] One of them, Pierre Adolphe Piorry (1794–1879), argued that attention should be especially directed to hypertrophy of the left ventricle of the heart, while François Joseph Victor Broussais (1772–1835) and Pierre Charles Alexandre Louis (1787–1872), the father of 'numerical medicine', expressed their belief that *ramollissement* and haemorrhage of the brain were completely different conditions.

The role of heart disease was also noted in London. Hypertrophy, dilatation, or valvular disease occurred in no less than three-fifths of 132 patients with apoplexy and sudden hemiplegia in published series tabulated by George Burrows (1771–1846),[77] in his book about the cerebral circulation.[78] Incidentally, the main purpose of Burrows' text was to revive the notion of cerebral congestion and to contest, supported by experiments in rabbits, the Monro–Kellie hypothesis of a constant blood volume in the skull.[79] Another review of the literature by William Boyd Mushet (n.d.) also implicated hypertrophy of the heart as an important causal factor; his account was more complete, but also more complex, if only by including cases of 'apoplexy' unrelated to the head.[80] But at least Mushet summarized eight 'unselected' case histories from his own practice to support his view.[81] A contrasting result appeared in Berlin, chronicled by the young Albert Eulenburg (1840–1917);[82] he found hypertrophy of the heart in only a minority (9 out of 42) of published patients with intracerebral haemorrhage.[83]

William Senhouse Kirkes (1823–1864),[84] an assistant physician in St Bartholomew's Hospital, drew attention to the role of kidney disease in producing hypertrophy of the heart. Of 22 patients who had died of sanguineous apoplexy, one of whom was a young girl, 14 showed this feature – in all but one predominantly of the left ventricle.[85] In only four patients of this series, valvular disease could account for enlargement of the heart. The renal degeneration amounted to a 'small, hard, shrunken and granular condition'. Retention of urine, Kirkes reasoned, led to thickening of the walls of the left ventricle; then the resulting increase in pressure caused damage to the vessels of the brain, evidenced by atherosclerosis and eventually by rupture.

[75] Rochoux (1836), L'hypertrophie du coeur.
[76] Anonymous (1836), Discussion du mémoire de M. Rochoux.
[77] Hirsch (1884–8), *Biographisches Lexikon*, vol. I, 629.
[78] Burrows (1846), *Disorders of the Cerebral Circulation*, 105–25.
[79] Monro (1783), *Structure and Function of the Nervous System*, 5.
[80] Copeman (1845), *A Collection of Cases of Apoplexy*.
[81] Mushet (1866), *A Practical Treatise on Apoplexy*, 42–60.
[82] Hirsch (1884–8), *Biographisches Lexikon*, vol. II, 313.
[83] Eulenburg (1862), Herzhypertrophie und Erkrankungen der Hirnarterien.
[84] Hirsch (1884–8), *Biographisches Lexikon*, vol. III, 481.
[85] Kirkes (1855), On apoplexy in relation to chronic renal disease.

DEGENERATION OF ARTERIOLES

Apart from hypertrophy of the heart or intrinsic abnormalities of blood, a degenerative process affecting small arteries was also high on the list of factors implicated in the pathogenesis of brain haemorrhage. Different research approaches went in this direction.

Moritz Romberg explained, in 1820, the preferential occurrence of extravasation in the corpus striatum and thalamus by pointing out that small vessels in this area directly branched out from large vessels, without the gradual tapering of calibre that typified the arterial system on the surface of the brain. Romberg went even further, by demonstrating the fragility of the deep arterioles by injection experiments in cadavers.[86]

James Paget (1814–1899), a physician at St Bartholomew's Hospital in London, wrote in 1850 that on microscopic examination of the brain in patients with cerebral haemorrhage, but also in those with primary softening, he had seen abnormalities surrounding the outer surface of blood vessels, especially small ones. They consisted of 'minute, shining, black-edged particles, like molecules of oil'; as these particles were greater in number, they tended to conglomerate into larger drops, while the outer layer of the vessels became fainter.[87]

Some 15 years later, the issue of structural changes in small brain arterioles of patients with intracerebral haemorrhage was again taken up, in the Salpêtrière.

The Diverse Origin of Cellular Elements around Arterioles

The assistant physician Charles Jacques Bouchard (1837–1915)[88] (Box 5.3) obtained his doctorate in 1866 with a thesis entitled *Study of some Aspects of the Pathogenesis of intracerebral Haemorrhages*. He made it clear from the beginning that he excluded haemorrhages from aneurysmal dilatations of large arteries, and also haemorrhages secondary to venous occlusions.[89] His mentor in this study was Jean-Martin Charcot (1825–1893) (Box 7.2, p. 229), who will figure even more prominently in the chapters on brain softening.

First of all, Bouchard was able to explain Paget's finding of 'fatty degeneration'. He could build on the discovery of Charles-Philippe Robin (1821–1885) that larger capillaries and smaller arterioles in the brain are enveloped by a transparent sleeve; the intervening space was filled with 'lymph' and nuclei, presumably belonging to a variety of white cells.[90] He showed that in large brain lesions, through haemorrhage or otherwise, these spaces became more

[86] Romberg (1820), Ueber den Schlagfluss, 451.
[87] Paget (1850), Degeneration of small blood vessels.
[88] Loeper (1947), Bouchard; Contrepois (2002), The example of Charles Bouchard.
[89] Bouchard (1866), La pathogénie des hémorragies cérébrales, 7.
[90] Robin (1859), La structure des capillaires de l'encéphale, 543–8.

Box 5.3 Charles Bouchard (1837–1915).

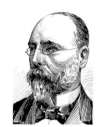

Bouchard was born in Montier-en-Der (Haute-Marne). His father Jean-Baptiste, a liberal and republican, was head of a secondary school but lost his job after the *coup d'état* of President Louis-Napoléon in 1851. The family moved to Lyon, where his father found employment as a bookkeeper and his mother Céline Pennet ran a haberdashery shop. Charles attended the medical school in Lyon; his excellent results earned him a six-month training position in Paris, where he followed the courses of Charles Robin (1821–1885) and bought a microscope. Back in Lyon, he worked as a clinical assistant; he could read German and was aware of Virchow's work.

In 1862, Bouchard came out first in the competition for internships at the Parisian hospitals; after stints at the Pitié and the Charité, he moved to the Salpêtrière, where Charcot, his senior by twelve years, spotted his talents and advised him to investigate the origin of intracerebral haemorrhages as a subject for his thesis (1866). He then successfully competed in the examination for the rank of *médecin agrégé*, fulfilled positions as *chef de clinique* and administrative chief of the Parisian hospitals, before assuming positions as senior clinician, first at the Pitié and later at the Lariboisière. At both hospitals, he set up laboratories for chemical and microscopical analysis of body fluids; later he favoured the inclusion of bacteriology into clinical thinking and performed experiments with antiseptic agents. Bouchard was also an active esperantist.

In 1879, he was appointed Professor of Pathology and General Therapeutics, a chair he would hold until 1910. In 1895, the first edition of his *Traité de Pathologie générale* appeared; he also wrote a textbook of medical radiology, following Röntgen's discovery of X-rays in 1896. At around the turn of the century, Bouchard had great influence on academic medicine in Paris. This became evident in 1892, when he gained the upper hand over Charcot on the issue of whose candidate was to obtain the position of *médecin agrégé*; Charcot's defeated candidate Joseph Babinski was to continue his career outside academia.

In 1875, Bouchard married Hélène-Henriette Ruffer; they had no children. He died in Lyon after a protracted illness following an automobile accident.

---

densely packed with elements of blood and debris of nerve tissue.[91] In other words, Paget's 'fatty particles' were an effect of brain damage, not part of its cause. Bouchard went in search of other structural changes in small arteries, inflammatory or otherwise, that might be causally related to subsequent vessel rupture.

A Lead from Virchow

Bouchard and Charcot had been alerted to changes in the wall of arterioles by a publication of Rudolf Virchow (1821–1902) (Box 7.1, p. 223), who had

---

[91] Bouchard (1866), La pathogénie des hémorrhagies cérébrales, 43–8.

reported widening of arterioles, capillaries, and veins in a variety of organs.[92] Virchow distinguished five types of widening and reordered the findings of earlier observers according to his new classification. The third type he defined was 'ampullary ectasia', a term he borrowed from Cruveilhier.[93] So far, Virchow had found these local bulges only in small arterioles of the pial membrane covering the brain, especially in furrows between the cortical convolutions, and only in vessels smaller than about 0.125 millimetres.[94] To the naked eye, these focal dilatations were just red specks. On microscopic examination, they proved to be true aneurysms, in the sense that the wall still contained all layers (intimal, muscular, and adventitial), but much rarefied. Such changes were most notable in the muscular layer, recognizable by its circular fibres and also by its nuclei, especially after immersion in acetic acid. In the widened segments, the fibres were further apart or they had even disappeared (Figure 5.6); the brain tissue around the 'ampullary ectasias' did not show any manifestations of disease. 'At most,' Virchow wrote, 'one might see these shapes as the beginning of extravasations, of sanguineous Apoplexy.'

Miliary Aneurysms and Periarteritis

The question Bouchard tried to answer was whether such dilatations might also occur in the deep regions of the brain where most haemorrhages occurred. When he used a jet of water to rinse the part of the brain with the haemorrhagic lesion, the relevant vascular structures disappeared together with the debris. And even if an arteriole showed a rent of its wall, it was impossible to determine whether this was the cause or the effect of the haemorrhage. He therefore changed to a different method: suspending the affected portion of the brain in water, regularly refreshed.[95]

And indeed, Bouchard found Virchow's 'granules' or 'ampullary ectasias' also in the region of the fatal haemorrhages, in seven consecutive patients. They occurred mostly in the striate body or the thalamus; their average size was comparable with that of hemp seed. His mentor must have been rather closely involved, since Charcot personally made the drawings for the thesis. Bouchard regarded these dilatations, characterized by an increase of nuclei in their walls and in their 'lymphatic sleeves', as the primary disease process – a 'periarteritis', a term he borrowed from Rokitansky.

---

[92] Virchow (1851), Ueber die Erweiterung kleinerer Gefässe.
[93] Cruveilhier (1829–42), *Anatomie pathologique*, livr. xxxv, planche v, fig. 1; this concerned a vein.
[94] Virchow (1851), Ueber die Erweiterung kleinerer Gefässe, 442–4. Virchow wrote: '½ Linie', probably similar to the Parisian *ligne*.
[95] Bouchard (1866), La pathogénie des hémorrhagies cérébrales, 61–3.

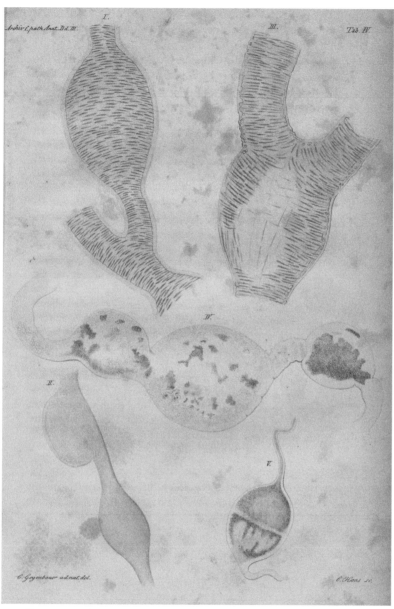

5.6 Illustrations of 'ampullary ectasia' of small arteries in the cortex of the brain (Virchow, 1851). The author did not add separate legends but referred to them in the text; these comments are paraphrased below.

   I. Dilatation over the entire circumference of the vessel (the stripes represent muscle fibres in the middle layer).
  II. Dilatation of only a part of the vessel's circumference.
 III. Disappearance of the muscle layer in a dilated part of the vessel.
 IV. String of dilatations, in the form of a rosary.
  V. Fatty material, partly filling the dilated area (lower half).

This generalised alteration in the entire arterial system of the brain is particularly manifest in small arteries. [...] It essentially consists in a marked and sometimes enormous increase of nuclei in arterial walls and in the lymphatic sheath, and atrophy of the muscular layer.[96]

Bouchard clearly distinguished this alteration from atheromatous changes in larger arteries; the two types of change often coincided, but not necessarily.[97]

Two years later, Charcot and Bouchard published a journal article about the same subject, in three instalments. The title was *New Investigations about intracerebral Haemorrhage.*[98] The 'newness' did not apply to Bouchard's thesis, but to the previous scientific literature about dilatations of small arteries. These had dealt with morphological changes per se, whereas the authors wished to point out the possibly causal relationship between intracerebral haemorrhage and the changes they now called 'miliary aneurysms'. The number of patients with spontaneous intracerebral haemorrhage, recent or in the past, in whom they found miliary aneurysms post-mortem, had now increased to 84 (77 from personal observations). It is highly probable that Charcot, who produced new drawings for the article (Figure 5.7), wished to claim his part in the discovery. Much later, Charcot and Bouchard were to fall out with each other, but for different reasons than their collaboration in this project.[99]

In the reasoning of Charcot and Bouchard, only miliary aneurysms satisfied their criterion for causality, in that they were looking for a necessary cause – a characteristic that was always present. This could not be said of other causes that had been suggested in the past: increased pressure, preceding changes in brain tissue, or atheromatous changes in the arterial wall.

We have already done our best on other occasions to show that some of these purported causes do not exist, that the influence of other ones is debatable, and that others contribute only in an accessory fashion, as ancillary factors. None of them shows sufficient properties of generality to be regarded as the true pathogenetic process of – we will not say all brain haemorrhages, but at least the great majority.[100]

They explicitly played down the role of atherosclerosis, not only because the correlation was incomplete, but also because they postulated the primary changes in the vessel wall did not occur at the inner, but at the outer layer – *periarteritis*:

---

[96] Bouchard (1866), La pathogénie des hémorrhagies cérébrales, 91.
[97] Bouchard (1866), La pathogénie des hémorrhagies cérébrales, 92–4.
[98] Charcot and Bouchard (1868), Nouvelles recherches sur l'hémorrhagie cérébrale.
[99] Iragui (1986), The Charcot–Bouchard controversy.
[100] Charcot and Bouchard (1868), Nouvelles recherches sur l'hémorrhagie cérébrale, 111.

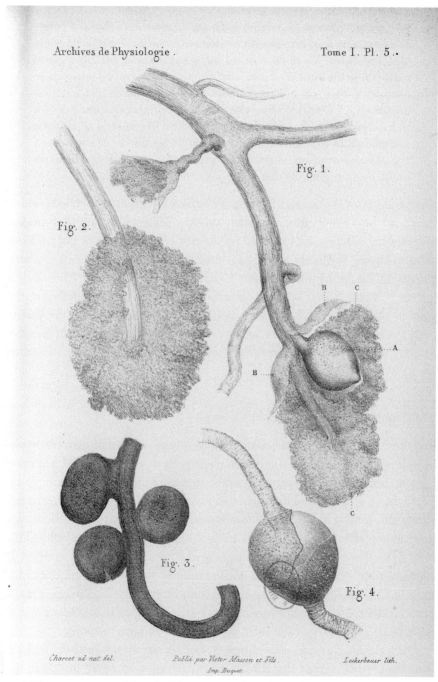

5.7 Miliary aneurysms, with and without surrounding clots (Charcot and Bouchard, 1868; original drawings by Charcot). The illustration has no legends. 'Fig. 1' and 'Fig. 2' also appeared earlier in Bouchard's thesis of 1866, in a slightly different form. The explanations there are as follows:

1. (A) Ruptured aneurysm in a haemorrhagic lesion. (C) The clot, having stretched and ruptured the lymphatic sleeve (B), is mixed with the mass of blood in the lesion.
2. Vessel that has ruptured secondarily, in a recent haemorrhagic lesion and crowned by a clot that initially gave the impression of an aneurysm.

Source: Courtesy of the *Bibliothèque nationale de France*, Paris.

The miliary aneurysms can exist and often do exist, sometimes in considerable number, independently from any atheromatous lesion of [arter-
ies of] the base or of branches distributed across the meninges; in the same
way, one meets the most marked atheroma without finding a single
aneurysm in the brain. But these two different alterations do not exclude
each other, they are not antagonistic, they can coincide and often do
coincide. [. . .] Certainly, these two essentially different alterations do not
lack a certain analogy; both result from arteritis; but whereas atheroma is
the product of an endarteritis, the miliary aneurysms are produced as a
complication of a periarteritis, diffuse periarteritis, the study of which, we
think, ought to precede that of the miliary aneurysms.[101]

From then on, Charcot and Bouchard's miliary aneurysms, or 'micro-aneurysms', as they were often renamed, quickly became part of the standard
neurological folklore, as evidenced by the first edition (1892) of the textbook
of medicine by William Osler (1849–1919)[102] and by the textbook on brain
diseases of the influential Professor Constantin von Monakow from Zurich
(1897).[103] Though later scrutiny identified earlier descriptions of tiny aneurysms in the brain,[104] Charcot and Bouchard were undoubtedly the first to
study the subject systematically and to propose a causal relation with haemorrhage. Their publication received much attention, but the reactions
were mixed.

The Charcot–Bouchard Hypothesis Contested

In a flood of subsequent articles, up to 1960, physician–pathologists recounted
how they had scrutinized the brains of patients in the vicinity of a massive
intracerebral haemorrhage, usually in the region of the basal ganglia or in the
pons. Most original publications were from German-speaking countries,
where the leading light of Virchow had resulted in many departments and
journals devoted to pathological anatomy. Often the new findings differed not
only from those of Charcot and Bouchard, but also from one another. In
addition, new techniques evolved for the microscopic study of tissue sections:
fixation in formalin, embedding in colloidin or paraffin, a growing array of
stains, and serial sectioning of thin slices. Since details of that kind are out of
place here, a summary of the main conclusions will have to suffice.

The primary question was whether miliary aneurysms actually existed.
Almost everyone agreed that dilatations of arterioles occurred, but there was

[101] Charcot and Bouchard (1868), Nouvelles recherches sur l'hémorrhagie cérébrale, 117.
[102] Osler (1892), *The Principles and Practice of Medicine*, 871.
[103] von Monakow (1897), *Gehirnpathologie*, 687–91.
[104] Gull (1859), Cases of aneurisms of cerebral vessels, 298; Meynert (1864), Gefässentartungen;
       Heschl (1865), Capillar-aneurysmen im Pons Varoli.

disagreement on the definition of the term 'aneurysm'. Some argued that only dilatations containing all three layers of the wall were true aneurysms and that other outpouchings should be called dissecting aneurysms;[105] others insisted that true aneurysms should have a circumscribed gap in the elastic layer.[106] Lastly, several authors were happy to use the name of aneurysm for any focal widening, as long as it contained a lumen. But the role of the lumen was another contentious issue – some globules were completely filled with clotted red blood cells, not only inside the vessel wall, or at least some of its layers, but also outside it, in the perivascular space, or even within brain tissue.[107] Such extramural mini-haematomas, or 'tiny blood bags' or *Blutsäckchen*, as Hilde Lindemann called them, were thus, in fact, spurious aneurysms.

An equally controversial issue had to do with logic instead of microscopy. If Charcot and Bouchard had always found small aneurysms, or at least arteriolar globules, in patients with massive intracerebral haemorrhage, this meant there was some kind of weakness in the vessel wall. But this did not necessarily imply, several researchers argued, that the haemorrhage occurred after the formation of the micro-aneurysm, and not before.[108] The cause-or-effect problem kept cropping up: several pathologists argued that many lesions, especially dissecting micro-aneurysms and extravasation outside the arteriolar wall, might be secondary phenomena. The true course of events in the case of massive bleeding largely remained a matter of guesswork.

That degenerative changes in the arteriolar wall constituted the primary process leading to the eventual rupture of a small artery, or at least contributed to it, was almost universally accepted.[109] The Parisian 'periarteritis', however, found few adherents;[110] it 'was conspicuous by its absence', wrote the Philadelphian Aller G. Ellis (1868–1953), who worked in the laboratory of Professor Ludwig Pick (1868–1944) at the Friedrichshain Hospital in Berlin.[111] The main pathological changes, according to this duo, consisted of thickening of the intimal layer, in agreement with several investigators before them[112] and

[105] Weiss (1869), Pathogenese der Gehirnhämorrhagie, 35–6; Ellis (1909), Cerebral hemorrhage; Pick (1910), Miliare Aneurysmen.
[106] Eppinger (1888), Miliare Hirnarterieaneurysmen.
[107] Ellis (1909), Cerebral hemorrhage; Pick (1910), Miliare Aneurysmen; Unger (1911), Zur Lehre von den Aneurysmen; Lindemann (1924), Apoplektische Blutungen; Rühl (1927), Apoplektische Gehirnblutung; Green (1930), Miliary aneurysms; Staemmler (1936), Entstehung des Schlaganfalles; Beitzke (1936), Kleine Aneurysmen; Wolff (1937), Apoplektische Hirnblutung.
[108] Turner (1882), Cerebral haemorrhage; Löwenfeld (1886), *Spontane Hirnblutungen*, 85; Stein (1895), Ätiologie der Gehirnblutungen; Ellis (1909), Cerebral hemorrhage; Pick (1910), Miliare Aneurysmen; Shennan (1915), Miliary aneurysms; Beitzke (1936), Kleine Aneurysmen.
[109] Mendel (1891), Ueber die apoplexia cerebri sanguinea.
[110] Turner (1882), Cerebral haemorrhage.   [111] Ellis (1909), Cerebral hemorrhage.
[112] von Zenker (1872), Spontane Hirnhämorrhagien; Roth (1874), Ueber Gehirnapoplexie; Eichler (1878), Pathogenese der Hirnhämorrhagie; Löwenfeld (1886), *Spontane Hirnblutungen*.

with numerous later studies already cited. These intimal changes were accompanied by atrophy and fatty infiltration of the muscular layer. Several studies emphasized the relationship between these changes and hypertension.[113] Different names were chosen for the fatty changes, but 'hyalinosis' became more and more common. The process seemed to occur only in brain vessels.[114] Most reports noted a coincidence with atherosclerosis of the larger arteries forming the circle of Willis; though the two degenerative lesions were morphologically different, a common origin was often proposed.[115] However, others thought the emphasis was too much on morphology.

FUNCTIONAL HYPOTHESES: HUMOURAL, NERVOUS, OR OTHER

Renal Toxins

William Rosenblath (1875–1935), Professor of Neurology in Marburg and practising in Cassel, came up with an idiosyncratic theory in 1918. To some extent, it leaned on Rochoux's earlier theory that brain softening preceded haemorrhagic lesions. Rosenblath envisaged the changes preceding haemorrhage as necrosis of nervous and vascular elements in many adjoining small foci, mediated by toxic factors, especially those produced by renal dysfunction. The many small haemorrhages in the necrotic spots, emanating mainly from capillaries and small veins, then merged, the idea was, to form a single, large haemorrhage.[116] He based his arguments entirely on evidence from microscopy; Rosenblath's terse description of macroscopical aspects suggests he did not strictly distinguish between primary haemorrhage and haemorrhagic softening.

Vasospasm

This same confusion may explain the hypothesis of multifocal necrosis followed by coalescence of small secondary haemorrhages, proposed in the 1920s and 1930s by Karl Westphal (1887–1951),[117] based in Frankfurt, later professor in Hannover. The difference with Rosenblath's theory is that

---

[113] Rühl (1927), Apoplektische Gehirnblutung; Staemmler (1936), Entstehung des Schlaganfalles; Feigin and Prose (1959), Hypertensive fibrinoid arteritis of the brain.
[114] Arab (1959), Hyalinose artériolaire cérébrale.
[115] von Zenker (1872), Spontane Hirnhämorrhagien; Eichler (1878), Pathogenese der Hirnhämorrhagie; Löwenfeld (1886), Spontane Hirnblutungen, 41–51; Ellis (1909), Cerebral hemorrhage; Pick (1910), Miliare Aneurysmen; Lindemann (1924), Apoplektische Blutungen, 42; Arab (1959), Hyalinose artériolaire cérébrale.
[116] Rosenblath (1918), Entstehung der Hirnblutung.
[117] Westphal and Bär (1926), Entstehung des Schlaganfalles.

Westphal explained the development of necrosis by means of vessel spasm, in turn evoked by hypertension.[118] The idea of vascular spasm in general came from Professor Gustav von Bergmann (1878–1955) in Frankfurt; he mainly applied it to internal organs, for example to explain peptic ulcers.[119] Westphal tried to bolster his own theory by showing that haemorrhages occurred after interruption of blood flow to the brain in rabbits, cats, and dogs.[120] Other voices cautioned not to lose sight of the distinction between primary rupture and haemorrhage secondary to softening,[121] and argued that mechanical factors were sufficient to explain vessel rupture.[122] Nevertheless, the idea of vasospasm appealed to several colleagues, wholly or partly.[123] Later on, Westphal proposed that lactic acid was an important intermediary factor through which vessel spasm caused tissue necrosis.[124] Excessive vascular sensitivity and spasm, followed by multifocal ischaemia and confluent haemorrhages, were also the explanation offered by Philipp Schwartz (1894–1977), who practised in five countries in the course of his life.[125] The specific element in his reasoning is that he attributed the spastic reactions of brain vessels to nervous impulses from afar.[126]

Rochoux Revived

In New York, in 1927, Joseph H. Globus (1885–1952), writing with his colleague Strauss, more or less resurrected Rochoux's old idea about the pathogenesis of intracerebral haemorrhage, though with a twist:

> [...] spontaneous massive cerebral hemorrhage is a terminal phase in a sequence of events which have their beginning in a generalized or somewhat localized disease of the cerebral vessels and which results in the closure of one or more of such vessels in a given, circumscribed area. This leads to the creation of an ischemic zone and a consequent focal encephalomalacia. [...] In the presence of a diseased blood vessel and increased vascular tension, a reduction in the consistency of the

[118] Westphal (1926a), Entstehung des Schlaganfalles; Westphal (1932), Apoplexia sanguinea.
[119] von Bergmann (1913), Das spasmogene Ulcus pepticum.
[120] Westphal (1926b), Entstehung des Schlaganfalles.
[121] Hiller (1935), Zirkulationsstörungen im Gehirn.
[122] Wolff (1932a), Apoplektische Hirnblutungen; Wolff (1932b), Apoplektische Hirnblutungen; Nordmann (1937), Spontanblutungen im Gehirn.
[123] Neubürger (1926), Funktionellen Gefässstörungen; Jaffé (1927), Hypertonus und Apoplexie; Böhne (1931), Hirnerweichung in der Hirnblutung; Fischer-Wasels (1933), Funktionellen Störungen des Kreislaufs; Büchner (1936), Pathogenese der Hochdruckapoplexie; Wolff (1937), Apoplektische Hirnblutung [the author had adapted his earlier view].
[124] Westphal (1937), Spontanblutungen des Gehirns.
[125] Hürlimann (2013), Das Vermächtnis der Philipp Schwartz.
[126] Schwartz (1930b), Apoplektische Schädigungen; Schwartz (1930a), *Schlaganfälle des Gehirns*, later published as Schwartz (1961), *Cerebral Apoplexy*.

surrounding tissue of the brain is an essential precursor to the rupture of
the vessel wall and the unhindered escape of blood.[127]

More than 20 years later, Globus presented his theory at a meeting of the
American Association of Neuropathologists, now supplemented by experiments in dogs. He had clamped their middle cerebral artery for some time and
found an area of softening in surviving animals; in a second series, he produced
haemorrhage in the region of softening by raising the blood pressure through
administration of catecholamines.[128] In the discussion, he met with considerable opposition. Especially Dr Ilya Mark Scheinker (1902–1954), from
Cincinnati,[129] explained in no uncertain terms that the speaker had not
produced haemorrhages, but red infarcts. According to Dr Scheinker's own
theory about spontaneous brain haemorrhages, venous congestion was the key
phenomenon.[130]

  In the end, the 'theory of prior occlusion' was buried, but the vasospastic
theory petered out more slowly. In 1940, Anders and Eicke, though recognizing the importance of hyaline changes of the vessel wall, attributed this
phenomenon to spasm and denied any relation with atherosclerosis.[131]

BLOOD PRESSURE

Despite the overriding interest in the morphological changes of terminal
arterioles, several physicians were aware that their pathogenesis should not
be dismissed as mere 'ageing' or 'degeneration'. Surely, the resistance of the
vessel walls could be decreased. But resistance to what? Soon after the discovery of miliary aneurysms, Professor Moritz Roth (1839–1914) in Basel drew
again attention to the factor of 'blood pressure'.[132] But how to get a grip on
this aspect?

Measuring Blood Pressure

In the entire nineteenth century, the force exerted by blood on the arterial
wall remained a merely theoretical notion. A large decrease or increase in this
tension was thought to be harmful, but no other measure existed than feeling
the pulse. Among the instruments devised to record pulse movements at the
wrist by mechanical means, instead of the existing and confusing vocabulary

---

[127] Globus and Strauss (1927), Cerebral hemorrhage and preexisting softening, 238.
[128] Globus, *et al.* (1949), Focal cerebral hemorrhage. The final article was more guarded: Globus
       and Epstein (1953), Massive cerebral hemorrhage.
[129] Zeidman, *et al.* (2016), Ilya Mark Scheinker.
[130] Scheinker (1945), Changes in cerebral veins.
[131] Anders and Eicke (1940), Die Gehirngefässe beim Hochdruck.
[132] Roth (1874), Ueber Gehirnapoplexie, 148.

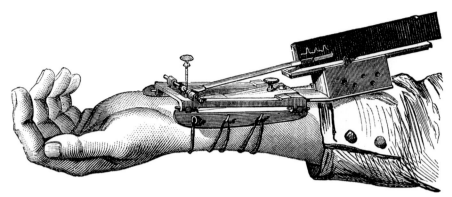

5.8 Instrument for recording movements of the radial artery at the wrist (Marey, 1860).

for describing pulse characteristics, was the 'sphygmograph' of Étienne Jules Marey (1830–1904), a pioneer in recording biological movements (Figure 5.8).[133] Nevertheless, at the beginning of the twentieth century, monitoring during operations was still usually performed by mere palpation.[134]

In 1896, Scipione Riva-Rocci (1863–1937), an assistant physician for internal diseases in Turin, published his idea for measuring blood pressure by temporarily occluding the artery upstream, in the upper arm, by means of an inflatable cuff, adapted from a bicycle tube. To begin with, the rubber cuff was inflated by means of a balloon; both the cuff and the balloon were connected to a manometer. The pressure in the cuff was expressed as the height (in millimetres) of the column of mercury in the manometer. When the pressure was increased to a level at which pulsation at the wrist was no longer palpable, the air was slowly allowed to escape, until pulsations at the wrist returned; that level corresponded to the peak (systole) of the blood pressure upstream, in the brachial artery. Riva-Rocci's publication, in Italian, attracted little attention.[135] Yet the American neurosurgeon and bibliophile Harvey Cushing (1869–1939) somehow got wind of the invention and, in 1903, visited Riva-Rocci, who in the meantime had followed his chief to Pavia. Cushing was quick to introduce the method in North America (Figure 5.9).[136]

In 1905, the Russian army surgeon Nikolai Korotkoff (1874–1920) introduced a modification of the method; he replaced palpation of the radial artery by picking up the sounds of blood rushing through a narrow passage, by means of a stethoscope placed at the crook of the elbow. This method was more sensitive than palpation and also allowed determination of the pressure at the moment the

[133] Marey (1860), *Recherches sur le pouls*.
[134] Cushing (1903), On routine determinations of arterial tension.
[135] Riva-Rocci (1896–7), Un nuovo sfigmomanometro. English translation in: Zanchetti and Mancia (1996), The centenary of blood pressure measurement.
[136] Cushing (1903), On routine determinations of arterial tension.

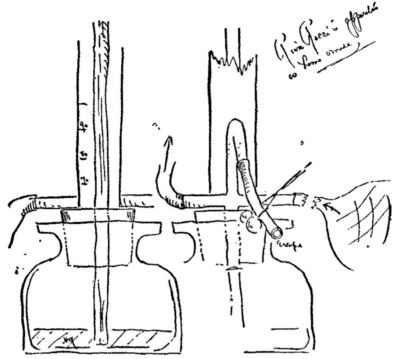

5.9 Sketch of Riva-Rocci's manometer, made by Harvey Cushing in his diary of 6 May 1901
(Fulton, 1946). The drawing on the left shows a view from the front, and the one on the right
that from behind. The apparatus is constructed from a glass jar, covered by a cork; at the bottom
is a layer of mercury. A glass tube is fitted through the cork and has an open end in the layer of
mercury. Above the cork, the tube is attached to a support with calibration in millimetres.
Behind the support is a four-armed tube. Its lower end also runs through the cork and ends in
the air chamber of the manometer. The horizontal branches of the tube are attached to the
inflatable cuff (not shown) and a balloon (partly visible). The upper end is connected to a rubber
tube that can be closed off with a clamp. When the clamp is released, air can escape in a
controlled fashion.

sounds disappeared – the diastolic pressure.[137] Soon the industry devised com-
mercially available instruments. The column of mercury remained a traditional
feature until the last decades of the twentieth century; the calibration of today's
digitalized gauges still corresponds to millimetres of mercury.

For a long time, it remained controversial as to whether high blood pressure
was a distinct disease ('essential hypertension') or just one end of the distribution curve in the general population. Eventually, population studies vindicated
the conception of George Pickering (1904–1980), formulated in 1955:

> What is currently designated essential hypertension represents that
> section of the population having arterial pressures above an arbitrarily

---

[137] Korotkoff (1905), Methods of blood pressure measurement. Facsimile and translation:
Shlyakhto and Conrady (2005), Korotkoff sounds.

defined value, and having no other disease to which the high pressure can
be attributed. If secondary hypertension is excluded, there is no evidence
that high pressure is qualitatively different from normal arterial pressure:
the difference it not one of kind but of degree.[138]

From then on, several epidemiological studies addressed the relation between
hypertension and intracerebral bleeding.

Hypertension and Brain Haemorrhage

Population studies of disease became more common in the twentieth century
but could not distinguish between intracerebral haemorrhage and ischaemic
softening. Given the diagnostic uncertainty, all types of cerebrovascular disease
had to be taken together. In contrast, the diagnosis of coronary heart disease
(angina pectoris or myocardial infarction) was much more straightforward in
the 1950s. A pivotal population-based study in the community of
Framingham, Massachusetts, uncovered the relation of cardiovascular disease
with blood pressure and with other potentially relevant biological variables,
newly called 'factors of risk'. Among persons aged 45 to 59 years on entry, both
men and women, blood pressures, systolic and diastolic, were significantly
higher in those who went on to develop coronary disease during a six-year
period than in the entire population; each increment of blood pressure corresponded to a higher rate of coronary heart disease,[139] or cardiovascular disease
in general.[140]

Analogous results for cerebrovascular disease might be expected. And
indeed, after 12 years of follow-up, a significant relationship emerged between
blood pressure and 'apoplexy'.[141] Probably, the majority of these cerebrovascular diseases must have been caused by atherothrombotic, or at least ischaemic, lesions, a distinction that had become well recognized. Yet, to what
extent the harmful effect of raised blood pressure applied to intracerebral
haemorrhages was still an open question.

Hypertension and Radiological Imaging of Micro-aneurysms

A new approach was to study the relation between blood pressure and micro-
aneurysms in whole sections of the brain. Ralph Ross Russell (1928–)
(Box 10.2, p. 331), later consultant at the National Hospital for Neurology
and Neurosurgery in London, developed a technique of micro-angiography,

---

[138] Pickering (1955), *High Blood Pressure*, 183.
[139] Kannel, *et al.* (1961), Factors of risk in coronary heart disease.
[140] Kannel (1975), Role of blood pressure in cardiovascular disease.
[141] Dawber, *et al.* (1965), An epidemiologic study of apoplexy ('strokes').

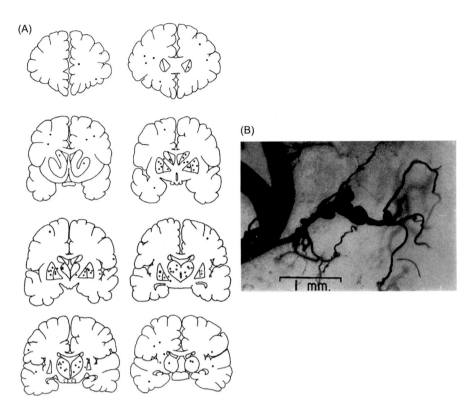

5.10 Location of small aneurysms of lenticulo-striate arteries (Ross Russell, 1963). (A) Distribution of aneurysms in 16 hypertensive subjects; the brainstem and the cerebellum were not studied. (B) Area with multiple aneurysms.

during his stay at the Mallory Institute of Pathology in Boston. In 54 brain specimens, he injected a mixture of barium sulphate and gelatine into the internal carotid artery, on both sides. After fixation of the brain in formalin, slides were cut in a coronal direction and X-rayed; the films were studied by microscope. In all but one of the 16 patients classified as hypertensive, he found small saccular dilatations, against only one of the other 38 patients (Figure 5.10, right).[142] Hypertension was defined as a diastolic value above 110 millimetres; these were retrieved from the case notes (penultimate values). The number of aneurysms per hypertensive individual ranged between 1 and about 20; their location was most commonly the region of putamen, pallidum, and thalamus, and to a lesser extent the caudate nucleus, internal capsule, centrum semiovale, and cortical grey matter (Figure 5.10, A).

A similar, but larger study from Manchester compared the brains of 100 hypertensive patients with those of 100 control subjects and largely

---

[142] Ross Russell (1963), Intracerebral aneurysms; Compston (2005), 'Observations on intracranial aneurysms'. By R. W. Ross Russell.

confirmed Ross Russell's findings;[143] small aneurysms occurred also in the subcortical white matter and the brainstem, and less often in the cerebellum.

Four Types of Micro-aneurysms

In the early 1970s, in Boston, C. Miller Fisher (1913–2012) (Box 8.3, p. 275), familiar with most of the earlier reports cited above, once more used micro-scopy to investigate the origin of spontaneous brain haemorrhage. Fisher scrutinized 100 tissue blocks from the pons, basal ganglia, or cerebral cortex, taken from 20 hypertensive patients with small strokes, massive brain haemor-rhage, or both. Not wishing to be censorious about the designation of 'aneurysm', he distinguished three types of arteriolar dilatations and one non-aneurysmal structure. 'Together,' he wrote, 'they probably account for all of the different kinds of miliary aneurysms reported in the past 100 years.'[144]

The first type, that of 'miliary saccular aneurysms', was represented by tiny, narrow-mouthed outpouchings on small penetrating brain arteries. Their shape was circular in cross-section and smoothly rounded, often, but not always, arising at bifurcations and protruding without a neck. They usually occurred in a haemorrhage-free zone of the brain and never in the vicinity of major bleeding. The parent vessel was not necessarily normal, but patent, and did not show hyalinosis. The wall of the aneurysm consisted mostly of thin collagenous tissue, lined on the inside by fibrin and mural thrombus, without an intimal layer. Fisher supposed that the outpouchings shown by Ross Russell were often of this type; he did not regard them as a likely source of major bleeding, given the lining with thrombus and their small size, with parent vessels in the order of 15 microns.

The second type he called 'miliary aneurysms with lipohyalinosis'. Fisher preferred the term 'lipohyalinosis' for the well-known fatty changes in the arterial wall, to indicate the combination of fibrin and fat-filled macrophages. These outpouchings occurred by far most often in the cortex. Typically focal, occurring where the elastic and muscular layers lose their integrity, they extended over a distance of twice or thrice, sometimes up to 10 times, the diameter of the uninvolved segment of the vessel, with the width measuring 0.5–1.5 millimetres. Sometimes whorls of reactive connective tissue occluded the lumen, and sometimes there was modest extravasation. Fisher thought these small dilatations might indirectly contribute to massive bleeding. A year later, researchers in Maebashi, Japan, were much less hesitant; they used the term 'plasmatic arterionecrosis'.[145]

---

[143] Cole and Yates (1967), Intracerebral micro-aneurysms.
[144] Fisher (1972), Cerebral miliary aneurysms in hypertension, 313.
[145] Ooneda, et al. (1973), Hypertensive intracerebral hemorrhage.

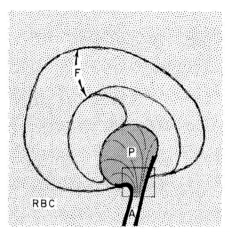

5.11 Diagram of a typical 'bleeding globe' (Fisher, 1971). A, ruptured artery, 100 microns in diameter; P, platelet aggregation; F, fibrin strands; RBC, red blood cell mass. *Source:* By permission of the *Journal of Neuropathology and Experimental Neurology.*

Fisher's third type, consisting of so-called 'asymmetric fusiform miliary aneurysms', was definitely rare: he found only two examples. The dilated lumina contained recent thrombi that blocked the exit. The walls were very thin and ill-defined. Thrombotic occlusion of these two aneurysms had resulted in lacunar infarction (see Chapter 10) in the subcortical central white matter.

The fourth type of dilatation Fisher identified was a false aneurysm, because it was formed by blood elements outside the vessel wall, probably identical to the mini-haematomas often described decades before. Hilde Lindemann had called them *Blutsäckchen* (tiny bags of blood),[146] but Fisher chose to use the term 'bleeding globules' or 'fibrin globes'.[147] They represented bleeding from a small artery, 100–200 microns in diameter. Each consisted of a mass of red blood cells, enveloped in concentric rings of fibrin. The fibrin rings connected the globular body to the parent artery. At the site of the breach, a clump of platelets might protrude into the surrounding red blood cells (Figure 5.11). Intriguingly, these lesions were found only in the vicinity of large haemorrhages. Fisher supposed that 'fibrin globes' represented many of Charcot and Bouchard's miliary aneurysms.[148]

The Fatal Breach Identified?

Fisher devoted a separate study to the brain of a 74-year-old man with long-standing hypertension and finally a fatal haemorrhage in the pons; he had

---

[146] Lindemann (1924), Apoplektische Blutungen.
[147] Fisher attributed the term to 'S. Matuoka' (1952), for S. Matsuoka; his reference could not be retrieved.
[148] Fisher (1972), Cerebral miliary aneurysms in hypertension, 315.

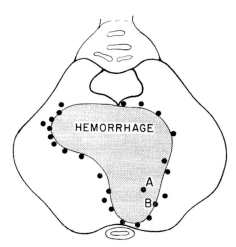

5.12 Ruptured arterioles (pseudoaneurysms) around a spontaneous pontine haemorrhage in a hypertensive patient (Fisher, 1971). Arteries A and B were potential sites of origin of the main haemorrhage, according to Fisher. His own legend reads: 'Diagram to show in one plane the sites of ruptured arteries. At A the artery involved was 150 microns in diameter and at B 200 microns. The fibrin globes at both A and B were 5 mm in diameter'. Source: By permission of the *Journal of Neuropathology and Experimental Neurology*.

become unconscious half an hour after the first symptoms and died four hours later. Around the outer borders of the haemorrhage, Fisher found as many as 24 definite and ten possible 'bleeding globes'.[149] Two of the globes were large enough to suspect they might have accounted for most of the main haemorrhage (Figure 5.12). Fisher regarded the other arterial lesions as secondary to the mechanical force of the expanding haemorrhage; such an avalanche effect had been previously proposed, among others, by Hermann Beitzke (1875–1953).[150] Near the suspected site of rupture, the wall of the arteriole usually showed hyalinization, as well as absence of elastic and muscular layers.

To conclude, if massive brain haemorrhage results from the decreased resistance and integrity of the arterial wall, and if this weakening is, in turn, caused by fatty depositions and concomitant degenerative changes, and if these alterations are again attributed to high blood pressure, the next question is: what caused the increased pressure? Some imbalance in the internal homeostasis? A liberal intake of salt? Another environmental factor? And what about people of the same age with similarly high blood pressures who remain free from brain haemorrhage? Causality becomes more and more nebulous as one attempts to reconstruct the chain of events backwards.

[149] Fisher (1971), Hypertensive cerebral haemorrhage.
[150] Beitzke (1936), Kleine Aneurysmen.

SIX

RAMOLLISSEMENT

SUMMARY

Rochoux had equated 'apoplexy' with intracerebral haemorrhage, but he also reported a few rare and unexplained cases of softening, 'simulating apoplexy'. Others tentatively proposed 'essential softening' as a separate disease. Rostan in 1820 made this a postulate, but since his starting point was softening of brain tissue, he included patients in whom the state of 'apoplexy' represented not the onset, but an aggravation of pre-existing illness. He interpreted non-focal premonitory symptoms as the initial stage of the disease; this was followed by a phase of focal deficits. Rostan explicitly opposed the idea that softening was an inflammatory condition, a hypothesis to which Lallemand and others adhered, following Broussais' popular 'irritation theory'. Fuchs, insisting on paralysis as the essential feature, excluded inflammation as the cause of any form of 'encephalomalacia'.

A nutritional disorder, comparable to 'senile gangrene', was the explanation Rostan proposed somewhat later. Abercrombie, following his lead, explicitly distinguished two forms of softening: one inflammatory, the other resulting from arterial disease; the 'gangrenous' form was manifested by sudden hemiplegia. Closer study of softened areas indeed seemed to favour a vascular origin (Bright, Carswell). Despite demonstration of local arterial occlusions (Hasse, Bouchut), the theory of inflammation remained alive as long as reports of softening included patients with progressive disease (Durand-Fardel) or even diseases with predominantly mental symptoms, especially general paralysis of the insane (Laborde).

Jean-André Rochoux had equated apoplexy with haemorrhage within the brain. Whenever he encountered serous effusion or areas of softening in his dissections, he regarded such lesions as complications of haemorrhage. In this way, he had explained everything. Almost.

A DISEASE SIMULATING APOPLEXY

In his first book, Rochoux listed, in the chapter on the differential diagnosis of apoplexy, conditions where the clinical distinction was relatively easy, but he also mentioned rare patients in whom the distinction from haemorrhage was difficult.[1] Actually, in two cases, it was impossible. Both were women; they had become suddenly hemiplegic without warning and subsequently died within a few weeks, but failed to show blood in the brain. One of these two stories is the following.

> Louise Rathienne, 47 years old, from Blaisy (Côte d'Or), unmarried, with a bilious-sanguineous constitution, large, well-built, brunette, with a remarkable embonpoint, had been troubled for about two years by episodes of coughing and oppression, especially at night, had been less healthy than usual for the last three months and had lost weight. Otherwise, she had noted nothing remarkable when, on 25 December, she suddenly lost consciousness; this lasted for about one hour. She then came round and appeared hemiplegic on the left side, showing a mild degree of delirium and difficulty of articulation; she was hardly understandable. After about eight days the delirium disappeared and another five or six days later, she was able to move her left leg a little. [...]
>
> On 18 January 18, the day of her admission to the 'Maison de la Santé', her condition was as follows: severe weakness of the left leg and paralysis of the left arm, but fluent and clear articulation; little sleep, sometimes headache, abdomen tight, pulse slow. Daily stools. [*Up to 1 March, the day of her death, ten brief interim reports documented her course: coughing more and more frequent, sputum sometimes tinged with blood, chest pain, increasing weakness; on 29 February loss of consciousness, high pulse rate, stertorous breathing, wide pupils with slow contraction, death*].
>
> *Dissection of the skull:* The dura contained much blood in its vessels. The right corpus striatum showed three or four irregular cavities, each of which might contain a fingertip, traversed by filamentous debris and filled by a yellow fluid, with a touch of ochre. The hemisphere on this side was markedly soft, especially in its anterior part. The rest of the brain and the cerebellum were firmer than usual. [*Chest: one half of the mitral valve was cartilaginous and flattened. The lungs were engorged with blood,*

---

[1] Rochoux (1814), *Recherches sur l'Apoplexie*, 164–90.

especially at their base and posterior border; many adhesions with the pleura, especially on the right side].[2]

'This is truly a disorder,' Rochoux wrote in closing, 'that has shown in its course extensive similarities with an attack of severe apoplexy.' For him, it remained a mystery; despite the patient's survival for nine weeks, he could not classify the lesion as a 'complication'. In the other patient with a similar story and brain lesion, 61-year-old Anne Fauché, the interval between apoplexy and death was even shorter, two to three weeks.[3]

In the second edition of his book (1833), Rochoux cited two more reports of 'softening simulating apoplexy', both from other sources,[4] but again he offered no thoughts about its cause. Still, by 1833, he regarded it as a true entity and did not fail to point out that he had been the first to describe it.[5]

Something was in the air. In the course of time, softening of brain tissue had been explained as a toxic phenomenon (Willis), or as serous apoplexy (Wepfer, Valsalva and Morgagni, Stoll, Portal). But given the avalanche of post-mortem studies in early nineteenth-century Paris, it was inevitable that someone else would recognize it as a separate category of disease. The riddle of Rochoux's two patients with 'apoplexy-like softening' set others thinking. In 1818, the young Isidore Bricheteau (1789–1861) wrote that, as a student at the *Hôtel-Dieu*, he had heard Professor Joseph Récamier (1774–1852) say that *ramollissement du cerveau* was a disease in its own right;[6] Bricheteau tried to support the idea with two personal – but rather unconvincing – cases.[7] In 1819, the even younger Étienne Moulin (1795–1871) interpreted Rochoux's enigmatic cases as *ramollissement essentielle*.[8] Finally, in 1820, another eager young physician took the matter further.

BRAIN SOFTENING – A SEPARATE DISEASE ENTITY

His name was Léon Rostan (1790–1866) (Box 6.1).[9] He did not merely *suggest* that brain softening might be a disease condition on its own, as Moulin and Bricheteau had done, he explicitly claimed it, straightaway with the title of his book *Investigations on a still little-known Malady, which has received the Name*

---

[2] Rochoux (1814), *Recherches sur l'Apoplexie*, 170–5.

[3] Rochoux (1814), *Recherches sur l'Apoplexie*, 175–7.

[4] Rochoux (1833), *Recherches sur l'Apoplexie*, 315–33. One new case Rochoux had borrowed from Rostan's book of 1820 (see below, 49–53), and the other from London (Ward (1824), Softening of the brain), translated in a French periodical (Anonymous (1824), Hémiplégie).

[5] Rochoux (1833), *Recherches sur l'Apoplexie*, 326.

[6] Hirsch (1884–8), *Biographisches Lexikon*, vol. IV, 683–4.

[7] Bricheteau (1818), Considérations et observations sur l'apoplexie, 301–5.

[8] Moulin (1819), *Traité de l'Apoplexie*, 101–3.

[9] Monneret, *et al.* (1866), Discours aux obsèques; Hirsch (1884–8), *Biographisches Lexikon*, vol. V, 90.

Box 6.1 Léon Rostan (1790–1866).

Rostan was born in Saint-Maximim (Provence) and studied medicine in Marseille and Paris. Appointed as *interne des hôpitaux* in 1809, he graduated three years later with a thesis on 'charlatanism'. He continued as an assistant physician in the Salpêtrière, where he participated in dealing with an epidemic of typhus during the foreign occupation after the battle of Waterloo, until he contracted the disease himself. He became a full physician in 1819. A year later, he published his seminal book on brain softening. At the Salpêtrière, he was a passionate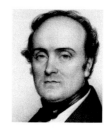
teacher, publishing a didactic course on the principles of medicine in three volumes, *Cours de médecine clinique* (1826). He was attentive and kind with patients, hospital employees, and also students, but he hated vague expressions.

In 1833, he was appointed Professor of Medicine at the Faculty of Medicine of the *Collège de France*. He published extensively on a variety of medical subjects, mainly in journals. Rostan was an outspoken anti-vitalist, denying any principle of life that could not be related to material origins. The balance between health and disease depended first of all, he believed, on organs; functions and fluids were secondary. He published these views in his *Exposé des principes de l'organicisme* (1846, twice republished). His view was opposed by François-Joseph-Victor Broussais (1772–1832), a physician at the military hospital of Val-de-Grace and, in 1831, Professor of Pathology; Broussais attributed most diseases to functional disturbances such as irritation and inflammation. Rostan retired in 1864, aged 73 years. He was happily married and had a daughter on whom he doted.

Softening of the Brain (*ramollissement du cerveau*). He supported his assertion with 22 case reports from the Salpêtrière, the Parisian hospital annex poorhouse for women.

'A Still Little-Known Malady'

In his introduction, Rostan recounted how, nine years before, as a young resident, he had found softening of the brain in a patient with apoplexy in whom the chief had confidently predicted the presence of extravasated blood. Colleagues and teachers with whom he discussed the case had offered all sorts of unsatisfactory explanations. The question had never left him,[10] and in the end, he had convinced himself that 'softening of the brain' was a separate disease entity. Of course, brain softening could surround areas of intracerebral haemorrhage, as Rochoux and others had shown. Yet, Rostan repeatedly found it without previous extravasation.

With regard to the 'nature' of softening, Rostan firmly denied it was inflammation, at least in the patients he presented, while admitting that

---

[10] Rostan (1820), *Ramollissement du Cerveau*, 7–9.

inflammation could cause softening in other cases.[11] Softened tissue was often red and swollen, and so shared some of the four classical characteristics of inflammation (*rubor, tumor, calor, dolor* – redness, swelling, warmth, pain), but not all of them were present, and not even in all patients. Furthermore, Rostan pointed out, the symptoms of softening, such as paralysis and numbness, were negative rather than positive. Also, the predilection of brain softening for the aged was at odds with such a categorical explanation.

Other physicians, however, explained all forms of brain softening as a form of inflammation. Following the heyday of pathological anatomy, with pioneers such as Laennec, Corvisart, Bayle, and Louis, many physicians had become impressed by the 'physiological' approach of François-Joseph-Victor Broussais (1772–1838);[12] he criticized the 'ontological' classification of diseases and emphasized function rather than form. He assigned a key role to the factor of irritation, which, he thought, might in turn lead to inflammation – in any organ, but particularly in the gastrointestinal tract. Modern readers tend to associate the term 'inflammation' with infectious agents, but in its wide, pre-1870s meaning, the term referred to a variety of environmental factors.

Despite all efforts, Rostan had to admit the true cause of softening was unknown. A few predisposing factors might favour its occurrence: old age, heat and cold, emotions, etc. – factors it again shared with intracerebral haemorrhage.[13] Yet he was convinced that 'different causes must have different effects',[14] even though the residual functional deficits of softening and haemorrhage were identical. And since effective treatment was impossible without an accurate diagnosis,[15] Rostan set out to find characteristic symptoms that might distinguish softening from haemorrhage.

A Search for Specific Symptoms

Perhaps the similarity between the clinical features of softening and those of extravasation, Rostan reasoned, applied only to the climax, with focal deficits such as hemiplegia. He therefore aimed his search for cause-specific symptoms at an earlier phase. His belief in such symptoms may well have been inspired, though he did not put it in writing, by a hunch that the process of *ramollissement*, brain tissue losing its consistency and colour, could not take place in a few seconds or minutes, as it does with rupture of an artery. At any rate, he divided the symptoms of brain softening into two stages.

[11] Rostan (1820), *Ramollissement du Cerveau*, 101–4.
[12] Albury (2007), François-Joseph-Victor Broussais.
[13] Rostan (1820), *Ramollissement du Cerveau*, 107–9.
[14] Rostan (1820), *Ramollissement du Cerveau*, 9.
[15] Rostan (1820), *Ramollissement du Cerveau*, 109–11.

The first stage, Rostan wrote, consisted of preliminary symptoms of a rather general nature. Only the second phase consisted of focal deficits, reflecting a local lesion in the brain.[16] In fatal cases of haemorrhage, the course of the disease is always faster than with softening, Rostan argued. In contrast, mild haemorrhages might be followed by survival or even recovery, something that, in his opinion, never occurred in softening, which he associated with an inexorably fatal course. But there are cases, he had to concede, where distinction between softening and haemorrhage is difficult.[17]

Of what kind were these preliminary symptoms to which Rostan attributed such an important role in the accurate diagnosis of softening? The list is long and disconcertingly non-specific: headache, dizziness, mental slowing, sleepiness, pins and needles, stiffness or numbness of limbs, agitation, memory problems, visual disturbances, buzzing of the ears, loss of appetite, thirst, nausea, abdominal pain, constipation, frequent voiding of urine, slowing of the pulse.[18] Given this wide range, it is not surprising that prior symptoms were so common. Also, it should be kept in mind that many of the women with *ramollissement* had already been admitted to the asylum department of the Salpêtrière, for the very reason they could no longer be cared for at home. Nevertheless, Rostan argued, it is especially in retrospect, after the functional deficits of the second phase, that the significance of preceding symptoms could be fully appreciated. With regard to headache, there was a particular sign to which he attached special importance: patients with hemiplegia as a result of softening often moved their unaffected hand to the front or to the side of their head. He regarded this phenomenon as almost pathognomonic for softening and repeatedly drew attention to it in reports about individual patients. Rostan was well aware of possible bias in his observations:

> I have taken all possible precautions against being guided by preconceived opinions. To avoid colouring my observations through my manner of reasoning, I have not wished to collect these myself; I have entrusted them to pupils – intelligent, well-educated and trained. I prefer the risk of losing a few details which might have been useful in painting the picture I am about to draw, above the risk of being under the offensive suspicion that I have tampered with the truth.[19]

And indeed, every report but one of the 22 cases has a footnote with the name of the assistant physician who wrote the report. Yet, inevitably, the assistants were taught to adopt Rostan's approach.

[16] Rostan (1820), *Ramollissement du Cerveau*, 12–22.
[17] Rostan (1820), *Ramollissement du Cerveau*, 152–6.
[18] Rostan (1820), *Ramollissement du Cerveau*, 11–16.
[19] Rostan (1820), *Ramollissement du Cerveau*, 5–6.

Pathology as a Leading Criterion

It is important to understand Rostan's 'programme' before one starts wondering why the symptoms in most of his 22 case reports are so different from Rochoux's stories of Louise Rathienne, or that of Anne Fauché, both comfortably recognizable in the twenty-first century. Rostan's starting point was local softening on dissection of the brain, not attributable to inflammation – at least in his opinion; he did not specify his criteria, but a two-stage disease course must have favoured the diagnosis. As a result, only three of the 22 case histories in Rostan's series fitted into the profile of non-haemorrhagic apoplexy.[20] Two other patients had a tumour;[21] Rostan included them to illustrate his point that softening could sometimes result from diseases other than haemorrhage. Of the 17 remaining patients, there were seven in whom Rostan regarded the course of the disease as 'regular', in that it broadly represented the two stages he had outlined. To clarify his 'ideal model' of softening, the following case report – the very first in the book – follows in an almost complete form, with Rostan's own italics and changes of tense:

> Marie-Génevieve-Angélique Dassonville, widow of Moissonnet, aged 70 years, with a dry constitution, suffers for the last year from *attacks of numbness in the lower limbs*. These have come on without known cause and have worsened to such an extent that she is limited in their use. Indeed, Dassonville drags her legs when she walks, especially on the *left*; this is also the side on which she especially experiences the numbness. Both legs have in no way lost their sensitivity; the patient feels pain when one pinches them. [...]
>
> The cause of this numbness seems to have also affected the mental capacities of the patient, since she sometimes goes to the dormitory because '*her brain is out of order*'. Yet her hearing is good and she responds quite well to questions put to her, but she rarely participates in conversations of her companions and it seems her mind is no longer able to remain on the same subject for some time.
>
> In the first days of July 1819, Dassonville experiences *heaviness in the head*, accompanied by *dizzy spells*. [...] The headaches then worsened and were complicated by some gastric trouble. She was admitted to the infirmary on August 1. She presented the following characteristics: general weakness, headache, loss of appetite, dry mouth, tongue red and dry, abdomen supple and not painful, constipation, skin warm and slightly humid, rapid pulse, breathing unimpaired, no cough. A few hours after admission, an attack of *delirium*, so that one has to apply a straitjacket. She did not speak, but moved her arms around and tried to get out of bed.

[20] Rostan (1820), *Ramollissement du Cerveau*, 46–9 (case VIII), 71–5 (case XVI), and 78–80 (case XVIII).

[21] Rostan (1820), *Ramollissement du Cerveau*, 84–90.

The delirium lasted a few hours, came back on the day after and on two more days, but was less prolonged.

On August 5, the delirium did not return but was replaced by calmness, or rather a kind of remarkable disinterest. She lies on her back, almost completely immobile, her head bent backwards, her face slightly turned to the right, the eyes open and turned slightly upwards, the jaws together but the lips opened, arms and lower limbs extended. This is the position the patient stays in and maintains up to her death. She speaks only when asked a question, but even then the response is slow and incomplete. [...] On August 8, *when the patient was asked about headache, she always answered in the affirmative.* I asked to show me the site of the pain with her hand; only when the question was clearly repeated three or four times, she slowly lifted her right hand from the bed, staying immobile otherwise, put it on the top of her head, then strayed to the front and let it drop. [...] On August 11 and 12, face feverish. She died on the 15th.[22]

In this patient, Rostan's 'first phase' of the illness included a variety of symptoms. In contrast, focal signs, constituting Rostan's second phase, were not at all prominent. In the seven patients Rostan regarded as representative for *ramollissement*, the course of the second phase had been gradual, stepwise, or unclear; this was also the case in all but 6 of the 15 other patients, in whom he found the course less typical or 'complicated'. Hemiplegia was absent in 4 of his 22 cases, and in three others, only the arm was affected.

At this time, physical examination was still unhelpful in the diagnosis of brain disease; in the 1820s, when auscultation and percussion of the chest had already been adopted, a system for the examination of the nervous system had yet to be developed, the more so in patients with an impaired level of consciousness. Only the contractibility of the pupils might be tested, if needed with the help of a candle. Loss of speech was called 'paralysis of the tongue'; it was not until 40 years later that Paul Broca (1824–1880) showed the relationship between language and the lower part of the left frontal lobe. The findings on dissection of Ms Dassonville's brain, a fortnight after her admission to hospital, were far more eloquent than the description of her symptoms:

One can easily lift the arachnoid membrane from all regions of the brain without taking along portions of the brain itself, except the interior middle and superior parts of the *right* hemisphere. [...] The cortical layer had merged with medullary substance, both in state of softening, to such a degree that they showed the aspect of a greyish pulp. Here the convolutions, very marked everywhere else in the brain, had become indistinguishable in an area with a circumference of three-and-a-half to four inches [*pouces*]. Its border was not sharply demarcated and extended

[22] Rostan (1820), *Ramollissement du Cerveau*, 22–5. Report written by 'Mr Bardin, hospital resident of the first class'.

further forwards than backwards and occupied almost the entire portion of the brain serving as the floor of the lateral ventricle. The corpus striatum on the right side showed a pink colour that was not at all seen on the other side; for the rest, the feel of its consistency was not different. The right thalamus was also softened, but to a mild degree. [... The lesion] was not enclosed in a membrane. [...] The left hemisphere of the brain was entirely normal.[23]

In summary, this patient ended up in Rostan's series because of partial softening of her brain, despite the absence of an 'apoplectic' onset. In some of the other dissections, even the morphological abnormalities were equivocal, for example a 'gelatinous aspect' of the surface or softening in both hemispheres.[24]

Thus, primary softening of brain tissue might be an undeniable phenomenon, but its cause remained unknown and its clinical manifestations poorly defined. No wonder there were dissenting interpretations.

Partisans of Inflammation

Among the supporters of Broussais' belief in inflammation as a principal cause of disease was Claude François Lallemand (1790–1854).[25] He had been trained in the Hôtel-Dieu under Guillaume Dupuytren (1777–1835) and Joseph Récamier (1774–1852); in 1819, he became Professor of Medicine in Montpellier. One year later, the same year in which Rostan's book appeared, Lallemand published the first part of what was to become a three-volume book on the pathological anatomy of brain diseases. Following the example of no less a person than Morgagni, he divided the subject into 'letters'; the first was about softening.

Lallemand began with a series of case reports,[26] as Rochoux and Rostan had done. Of the 21 cases, only eight were new observations from the Hôtel-Dieu; the others he borrowed from Morgagni, Bricheteau, and Rochoux (the problematic case of Anne Fauché!), and from a thesis of a young colleague – all profusely interspersed with his own comments. The range of clinical and anatomical findings in Lallemand's eight personal cases was as wide as in Rostan's series. A single example helps to understand the diversity; in several instances, the reader remains puzzled, despite the advantage of hindsight:

Anne Benoît, 54 years, with a strong and plethoric constitution, a considerable embonpoint though petite, and a thick, short neck, had

[23] Rostan (1820), Ramollissement du Cerveau, 25–7.
[24] Rostan (1820), Ramollissement du Cerveau, 96–101.
[25] Poirier (2010), Claude François Lallemand (1790–1854).
[26] Lallemand (1820–34), Recherches anatomopathologiques sur l'Encéphale, vol. 1, 3–72.

been irregular in her periods, despite a sanguineous temperament. [...] In 1814, at the age of 51, she had an unusually strong episode of cerebral congestion, during which everything seemed to turn around her, and everything she looked at seemed to have a red colour. [...] On November 27, 1817 she had an even stronger attack of congestion, in which she had a feeling of tight oppression, with buzzing of the ears; she lost consciousness for a few moments [*treatment*].

The next day she was admitted to the Hôtel-Dieu. I found her in deep coma, with eyes closed, but when the patient was roused she opened her right eye while the left one remained closed. She responded with difficulty; her tongue sounded slurred, as in the initial phase of inebriation; yet one could easily gather that she complained about weakness and numbness of her right limbs. [...] Directly after venesection [*from the jugular vein*] strong convulsive movements occurred, in the limb muscles on the right and the muscles of the face on the left, for a quarter of an hour. [...] On the next day the convulsions recurred several times; the patient no longer responded. [...] She died on the evening of the fourth day.

Dissection. The arachnoid is thick, red, injected. I could take it off on each side as a whole, without rupture; when it had been washed, it was completely opaque. [...] Brown discolouration and softening of the central right thalamus, with a diameter of about half an inch. Opposite this softening, the surface of the same thalamus, within the right ventricle, showed a kind of soft rind, a recent pseudo-membrane, about half an inch of thickness,[27] which adhered to the opposite surface of the septum pellucidum. On the left side, several areas of the corpus striatum and the pons also showed softening.[28]

The clinical and anatomical spectrum of 'softening' was broad indeed. Like Rostan, Lallemand preferred to regard *ramollissement* as a gradual process, though he did not distinguish phases. Accordingly, the onset of paralysis or loss of speech in Lallemand's personal observations was more often gradual or stepwise (four patients) than sudden (three); in the eighth patient, the cause was trauma.

Lallemand, having joined the Broussais bandwagon, urged that softening was always an inflammatory process. Moreover, he argued that primary softening and primary haemorrhage in the brain were closely related, both being complications of congestion – overfilling of cerebral vessels. According to this view, the irritation caused by cerebral congestion could evolve either into haemorrhage (rapid onset, erratic course, discrete ending) or into

---

[27] 'cinq ou six lignes'.
[28] Lallemand (1820–34), *Recherches anatomopathologiques sur l'Encéphale*, vol. I, 47–52.

softening (slow, regular, progressive).[29] Haemorrhage and softening are intimately related, Lallemand insisted, in that softening can be followed by different degrees of extravasation.[30]

Lallemand had more strings to his bow to support his idea of inflammation as the underlying process in cerebral softening, over and above the hypothetical role of 'irritation' and the interconnectedness with haemorrhage. In his second 'letter', he reproduced almost 30 case histories where brain dissection had shown purulent lesions, about as equally often from the *Hôtel-Dieu* as cited from others. Almost invariably the inflammation also involved the arachnoid membrane, with adhesions. A purulent abscess was nothing else, he proposed, but the final stage of softening, in which brain tissue had first been infiltrated with blood (red-brown) and was then transformed into pus (coloured off-white, at least in the grey matter).[31]

'Encephalomalacia': Sudden Paralysis, Never Inflammation

In 1838, Conrad Heinrich Fuchs (1803–1855) (Box 6.2),[32] Professor of Medicine at the University of Würzburg, and later in Göttingen, published a book on brain softening, 'encephalomalacia', with his personal observations and opinions; he had read Rostan and Lallemand.[33] Fuchs listed 11 patients, with extensive details on symptoms and on findings at autopsy. He came down on the side of Rostan: he never found purulent matter or other changes suggesting an inflammatory disorder and he even flatly denied that inflammation could ever explain brain softening.[34] It is therefore not surprising to read that in Fuchs' patients, sudden hemiplegia was almost invariably the first manifestation of disease.[35] Prodromal symptoms, if occurring at all, were diverse; especially headache was rather uncommon in Fuchs' view, whereas Rostan had put great emphasis on this feature.[36] On the other hand, several of Fuchs' patients had reported preceding episodes of temporary weakness of the arm and leg on the side that later became paralytic, something he had never heard in patients with 'sanguineous apoplexy'.[37]

---

[29] Lallemand (1820–34), *Recherches anatomopathologiques sur l'Encéphale*, vol. 1, 96–100.
[30] Lallemand (1820–34), *Recherches anatomopathologiques sur l'Encéphale*, vol. 1, 73–5.
[31] Lallemand (1820–34), *Recherches anatomopathologiques sur l'Encéphale*, vol. 1, 199–207.
[32] Husemann (1878), Konrad Heinrich Fuchs; Anonymous (2013), Kein Gauß drin.
[33] Rostan's book (2nd edn, 1823) had been translated in German (Rostan (1824), *Erweichung des Gehirns*). Conversely, a review of Fuchs' book had appeared in Paris (Anonymous (1840), Ramollissement du cerveau).
[34] Fuchs (1838), *Beobachtungen über Gehirnerweichung*, 4 and 237.
[35] Fuchs (1838), *Beobachtungen über Gehirnerweichung*, 98–9.
[36] Fuchs (1838), *Beobachtungen über Gehirnerweichung*, 91–5.
[37] Fuchs (1838), *Beobachtungen über Gehirnerweichung*, 96 and 123.

Box 6.2 Conrad Heinrich Fuchs (1803–1855).

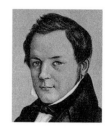

Fuchs was born in Bamberg and studied medicine at the Julius-Maximilian University in Würzburg. From 1825 to 1829, he was assistant physician there, under Johann Lukas Schönlein (1793–1864), an internist, pathologist, and paleobotanist. For the next two years, Fuchs visited hospitals in France and northern Italy. In 1831, he obtained the doctoral title and was appointed Extraordinary Professor of Pathology in Würzburg, followed by a full chair in 1836.

There is no documentation that Fuchs ever married. When, for some reason, he was pressured to exchange his chair for that of therapeutics, he moved in 1838 to the University of Göttingen as Professor and Head of the Department of Medicine, at first together with Johann Wilhelm Heinrich Conradi (1780–1861), and after 1843 alone. He published extensively, for example his popular books *Nosology and Therapy* and *Diseases of the Skin*; his classification was 'naturalistic', with illnesses divided into families, genera, and species. An interest shared with Schönlein was the history of pathology; he also founded a collection of pathological–anatomical specimens. In 1853, he became a member of the Academy of Science in Göttingen. After he had died at the young age of 52 years, his brain was preserved; it is presently at the Institute for Ethics and History of Medicine in Göttingen; in 2013, it emerged that Fuchs' brain had been inadvertently exchanged with that of the famous mathematician Carl Friedrich Gauß (1777–1855) who had died in the same year.

About the true cause of softening, Fuchs had to confess, he remained completely in the dark; he resorted, somewhat unwillingly, to terms like 'asthenia' and 'debilitating influences'.[38] Others went a bit further.

GANGRENE?

In 1823, Rostan produced a second edition of his book, three years after the first. In the introduction, he acknowledged favourable comments from abroad, in contrast to – unspecified – 'criticisms in France'.[39] New cases had been added, more than doubling the number of pages; most of them had 'regular' brain softening, at least in Rostan's eyes, in other words a gradual course of disease. Others he classified as 'simple' brain softening (a less gradual course), or as 'complicated' disease (concomitant diseases, mostly haemorrhage or a tumour), or as diseases that might be confused with softening. With regard to interpretations, Rostan stuck to his guns with regard to a non-inflammatory cause:

---

[38] Fuchs (1838), *Beobachtungen über Gehirnerweichung*, 176–89.
[39] Rostan (1823), *Recherches sur le Ramollissement du Cerveau*, x.

In most cases, the brain does not change colour, it is of a duller shade of white, shinier than in the normal state; surely, neither pus nor blood penetrates it. In other circumstances, the cerebral substance has a wine-red colour, presenting exactly the aspect of scorbutic stains or ecchymoses; in those cases, no sign of reaction has existed during the patient's life and the aspect is in no way that of inflamed tissue. It shows most likeness with scorbutic tissue; and as long as that is not considered an inflammatory condition, we shall be permitted to regard this state of the brain as different from phlegmasia.

Hardened Vessels

Yet, Rostan now wagered a cautious hypothesis on the true 'nature' of softening:

But what is its nature then? We might have abstained from a response to this question. But at any rate we believe we can say, with caution, and without fear of getting lost in the speculations we were just talking about,[40] that this change of the brain often seems to us a senile destruction, showing the most resemblance with gangrene of old age. Like that [condition], softening seems to us the disorganisation of the body part, because with this disease the vessels that should carry blood and life to the affected organ are hardened, not as a result of inflammation, but by advanced age.[41]

Whereas Rostan and Lallemand were at odds about the issue of whether *ramollissement* was always a form of inflammation or sometimes a disease in its own right, they agreed on including patients with progressive disease. As it turned out, this common ground they shared kept the controversy going. Fuchs had avoided the problem by limiting his selection – intuitively or by accident – to patients with sudden hemiplegia. It was a Scot who tried to resolve the entanglement.

Two Kinds of Softening

John Abercrombie (1780–1844) (Box 6.3) was 10 years older than Rostan and Lallemand. His main activity was not hospital-based, but in family practice, in Edinburgh.[42] Since he had direct contact with people at home, his case

---

[40] Earlier in the text (p. 168), Rostan had lambasted the reasoning: 'softening can be caused by inflammation, so it is always caused by inflammation'.

[41] Rostan (1823), *Recherches sur le Ramollissement du Cerveau*, 169–70.

[42] Royal College of Physicians of Edinburgh (www.rcpe.ac.uk/heritage/college-history/john-abercrombie); Hirsch (1884–8), *Biographisches Lexikon*, vol. I, 37–8.

Box 6.3 John Abercrombie (1780–1844).

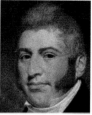

Abercrombie was born in Aberdeen. His father, a parish minister, greatly influenced his moral upbringing. In 1800, John attended Edinburgh University to study medicine; he obtained his MD three years later. After six months at St George's Hospital in London, he returned to Edinburgh, established a private practice, and became a Fellow of the Royal College of Surgeons of Edinburgh.

He devoted much of his time to the poor of Edinburgh. As one of the medical officers at the Royal Public Dispensary, he subdivided the poorer areas of the city into districts and allotted them to different students. In 1808, Abercrombie married the wealthy daughter of a manufacturer; they had seven daughters. In 1815, the New Town Dispensary was opened on Thistle Street, with Abercrombie as a senior surgeon. In 1821, he became a Fellow of the Royal College of Physicians. Despite a competitive atmosphere, his colleagues admired his mild and unassuming manners.

Abercrombie published extensively. Gradually he became the leading physician of his day in Edinburgh and also physician to the king in Scotland. He was a medical advisor and close friend of Sir Walter Scott. The University of Oxford conferred on him an honorary MD degree.

In the last decade of his life, Abercrombie espoused philosophical and religious topics. He wrote a number of essays, compiled as *Elements of Sacred Truth for the Young*. He donated widely to Edinburgh charities and societies. In 1841, he suffered a stroke, from which he largely recovered. On 14 November 1844, he was found dead in his room, on his way to a patient; autopsy showed a haemopericardium. The relatives donated his library of over 900 books to the Royal College of Surgeons of Edinburgh, and his extensive papers to the Royal College of Physicians of Edinburgh.

---

histories were more complete than those from large institutions. In 1828, Abercrombie published two treatises: *Pathological and Practical Researches on Diseases of the Brain and spinal Cord* and *Diseases of the Stomach, the intestinal Canal, the Liver, and other Viscera of the Abdomen*. Of brain disease, softening had his special interest. Abercrombie had read Rostan's work and compared it with his own; in the end, he provided a synthesis, which deserves to be reproduced *in extenso*:

> *Ramollissement* – A peculiar disorganization or softening of the brain, which has now received that name – a term adopted from the French to express the peculiar morbid appearance. It consists in a part of the cerebral substance being broken down into a soft pulpy mass, retaining its natural colour, but having lost its cohesion and consistence. It differs entirely from suppuration, having neither the colour nor the foetor of pus; but the white parts of the brain in which it is most commonly observed retain their pure milky whiteness. It may be found in any part of the brain [...]

When I formerly endeavoured to contribute something to the pathology of this remarkable affection, I had no hesitation in considering it as one of the results of inflammation of the cerebral substance. Since that time, it has been investigated with much attention by Mr Rostan and other French pathologists, and a different view of the nature of the affection has been strongly contended for by these eminent persons. They consider it as an affection of the brain entirely *sui generis*, and Mr Rostan, in particular, seems to look upon it as a peculiar and primary disease of the brain, though he admits it is sometimes the result of inflammation.

From all the facts which are now before us, in regard to this interesting affection, I think we are enabled to arrive at the conclusion, that it occurs under two modifications which differ essentially from each other. In the cases of Mr Rostan, the disorganisation was observed chiefly in the external parts of the brain; it occurred almost entirely in very old people, few of his cases being under sixty years of age, many of them seventy, seventy-five, and eighty. It was found in connection with attacks of a paralytic or apoplectic kind, many of them protracted; and was often found combined with extravasation of blood, or surrounding old apoplectic cysts. On the contrary, the affection which I had been anxious to investigate, was found chiefly in the dense central parts of the brain, the fornix, septum lucidum, and corpus callosum, or in the cerebral matter immediately surrounding the ventricles; and occurred in persons of various ages, but chiefly in young people and in children. [...]

When we compare the facts now alluded to, with the observations of Mr Rostan and his friends, I think we may arrive at a principle by which the apparent difference may be reconciled. The principle which I refer to is, that this peculiar softening of the cerebral matter is analogous to gangrene in other parts of the body; and that, like gangrene, it may arise from two very different causes; these are inflammation, and failure of the circulation from disease of the arteries. The former I believe to be the origin of the affection which I have described, and the latter to be the source of the appearances described by Mr Rostan. If this doctrine be admitted, the difficulty is removed; and I do not see any good objection to it. [...] It appears extremely probable that it may be the source of that particular condition of a part of the brain which terminates in the ramollissement of Mr Rostan, and indeed he distinctly points at this explanation of it.[43]

Though Abercrombie, in 1828, thus firmly supported Rostan's idea of a non-inflammatory form of brain softening, he made no attempts to reclassify some of Rostan's cases. What he did do was firmly label 'gangrenous softening' as a form of apoplexy.

---

[43] Abercrombie (1828), *Diseases of the Brain and the Spinal Cord*, 23–5.

As outlined in the previous chapter, Abercrombie divided apoplexy into three groups, according to the predominant symptom at onset: loss of consciousness, headache, or paralysis. Inevitably, the division often became blurred in the course of the disease, but grouping cases according to the first symptom was his preferred method of creating some order. Among Abercrombie's cases of apoplexy characterized by initial paralysis were two patients in whom dissection had shown softening as the primary lesion. The first one follows below. Abercrombie had described the story, more briefly, in an article published 10 years before;[44] at that time, he had regarded the lesion as inflammatory in nature, for want of better.[45] He now presented it once more, in the light of his fresh insight.

Apoplectic Paralysis, Caused by Softening

A man, aged 58, of a full habit and florid complexion, on the 7th of March, 1817, about nine o'clock in the morning, without any previous complaint, was found to have lost his speech. I saw him about half past ten, and found him walking about his room; he had the full use of all of his limbs; understood what was said to him, and answered by signs; he could put out his tongue freely, but could not articulate a word. He did not admit that he felt any uneasiness in his head, his pulse was natural and of good strength, and his face flushed. The usual remedies were employed through the day, without producing any change in the symptoms. In the morning of the 8th, he was found to be affected with perfect hemiplegia of the right side; and the tongue, when put out, was turned to the right side; he was still quite intelligent, but made no attempt at speech.

He now lay for a month without any change in the symptoms; he slept well in the night; in the day he was quite intelligent, and answered by signs, but continued entirely speechless. [...] About the 10th of May, he began to have violent pain in the paralytic limbs, and could not bear to have them moved in the gentlest fashion without screaming; nothing was to be seen about the limbs that accounted for the uneasiness. For about a fortnight he suffered constant pain; his strength sunk, and he lost appetite. He then had some vomiting, but not urgent; his pulse became feeble, and his features collapsed; and he died in the end of May, of gradual sinking, without coma. There had been no recovery of speech, or of the motion of the right side.

Dissection. On opening the head, there appeared a remarkable depression on the upper part of the left hemisphere of the brain, about two inches in length and somewhat less in breadth, the dura mater sinking into it to the depth of about half an inch. On removing the dura mater, the substance of the brain at this place was to a great extent broken down,

---

[44] Abercrombie (1818a), On apoplexy, 565–6.   [45] Abercrombie (1819), On paralysis, 7.

soft and pulpy; and this appearance extended along nearly the whole upper part of the left hemisphere.[46]

The second case report was more concise. A 60-year-old man, having experienced a few spells of numbness in his left arm, became hemiplegic on the left side a week later; this was unchanged for about a month. He then lost his speech, became comatose after a few hours, and died two days later. The outer part of the right hemisphere was 'in a state of complete ramollissement'.[47]

Abercrombie had killed two birds with a single stone. Firstly, he proposed that the non-inflammatory form of softening was a kind of gangrene, in keeping with the tentative suggestion in the second edition of Rostan's book, five years before. Secondly, Abercrombie accepted that 'gangrenous softening' was associated with a sudden onset of clinical deficits. In this way, he discarded the difficulty Rostan had created by his insistence on identifying two phases of disease and thereby including patients with a progressive, instead of a sudden, onset. Admittedly, Abercrombie reiterated many of the premonitory symptoms and the progressive course he had adopted from Rostan's account in his introduction to the two cases,[48] but at any rate, a sudden onset of hemiplegia was for him the key feature of softening, as it was for Fuchs; he thus transformed Rostan's *ramollissement* into a second form of apoplexy.

In Abercrombie's time, the known forms of gangrene, especially of the limbs, represented a gradual process. That dysfunction of the brain on interruption of its blood flow was infinitely faster than in tissues of other organs was not yet known in detail. Yet examples of syncope and strangulation may have suggested to Abercrombie that a similar, instantaneous loss of function might occur at a more restricted, local level in the brain. Whatever induced him to follow Rostan's hint and implicate 'disease of arteries', it was a fruitful idea. Rostan's and Abercrombie's suggestion of 'disease of the arteries' in relation to 'gangrene' was adopted some 15 years later by the London physician Edwards Crisp (1806–1882),[49] in one of his reports on brain disease in the *Lancet* of 1840.[50] Also, other physicians started to pay attention to the characteristics of the softened area, sometimes also of its blood supply.

A CLOSER LOOK AT SOFTENED BRAIN TISSUE

Gabriel Andral (1797–1876),[51] a physician at the Charité, became famous by authoring the *Clinique médicale*, a multi-volume handbook of internal medicine

---

[46] Abercrombie (1828), *Diseases of the Brain and the Spinal Cord*, 271–3.
[47] Abercrombie (1828), *Diseases of the Brain and the Spinal Cord*, 273.
[48] Abercrombie (1828), *Diseases of the Brain and the Spinal Cord*, 268–71.
[49] Dobson (1952), Dr. Edwards Crisp.   [50] Crisp (1840), Cases of cerebral disease, 865–7.
[51] Hirsch (1884–8), *Biographisches Lexikon*, vol. I, 136–8.

appearing between 1823 and 1833. The fifth and last volume dealt with diseases of the brain. The section on cerebral softening contained 33 case reports and an extensive discussion. He did not speculate about a single cause but emphasized that these were diverse:

> In showing us softening of the brain in all its forms, with regard to anatomy as well as to symptoms, the preceding observations have also shown that the diagnosis of this disorder is far from easy in most cases. The study of these separate facts seems extremely important to us, for the very reason that each of them presents a different aspect of the disease. How might a general description sufficiently reflect all these individualities?[52]

On reviewing the controversy between Rostan and Lallemand (he did not mention Abercrombie), Andral did not at all doubt that, in some cases, inflammation was the explanation; occasionally he even identified tubercles.[53] Yet he also strongly asserted the existence of a form of softening that was completely unrelated to inflammation.

Red and White Softening

In some lesions, Andral found 'white softening' (*ramollissement blanc*), with pale, *anaemic* tissue, often traversed by intact blood vessels and not at all like a purulent lesion. In other cases, the tissue was *hyperaemic*, diffusely or spotted; he regarded this variety as secondary infiltration by blood, not as the redness of inflammation.[54]

Andral found it impossible to distinguish between softening and haemorrhage on the basis of the patient's symptoms;[55] in particular, he could not confirm the relationship between headache and *ramollissement* on which Rostan had so strongly insisted.[56] Only the course of the disease offered something to hold on to. Within the group of patients with an acute onset, Andral distinguished two forms:[57] one resembled acute meningitis, beginning with headache or delirium, and the other mimicked cerebral haemorrhage – five patients with essentially sudden hemiplegia, with or without loss of consciousness or convulsions, perfectly fitted his model of 'essential', non-inflammatory softening.[58]

---

[52] Andral (1833), *Maladies de l'Encéphale*, 522.
[53] Andral (1833), *Maladies de l'Encéphale*, 503–6.
[54] Andral (1833), *Maladies de l'Encéphale*, 524–8.
[55] Andral (1833), *Maladies de l'Encéphale*, 539–82.
[56] Andral (1833), *Maladies de l'Encéphale*, 440 and 570–3.
[57] Andral (1833), *Maladies de l'Encéphale*, 584–5.
[58] Andral (1833), *Maladies de l'Encéphale*, 458–61 (case XVIII), 464–7 (case XIX), 476–89 (cases XXIII–XXV).

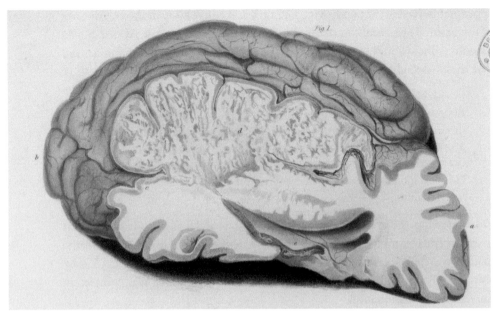

6.1 Softening, three to four weeks after the attack (Bright, 1931). Drawing by C. J Canton, engraving by W. T. Fry. The original legend is as follows:
'A portion of the middle and posterior lobes of the left hemisphere of the cerebrum. The section is made horizontally through the lateral ventricle. The medullary portion has assumed a broken curd-like appearance, while the cortical part has become yellow and disorganized.
a) the anterior; b) the posterior portion of the brain; c) a portion of the cortical substance, become diseased without any changed having taken place in the corresponding part of the medullary matter, appearing to render it probable that the disease had its commencement in the cortical substance; d) the softened portion of the medullary substance; e) the cavity of the lateral ventricle.'

Softening Illustrated

Richard Bright (1789–1858) (see Box 5.2, p. 160) from Guy's Hospital described the case of James Kennedy, 63 years of age. The story on admission was brief: he had suddenly collapsed, was paralysed on the right side, and had lost his speech. Later, having lapsed first into 'delirium coma', he died after three to four weeks. The findings on dissection were illustrated by a coloured engraving (Figure 6.1).

> The substance of the left hemisphere was obviously soft, particularly at its posterior and lateral part: and on attempting to separate the membranes, the cortical substance tore away with them. A slice being taken very superficially from the top of this hemisphere cut into a portion of the softened brain, showing the cortical substance of a yellowish fawn colour, and the brain itself broken down near the cortical substance, like curd. [...] The line of distinction between the healthy and diseased portions was decidedly marked by the dead white of that which was diseased.[59]

[59] Bright (1827–31), *Reports of Medical Cases*, vol. II, part 1, 177–9 and plate 14, Fig. 1.

Clearly this was an example of Andral's anaemic form of softening, without any secondary infiltration of blood. Bright's thoughts went in the same direction:

> It certainly produced in my mind an impression, that the proper supply of blood had been cut off by some change in the vessels of the pia mater, or some obstruction in their passage through the cineritious substance, and that in this way the death and disorganization of the brain had been produced.[60]

In a later article, Bright came back on the relationship between softening and 'thick lumps of atheromatous deposit' in the arteries at the base of the brain, but without referring to the local blood supply.[61]

'Capillary Apoplexy'

The serially published fascicles with lithographies of Jean Cruveilhier (1791–1874) (Box 6.4), Professor of Pathological Anatomy in Paris,[62] included examples of brain softening, but not of the bloodless form. His patients, mostly dissected within a few days of the attack, all showed what Andral called haemorrhagic infiltration or injection; in the example in Figure 6.2, red softening was limited to the cortex of several convolutions.[63] The disease histories were usually unknown, apart from the interval between the first symptoms and death. Cruveilhier made much of the combination of softening and bleeding, and devised a separate name for it: *apoplexie capillaire* – a term Andral considered infelicitous.[64]

Though Cruveilhier also practised as a physician, his conceptions of disease were dominated by morbid anatomy. In the course of time, having devoted three separate sections to 'capillary apoplexy' in what was to become his two-volume atlas,[65] he somewhat modified his views. In the twentieth instalment - the first appeared in 1829 and the fortieth and last in 1842 - he distinguished several shades of redness, depending on the degree of infiltration and the interval between apoplexy and death; the amaranth hue in Figure 6.2 was in the middle range.[66] Several years later, in the thirty-sixth instalment, Cruveilhier defined 'capillary apoplexy' as the middle of a continuum between, on the one hand, pure softening, grey-white in colour, and, on

[60] Bright (1827–31), *Reports of Medical Cases*, vol. II, part 1, 192.
[61] Bright (1836), Diseases of arteries and the brain, 21–5.
[62] Hannaway (2007), Jean Cruveilhier, 377–8; Hirsch (1884–8), *Biographisches Lexikon*, vol. II, 110–11.
[63] Cruveilhier (1829–42), *Anatomie pathologique*, vol. I, livraison XX, planche 4, figure 3.
[64] Andral (1833), *Maladies de l'Encéphale*, 528–9.
[65] Cruveilhier (1829–42), *Anatomie pathologique*, vol. I, livraisons XX, XXXIII, and XXXVI.
[66] Cruveilhier (1829–42), *Anatomie pathologique*, vol. I, livraison XX, 8.

> ## Box 6.4 Jean Cruveilhier (1791–1874).
>
> 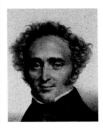 Cruveilhier was born in Limoges, where his father was a military surgeon. Pious by nature, Jean intended a future in the clergy, but at his father's insistence, he became a student of medicine in Paris, at the age of 19. He received much encouragement from the famous surgeon Guillaume Dupuytren (1777–1835), also a native of the Limousin region. However, disgusted by his first experiences with post-mortem dissections, Jean took refuge with the Priests of Saint-Sulpice, until his father forced him back into the fold. After graduation in 1816, with a thesis on 'Pathological anatomy in general and transformations and organic processes in particular', he returned to Limoges to take over his father's practice and to marry a banker's daughter, with whom he was to have seven daughters and a son.
>
> Encouraged by his father, he successfully entered the competition for an Extraordinary Professorship of Surgery in Montpellier. When he was still in doubt about this move, the minister of education, a priest he had met during his brief sojourn at Saint-Sulpice, invited him to apply for the chair of Descriptive Anatomy in Paris. He became the chosen candidate and gave his inaugural lecture in November 1825. A little more than a decade later, he moved to the chair of Pathological Anatomy, the first of its kind in France. He held this post for more than 30 years, besides hospital attachments at the Maternité, the Salpêtrière, and later also the Charité. He became the personal physician of Charles-Maurice de Talleyrand (1754–1838), at least towards the end of the life of this politician and diplomat.
>
> Among the several handbooks Cruveilhier published, the most famous is *Anatomie pathologique du Corps humain*. This treatise was not ordered in the traditional textbook fashion, but it consisted of 40 separate fascicles, serially appearing between 1829 and 1842. Every three or four months, subscribers received an instalment with four or five brief chapters about a variety of subjects (the prostate, the heart, exostoses, etc.), illustrated with up to six lithographic plates.

the other hand, massive extravasation of blood; he even suggested it could precede softening.[67]

Obliterated Arteries

Robert Carswell (1793–1857) (Box 6.5) appeared in Chapter 5 as a gifted pathologist producing his own drawings and lithographies.[68] In his chapter on haemorrhage – in different organs – he clearly distinguished in the brain a form of 'sanguineous exhalation' without vessel rupture, which he called 'vicarious or supplemental haemorrhage'.[69] In other words, he regarded the

---

[67] Cruveilhier (1829–42), *Anatomie pathologique*, vol. II, livraison XXXIII, 1–5.
[68] Payne (1887), Robert Carswell.
[69] Carswell (1838), *Pathological Anatomy*, section 'Haemorrhage' (there is no page numbering).

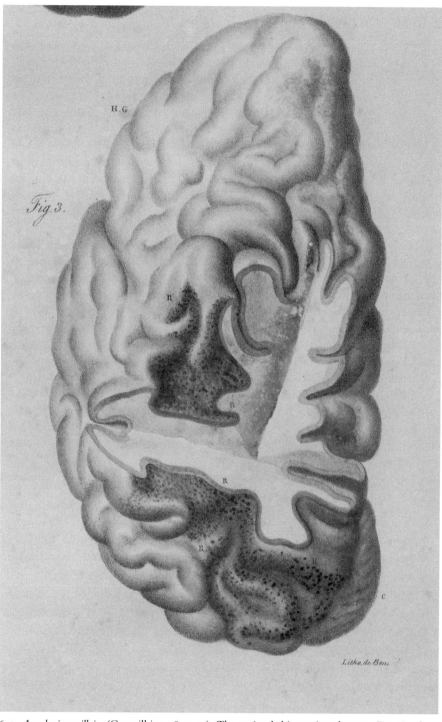

6.2 *Apoplexie capillaire* (Cruveilhier, 1827–42). The patient's history is unknown. Drawing by Antoine Chazal (1793–1854). Cruveilhier's legend reads: 'The figure represents the pink-red softening that forms the transition between wine-coloured and lilac hydrangea-coloured softening. The softening (R) is confined to the grey matter; there is diffuse spotting with blood.'

Box 6.5 Robert Carswell (1793–1857).

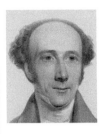

Carswell was born in Paisley, Scotland. He studied medicine at the University of Glasgow. As a student, he stood out by his drawing skills; John Thompson (Edinburgh) employed him to illustrate morbid anatomy. He pursued this activity on the continent and spent two years (1822–3) at hospitals of Paris and Lyon. Having obtained his MD degree in 1826 at the Marischal College, Aberdeen, he returned to Paris and resumed his studies in morbid anatomy under the celebrated Louis. Around 1828, appointed Professor of Pathological Anatomy at University College, London, he was commissioned to prepare a collection of pathological drawings before taking up his lectures. He therefore remained in Paris until 1831, when he had completed well over 1000 watercolour drawings of diseased structures. This collection is still preserved at University College.

Once having undertaken the duties of professorship in London, Carswell was also a physician at the University College Hospital. He did not, however, at once engage in practice but occupied himself with the preparation of his book on pathological anatomy, with illustrations from his large store of pathological drawings, transferred on stone by himself. This is the famous work on which his reputation rests, published in 1837 as *Illustrations of the elementary Forms of Disease*; the illustrations are unsurpassed in artistic merit and fidelity. Around 1836, Carswell entered private practice, but without much success.

As his health was failing, he resigned his professorship in 1840 and accepted an appointment as physician to the King of Belgium. The rest of his life was spent at Laeken, near Brussels, with official duties and charitable medical attendance on the poor, but interrupted by several journeys to the south because of poor health. Carswell made no further contributions to medical science. He was knighted in July 1850 by Queen Victoria for his services at the time when the former king Louis-Philippe had been in exile in the UK. Carswell was married to Marguerite Chardenot, who survived him; they had no children. He died on 15 June 1857, from chronic lung disease.

haemorrhagic component as a secondary phenomenon, with Bright and Andral. His own lithographic examples clearly showed such haemorrhagic changes, with yellow-brown or red-brown discoloration (Figure 6.3).[70]

Importantly, in the chapter on softening, Carswell emphasized the relationship with specific arterial lesions and he clearly distinguished inflammatory brain lesions from softening by occlusion of arteries. Recalling that Rostan had regarded softening as a disease *sui generis*, akin to *gangrena senilis*, whereas Lallemand maintained it was always the consequence of inflammation, Carswell wrote:

> This latter opinion, which is by far the most generally received one, is as far from the truth as the former is ambiguous and inconclusive. Indeed,

[70] Carswell (1838), *Pathological Anatomy*, section 'Softening', plate IV.

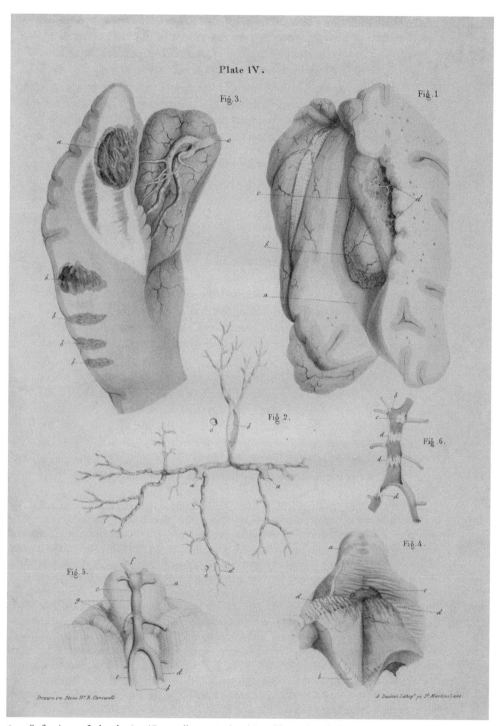

6.3 Softening of the brain (Carswell, 1838; he himself produced the watercolours and lithographs). His legends are as follows:

'Fig. 1 A portion of the right hemisphere; a, the lateral ventricle laid open; b, thalamus; c, corpus striatum of the right side. The upper half of this body was converted into a soft pulp of a pale straw and light brown colour, in which two small arteries, d, were seen ramifying. They were completely obliterated, and felt as firm to the touch as fine wires.

no pathologist who has investigated this subject has, so far as I know, furnished us with evidence that the real nature of this kind of softening, to which the brain is subject in the aged, has been ascertained. It has been conjectured to originate in ossification of the arteries, yet even M. Rostan, among the great number of cases of softening of the brain, the histories of which are detailed in his work, has not given a single case in which ossification and obliteration of the arteries of this organ are mentioned as having been observed at the autopsy.

Carswell filled this gap himself, by giving a precise description of the aspect and distribution of the arterial lesions, also in end arteries (Figure 6.3):

The obliteration of the arteries may depend on the presence of fibrous, cartilaginous, or osseous substances, formed in the interior of these vessels or between their coats. These accidental products may exist in the form of cylinders occupying the entire calibre of arteries of considerable size, and also the smaller branches; or they may form patches or small masses projecting internally, which obstruct the circulation of the blood. The cessation of the circulation in the diseased arteries probably takes place gradually, and a supply of the materials of nutrition being ultimately cut off from the portion of the brain to which these arteries are distributed, softening follows. [...]

If the obliteration be confined to a limited portion of an artery whose branches terminate in the softened part of the brain, the cause of the softening may be overlooked. In the case of obliteration of minute arteries, or of a single small arterial trunk, the softening is generally confined to a space not exceeding an inch or two inches in superficial extent; but if several large contiguous branches be obliterated, the extent of the softening is considerably increased, or occupies two or more

6.3 (cont.) Fig. 2 Represents the principal branches of the carotids, aa, in this case, in which the circulation was obstructed to a considerable extent, chiefly from fibrous substance contained within them. The situation of this substance is recognized by the pale spots seen on the external surface of the arteries. Two of these vessels are represented laid open at b and d, where the fibrous substance is seen attached to their lining membrane; c and e are transverse sections of the same vessels, nearly the whole calibre of which is seen to be occupied by this substance.
Fig. 3 A section of part of the left hemisphere of the brain, in which the same kind of softening is seen, accompanied with orange-brown discoloration. The softening and discoloration are almost entirely confined to the brown substance of the corpus striatum, a, and that of several of the convolutions, bbb. [...] c is the principal arterial trunk, some of the larger branches of which are obliterated, others obstructed by the presence of bony and fibrous formations; only two or three of the smallest branches are pervious.
Fig. 4 Softening of the pons Varolii; a, a transverse section of the pons; b, a longitudinal section of the medulla oblongata; c and dd softening of the brown and white substance. [...]
Fig. 5 The softening of the pons was the consequence of obstructed circulation in the basilary artery. a, the pons; b, the medulla oblongata; c, the basilary artery; d, left vertebral, e, right vertebral artery. [...]
Fig. 6 The morbid condition of the basilary and right vertebral arteries, ddd. [...]'

> distinct portions of the brain; and if the obliteration has taken place in the
> carotid or one of its principal divisions within the cranium, the greater
> part or the whole of a hemisphere may be softened.[71]

Carswell seemed on a plausible track. Yet not everyone agreed, especially not across the Channel. There were still influential proponents of the idea that inflammation explained not just some, but all forms of brain softening.

INFLAMMATION VERSUS ARTERIAL DISEASE: AN ONGOING DISPUTE

The Inflammation Hypothesis Revived

In 1843, a new book on cerebral softening appeared; its author was (Charles-Louis) Maxime Durand-Fardel (1815–1899). We met him in Chapter 5 with his hypothesis about a form of 'atrophy' as the origin of intracerebral haemorrhage; in later life, he shifted his attention to the salubrious effects of Vichy and other spas.[72] With 526 quarto pages and 128 case reports, mostly of patients from the Salpêtrière, his book is the largest text written on the subject in the nineteenth century. The 28-year-old physician dedicated it to his teachers Rochoux and Cruveilhier, although quite often his conclusions diverged from their views.

As had been the case with Lallemand, Durand-Fardel's approach resembled that of Rostan on the important point that the definition of cerebral softening was purely morphological: almost any kind of brain softening was included, excepted head trauma and plainly purulent affections. This led, once more, to the inclusion of patients with progressive, instead of acute, symptoms; the author even considered a stepwise disease course most characteristic, though not most common.[73]

But in another important aspect, central to Durand-Fardel's reasoning, he squarely opposed Rostan's point of view: without exception, he regarded all instances of cerebral softening as inflammatory in nature. He also contradicted Andral, in that he regarded the redness of softened brain tissue as an essential testimony;[74] accordingly, he was highly critical of the notion of 'white softening'.[75] In Durand-Fardel's reasoning, congestion of brain vessels was the primary factor initiating the inflammatory cascade.[76] This was not to say

---

[71] Carswell (1838), *Pathological Anatomy*, section 'Softening' (no numbering of pages).
[72] Hirsch (1884–8), *Biographisches Lexikon*, vol. II, 243.
[73] Durand-Fardel (1843), *Traité du Ramollissement du Cerveau*, 183–4.
[74] Durand-Fardel (1843), *Traité du Ramollissement du Cerveau*, 8–13.
[75] Durand-Fardel (1843), *Traité du Ramollissement du Cerveau*, 75 and 473–84.
[76] Durand-Fardel (1843), *Traité du Ramollissement du Cerveau*, 73–4, 159, and 450.

that such overfilling invariably ended up in softening; it could wear off, he argued.[77] Conversely, he maintained that hemiplegia could result from the congestive phase alone, before softening had even begun.[78]

As might be expected with such a mixed collection of patients, the author had to adopt several subgroups with regard to symptoms. Even in the 'chronic period', after 25 to 30 days, the anatomical abnormalities showed substantial variation. For example, softening could be found in both hemispheres.[79]

Durand-Fardel could not avoid discussing the 'gangrene hypothesis'.[80] He judged 'ossification' of arteries an improbable cause, since it was often absent and if not, it tended to occur in main trunks instead of in branches to areas where softening mostly occurred. Even though he identified a clot in the internal carotid artery and in some of its branches in two patients with acute onset of contralateral hemiplegia,[81] he dismissed this as, at most, a contributory factor. Also, he disqualified Carswell's suggestion that inflammatory and non-inflammatory forms of softening could be distinguished by the state of the arteries as 'logically untenable'.[82] More than 10 years later, Durand-Fardel published a book on diseases of the aged, with essentially unchanged conclusions about softening.[83]

Local Arterial Obstruction, Once More

Duran-Fardel's high-handed repudiation of arterial occlusion as a cause of brain softening did not remain uncontested. In 1846, Karl Ewald Hasse (1810–1902), Professor of Medicine and Pathology in Zürich,[84] reported his own experiences in a journal with the intriguing title *Zeitschrift für rationelle Medicin*. The journal had been founded two years before, appearing in Heidelberg and Leipzig; one of the editors was Jakob Henle (1809–1885), Professor of Anatomy and Physiology in Zürich; he had spent the 1830s as a research student under the wings of the influential Johannes Müller (1801–1858), in Bonn and Berlin.[85] In the opening article of the first volume, Henle had firmly stated his credentials:[86] medical science, he wrote, required empirical observations and should distance itself from the idealistic *Naturphilosophie*

[77] Durand-Fardel (1843), *Traité du Ramollissement du Cerveau*, 54.
[78] Durand-Fardel (1843), *Traité du Ramollissement du Cerveau*, 167.
[79] Durand-Fardel (1843), *Traité du Ramollissement du Cerveau*, 201–70.
[80] Durand-Fardel (1843), *Traité du Ramollissement du Cerveau*, 452–63.
[81] Durand-Fardel (1843), *Traité du Ramollissement du Cerveau*, 91 and 103.
[82] Durand-Fardel (1843), *Traité du Ramollissement du Cerveau*, 486–7.
[83] Durand-Fardel (1854), *Maladies des Vieillards*, 164–75.
[84] Hirsch (1884–8), *Biographisches Lexikon*, vol. II, 78.   [85] Otis (2007), *Müller's Lab*, 43–59.
[86] Henle (1844), Medizinische Wissenschaft und Empirie.

personified by Friedrich Wilhelm Joseph von Schelling (1775–1854), with its vitalist principles of 'irritability', 'sensitivity', and 'reproduction'.

In his article on softening, Hasse recalled that in his former position as Extraordinary Professor of Pathological Anatomy in Leipzig, he had seen several instances of softening in aged persons where this lesion was clearly related to occluded arteries. He had no more doubts on this point. Moreover, from the archives in Zurich, he had retrieved records of six more patients in whom focal softening of the brain was associated with occlusion of the corresponding arteries, most often the 'Sylvian' (middle cerebral) artery or its branches.[87] Clinical details were missing, but not in two other, recent examples, remarkable because of their young age, 39 and 40 years. They are the more relevant because, as in Carswell's earlier description, occlusion of the arterial supply to the softened brain region was not just implied, but actually demonstrated. One of these two cases follows almost in full:

> M.M., a 39-year-old, tall, obese and robust woman, reported to have been always healthy apart from minor illnesses, walked on June 17 from Regensburg to Zürich, under a blazing sun. In the countryside she was suddenly seized by a stroke, while she was talking to a woman she had met on the way. She collapsed in a state of unconsciousness and was completely paralysed on the left side. She partly recovered a few times on that same day, but soon reverted to her comatose status. Bloodletting and other measures were fruitless; she was therefore brought to the 'Cantonspital', on June 20. On examination she was completely unconscious, the pupils were slow, saliva flowed continuously from the left corner of the mouth, the jaws remained tightly closed. She often raised her right hand to grasp the region of her right temple; she was entirely paralysed on the left side. [...] She died at 8 o'clock in the evening, three days and eight hours after the attack.
>
> *Dissection*, 36 hours after death. [...] Several convolutions in the middle of the right hemisphere stand out somewhat from the surroundings; also, they are broader and flatter, while the furrows between them are obliterated. The colour of these convolutions is pale bluish red (the colour of hortensia); this colour extends through the entire cortical layer, which is softer than usual, very friable, and spotted by a multitude of small blood specks. The medullary substance under the softened convolutions is milk-white, also softer and more friable than usual, and spotted with fewer specks of blood. [...] The right intracranial carotid artery is filled with a black, tightly adherent clot, which extends to the branches supplying the softened parts. On the whole, the clots in these branches are even more tightly adherent to the wall of the arteries and their colour is more brown-red. [...] The heart large, fatty and limp, with much clotted blood in the considerably enlarged right ventricle. The mitral

---

[87] Hasse (1846), Verschliessung der Hirnarterien und Hirnerweichung, 93–5.

valve [is] thickened at its borders, one of the slips broadened, its tendinous chords thickened and shortened. The left ventricle [is] somewhat
dilated and hypertrophic.[88]

A relation between heart disease and arterial occlusion seems likely in this
young patient, even more in Hasse's second example, a 40-year-old woman
known to have endocarditis; softening of a large part of the left hemisphere
could be attributed to occlusion of the carotid system, in its intracranial and
extracranial parts.[89]

A few years earlier, Aristide-Jules Gély (1806–1861) from Nantes had
contributed the case history of a 55-year-old man with softening of one
hemisphere and occlusion of the 'Sylvian' and carotid arteries, but he explained
the relationship in a reverse manner, as an inflammatory process extending
from the brain to the arterial system.[90] The story was somewhat complicated
by previous head trauma – probably irrelevant – and by transient conjunctival
oedema on the side of the occlusion. Nonetheless, an anonymous commen-
tator in the *Gazette médicale* preferred to regard the intravascular clots as the
primary event.[91]

Other case histories provided more indirect evidence. In 1844, Robert
Bentley Todd (1809–1860) in London recounted the story of a 37-year-old
man who, while at dinner, was suddenly struck by severe pain in his back and
abdomen; two days later, his limbs and face on the left side became at first
weak and then paralysed; he died eleven days after the onset. Post-mortem
examination showed dissection of the aortic arch, which had obstructed the
origins of the innominate artery and part of the left common carotid and
subclavian arteries; the right hemisphere was bloodless, pale, and severely
softened.[92] In other cases, brain softening had occurred as a result of trauma
or carotid ligation, as the ultimate measure in treating aneurysmal dilatation or
stopping arterial bleeding.[93] These surgical complications received only moderate attention in medical circles, since they could be explained in
different ways.

A Lone Parisian

In meetings of the *Société médicale des hôpitaux de Paris*, candidates for membership were supposed to submit an essay – at least in the middle of the nineteenth

---

[88] Hasse (1846), Verschliessung der Hirnarterien und Hirnerweichung, 96–9.
[89] Hasse (1846), Verschliessung der Hirnarterien und Hirnerweichung, 99–103.
[90] Gély (1837), Inflammation de la carotide interne.   [91] Anonymous (1838), Inflammation.
[92] Todd (1844), White softening of the brain.
[93] Vincent (1829), Tying the common carotid artery; Sédillot (1842), Ligature du tronc
     carotidien; Chevers (1845), Obliteration of the carotid arteries.

century. One of these contributions in 1850 was *The Nature of senile Brain Softening*, by Eugène Bouchut (1818–1891). At the time, he was assistant physician at the *Hôtel-Dieu*;[94] later on, he was to acquire special expertise in diseases of children. Noting that the concept of inflammation was past the peak of its popularity, Bouchut wished to draw attention to the opinions of Abercrombie, Carswell, and Cruveilhier, who had all proposed that brain softening could result from arterial disease.[95] In his own patients with brain softening, he had found that the well-known cartilaginous or bony changes of arteries often led to narrowing of the vessel lumen. These abnormal depositions were located between the intimal and the muscle layer, sometimes rupturing to the surface, at least in the larger arteries. In addition, smaller arteries often contained blood clots that seemed fresh. Bouchut concluded that brain softening in the aged could indeed be regarded as a form of gangrene. Only the characteristic smell was missing – perhaps because the lesion was not exposed to ambient air, he thought.

The adjudicator assigned to the essay was Alfred Becquerel (1814–1862), active in many fields of medicine; he was to die of acute brain softening at a rather young age.[96] Though praising the rigour of Bouchut's study, Becquerel voiced reservations, for example because 'white softening' could not be explained as gangrene. As long as the hypothesis depended on induction and analogy, he judged, more chemical and microscopic research was still needed.[97]

Yet, the new evidence implying arterial occlusion, put forward by Hasse, Bouchut, and others, caused merely a few ripples in the ponds of established medical authority.

Divided Opinions

The amalgamation of patients with acute disease and those with a gradual course continued to be a major stumbling block on the path to understanding the pathogenesis of brain softening. At any rate, the 'inflammation faction' remained powerful. Apparently, only few pathologists were interested in the vascular system, apart from its capillaries. Opinions remained divided during the 1840 and 1850s, or were suspended. A few examples follow.

In 1844, Rochoux, nearing the age of 60, aligned himself with Durand-Fardel against the gangrene hypothesis.[98] Incidentally, in the same article, he

---

[94] Hirsch (1884–8), *Biographisches Lexikon*, vol. I, 537 (Bouchut's first name is incorrectly given as 'Ernest').

[95] Bouchut (1850), Mémoire sur la nature du ramollissement cérébrale sénile.

[96] Hirsch (1884–8), *Biographisches Lexikon*, vol. I, 358–9.

[97] Becquerel (1850), Rapport sur le mémoire présenté par M. E. Bouchut.

[98] Rochoux (1844), *Du Ramollissement du Cerveau*, 412–13.

once more advanced his theory that brain softening preceded apoplectic haemorrhage.[99]

In Vienna, inflammation was the favoured explanation. Carl von Rokitansky (1804–1878),[100] who had added new vigour to the local tradition of pathological anatomy established by de Haen and Stoll, emphatically stated that not only 'red softening' was an inflammatory disorder, but also was its rarer 'white' form.[101]

Scipion Pinel (1795–1859), son of the famous proto-psychiatrist Philippe Pinel (1745–1826), regarded softening in his textbook on brain diseases as inflammatory in the young and as 'asthenic' in the old.[102]

While the battle between proponents and antagonists of inflammation as the overall cause of brain softening continued, matters became even more muddled when studies of brain softening came to include patients with mental disease.

Brain Softening and General Paresis of the Insane

How did brain softening become associated with mental disease? By far the most common form of major psychiatric illness in the nineteenth century was general paresis of the insane, also called *dementia paralytica*. It had been recognized as a clinical entity at the end of the eighteenth century.[103] The association with genital syphilis, now common knowledge, was utterly unknown up to the 1860s, including the very period in which the pathogenesis of brain softening was being hotly discussed. In 1857, syphilis was implied for the first time as a cause of mental disease, in a psychiatric journal for German-speaking countries;[104] yet it took a few more decades before this relationship became generally accepted.

In the 1820s, in which also the early phase of the Rostan–Lallemand controversy took place, the young physician Antoine Laurent Jessé Bayle (1799–1858) had found evidence of inflammation ('arachnitis') in the brains of some patients with general paralysis. This disorder was common in the large asylum where he worked, in Charenton-St Maurice, for patients with chronic mental disorders from Paris and its surroundings. Bayle rashly extrapolated his findings on general paralysis to mental disorders in general,[105] a conjecture that did not fail to antagonize other psychiatrists, especially those groomed in the

---

[99] Rochoux (1844), *Du Ramollissement du Cerveau*, 268–82.
[100] Hirsch (1884–8), *Biographisches Lexikon*, vol. v, 63–7.
[101] Rokitansky (1844), *Handbuch der speciellen pathologischen Anatomie*, vol. i, 823–24.
[102] Pinel (1844), *Pathologie cérébrale*, 463–4.   [103] Haslam (1798), *Observations on Insanity*, 120.
[104] Esmarch and Jessen (1857), Syphilis und Geistesstörung.
[105] Bayle (1826), *Traité des Maladies du Cerveau*.

'moral psychiatry' founded by Philippe Pinel and Jean-Étienne Dominique Esquirol (1772–1840).

Bayle's colleague in psychiatry Louis-Florentin Calmeil (1798–1895) was more circumspect. In a book on general paralysis he published in 1826, he pointed out that inflammation of brain tissue ('chronic diffuse peri-encephalitis') was at least as important as that of its membranes, but he clearly distinguished these multifocal areas of softening from the unilateral lesions described by Morgagni and Rostan.[106]

'Necrobiosis of Old Age'

As late as in 1866, yet another book on brain softening appeared in which the author again tried to find a general explanation for all kinds of brain softening, regardless of the attending clinical features. Its author was Jean-Baptiste Vincent Laborde (1830–1903), a physician at the Bicêtre. Later in life, Laborde specialized in experimental physiology, toxicology, and comparative anatomy.[107]

Of the 10 personal case reports on which Laborde's conclusions rested, five suffered from general paresis or – in one case – delirium.[108] It is worth remembering that at the Bicêtre, all patients were male. The five other men had fallen victim to sudden hemiplegia, in one case two years before; nowhere in the book is this group discussed separately. Instead, a special section dealt with mental symptoms, features that, in the author's opinion, had not yet received proper attention.[109] A morphological characteristic he singled out was the simultaneous occurrence of partial softening in two regions: the cortical convolutions and the corresponding deep ganglia (corpus striatum and thalamus).[110]

Laborde's explanation of the pathogenesis of softening revolved around the circulation at the level of the smallest vessels. He claimed it all started with congestion, a view propounded earlier by Durand-Fardel; he thought the dilatation eventually damaged the capillaries, especially in the aged, resulting in extravasation and mechanical damage ('necrobiosis') of nervous tissue.[111] Laborde briefly considered embolism, which had been recognized meanwhile, but dismissed it in a footnote as irrelevant.[112]

---

[106] Calmeil (1826), *De la Paralysie considérée chez les Aliénés*, 348–9.
[107] Deniker (1903), J. V. Laborde; Poirier (2015), Le docteur Jean-Baptiste Vincent Laborde.
[108] Laborde (1866), *Le Ramollissement et la Congestion du Cerveau*, 1–28.
[109] Laborde (1866), *Le Ramollissement et la Congestion du Cerveau*, 271–327.
[110] Laborde (1866), *Le Ramollissement et la Congestion du Cerveau*, 29.
[111] Laborde (1866), *Le Ramollissement et la Congestion du Cerveau*, 208–9 and 231–5.
[112] Laborde (1866), *Le Ramollissement et la Congestion du Cerveau*, 221–2 and 227.

Microscopy of Cerebral Softening: More Heat than Light

Attempts to resolve the pathogenesis of brain softening extended to micro-scopy, but in vain. Laborde based his congestion hypothesis on tissue sections stained with early techniques; he found that capillaries at first dilated, then progressively disintegrated.[113]

Before that time, others had tried to resolve the issue without stains. Gottlieb Gluge (1812–1898), born in Westphalia and, in 1838, appointed Professor of Pathological Anatomy at the University of Brussels,[114] had found globules of aggregated blood cells and regarded these as evidence of inflam-mation at the capillary level.[115] John Hughes Bennett (1812–1875), a physician and an extra-academic teacher in Edinburgh,[116] had distinguished inflamma-tory softening, characterized by 'exudation granules, masses or corpuscles', from non-inflammatory softening, in which the nervous tubes were merely broken up into fragments. He associated non-inflammatory softening mostly with an acute onset of symptoms, but thought these changes occurred post-mortem.[117]

A Deadlock

In the middle of the nineteenth century, the understanding of *ramollissement* had run aground, in Paris and elsewhere. From whichever direction one approached the problem, confusion was the result. If the starting point was the presence of softened brain tissue (Rostan, Lallemand, Durand-Fardel), this made room for patients with an acute, as well as a gradual, onset of disease. If patients from institutions for mental disease (*dementia paralytica*) were included, as Laborde had done, the clinical heterogeneity of brain softening became even more baffling. Microscopical analysis merely increased the confusion.

If, instead, clinical criteria were used to distinguish patients with either hemiparesis or hemiplegia as the first symptom, the underlying pathological change could indeed turn out to be brain softening, but also haemorrhage or inflammatory disorders.

As physicians have learnt since, the only solution is to combine the clinical and pathological approach and to distinguish two kinds of softening, according to the manner of onset of the patient's symptoms. This is what Abercrombie, Andral, and Carswell had explicitly proposed, and Fuchs and Hasse in a more implicit fashion. But the factions who interpreted softening as an indivisible

[113] Laborde (1866), *Le Ramollissement et la Congestion du Cerveau*, xiv–v and 115–28.
[114] Zylberszac (1977), Gottlieb Gluge.
[115] Gluge (1840), Recherches microscopiques sur le ramollissement du cerveau.
[116] Hirsch (1884–8), *Biographisches Lexikon*, vol. I, 396–7.
[117] Bennett (1843), Inflammation of the nervous centres.

disorder were still too powerful and also too much preoccupied with defending the origin of softening in general as either inflammation or an idiopathic degenerative process. The confusion had also struck Adrien Proust (1834–1903), future Professor of Hygiene, as well as future father of the novelist Marcel Proust. In 1866, he submitted a thesis on the subject of *ramollissement* in the competition for the rank of *professeur agrégé*;[118] with wholehearted approval, he cited the verdict of his colleague Sigismund Jaccoud (1830–1913), who had lamented in a book review:

> What conclusion do we have to draw from facts so numerous and so diverse? It is clear: one should not regard them as the same thing. Trying to torture the facts in order to classify them under the same heading is an illogical attempt. It was possible to undertake this at a time when one was relatively poorly informed on the nature and the pathology of these different kinds of softening; by then one could regard it as a *morbid category*, and defend it with some semblance of reason. But today that is impossible, softening of the brain being an anatomical condition one encounters in the most disparate conditions of the brain, resulting from the most diverse events.[119]

It required the efforts of an ambitious 26-year-old farmer's son, born and reared near the Baltic Sea, to get things again moving.

---

[118] Proust (1866), Ramollissement du cerveau, 24.   [119] Jaccoud (1861), Bibliographie.

SEVEN

THROMBOSIS AND EMBOLISM

SUMMARY

In an early part of his career, Virchow established that intravascular clotting is unrelated to inflammation, and also that clots can be dislodged and carried along, until they become stuck (embolism). The young Charcot, on reading this, proposed embolism as the cause in some hitherto unexplained post-mortem findings; wider acceptance took time.

Once occlusion of brain arteries had been identified as a cause of sudden deficits such as hemiplegia, not only embolism, but also local arterial thrombosis was proposed as a potential cause (Bristowe, Lancereaux). The anatomical distinction between thrombosis and embolism proved difficult (Prévost and Cottard, Walker); in addition, suspected emboli might disappear. Not only the heart, but also the aorta was a potential source of embolism. It emerged in the second half of the nineteenth century that arterial lesions resulted not only from atherosclerosis, but also from syphilis, especially in young males.

If softening could not be attributed to embolism from the heart or aorta, nor to syphilitic arteritis, atherosclerosis was the suspected cause, particularly in older patients. The main arteries of the brain were most often suspected as the sites of atherothrombotic disease; yet the evidence for thrombosis at these locations was scarce.

Historians of science tend to distrust the term 'revolution', but the identification of disease processes associated with brain softening in the middle of the nineteenth century lays some claim to this epithet. To introduce yet another anathema: a single person was mainly responsible. His name is Rudolf Virchow (1821–1902) (Box 7.1), the 'little doctor', full of ambition and

Box 7.1 Rudolf Virchow (1821–1902).

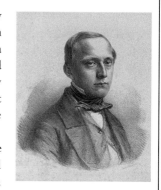

Rudolf Virchow was the first and only child of Carl Virchow and Johanna Maria Hesse, in Schivelbein (now Polish Swidwin), Pomerania. The family lived on farming. After a mix of primary school and private teaching, Rudolf attended the gymnasium in Köslin, as a boarder. Being a university student was expensive; with some help, he earned a place at the Pépinière, the school for military doctors in Berlin, where he lived more or less as a soldier.

By chance, Virchow, in 1846, became *Prosektor* at the University Hospital (Charité), instead of spending the usual eight-year stint with troops. Early in 1848, sent on a mission to report on an epidemic of typhus in upper Silesia, he ruffled some feathers by criticizing local authorities and calling for social reforms. His sympathy for democracy in that year of revolutions branded him a suspect when the state lashed back in 1849. Expecting disciplinary measures, Virchow accepted an offer from Würzburg to fill the first chair of Pathological Anatomy in the German states. There, he kept far from politics; he published extensively, mostly in a new journal he and Reinhardt had founded in 1847, *Archiv für pathologische Anatomie und Physiologie und klinische Medicin*. In 1850, he married 18-year-old Rose Mayer, the daughter of a gynaecologist he had befriended in Berlin. They were to have six children.

In 1856, the faculty in Berlin called him back; Virchow's fame now outweighed his liberal past. Promises included not only a chair for Pathological Anatomy, but also a separate institute, as in Würzburg. His book *Cellularpathologie* (1858; '*omnis cellula e cellula*', against Rokitansky's 'blastema' theory) earned much acclaim, though the cell theory was the work of Theodor Schwann (1810–1882) and Robert Remak (1815–1865).

After the 1860s, Virchow continued to flourish as the head of a growing institute, as a national and international icon of science, and as a politician. He was a delegate in the municipal council of Berlin (1859–1902), the Prussian parliament (1861–1902), and, following German unification, the Reichstag (1880–1891). He believed in rational solutions ('Politics is just like medicine, but on a large scale'). In 1865, he came at loggerheads with the Chancellor von Bismarck over military expenses and barely escaped a duel. He became highly interested in anthropology and co-founded societies for this discipline.

Virchow was initially ambivalent about Darwinism and critical of statistics and bacteriology; he was only gradually won over to contagionism. In the 1880s, he had to compete with Robert Koch, then another celebrity, over funds and cadavers. In that same period, he fiercely spoke out against antisemitism, then increasingly rearing its head. In January 1902, he broke his thigh bone on jumping from an electric streetcar. His health gradually deteriorated; he died in September of that same year. His funeral was a national event.

Source: Portrait: drawing made around 1849 by Ludwig Pietsch (1824–1911); courtesy of Rijksmuseum, Amsterdam.

self-confidence.[1] He figured briefly in the chapter about haemorrhage, because in 1851, he drew attention to local dilatation of arterioles at the brain surface. A few years before that more or less incidental finding, Virchow had made a head start in his career with another subject, soon after his appointment in 1846 as *Prosektor* at the Charité hospital in Berlin.

BLOOD VESSELS, CLOTTING, AND INFLAMMATION

At the time, pathological anatomy hardly existed as a discipline; only in Vienna, the university had just created a chair. The first problem the 25-year-old Virchow decided to tackle was the relation between coagulation and the accretions that were often found on the inner surface of arteries and veins. Often these changes were somewhat loosely called 'phlebitis' and 'arteritis', on the assumption that the clots resulted from an inflammatory process;[2] the paradigm of inflammation was still dominant in medicine. Virchow analysed these abnormalities of vessels in three parts: first coagulation, then lesions in veins, and finally those in arteries.

Coagulation

Fibrin (*Faserstoff*) was known only in the form of blood clots, once coagulation had occurred. A first question was whether there were different kinds of fibrin, as believed by, for instance, Carl Rokitansky (1804–1878; Vienna) and François Magendie (1783–1855; Paris). Virchow established there was only a single form of fibrin;[3] the chemical heterogeneity of its proteinaceous forms, he showed, was artefactual and merely resulted from differences in mechanical properties of clots.[4]

The formation of fibrin was thought to depend on some sort of soluble, protein-like pre-molecule, but it was an open question in which body fluids this precursor protein – or perhaps fibrin itself – could be found. Through series of experiments, Virchow established that fibrin itself never occurred in body fluids, but that circulating blood contained a close forerunner, for which he proposed the term 'fibrinogen';[5] a more distant precursor occurred in lymphatic fluids. Coagulation occurred by contact with uneven surfaces; oxygen enhanced the process[6] but was not indispensable.[7]

---

[1] Ackerknecht (1957), *Rudolf Virchow*; Goschler (2009), *Rudolf Virchow*.
[2] Rokitansky (1844), *Handbuch der speciellen pathologischen Anatomie*, vol. 1, 522–8.
[3] Virchow (1845), Faserstoff; form der Gerinnung.
[4] Virchow (1846a), Chemische Eigenschaften des Faserstoffs; Virchow (1846b), Physikalische Eigenschaften des Faserstoffs.
[5] Virchow (1846b), Physikalische Eigenschaften des Faserstoffs, 583.
[6] Virchow (1856c), Ursprung des Faserstoffs. Drafted in 1846, the report was published much later.
[7] Virchow (1847b), Zur pathologischen Physiologie des Bluts.

'Phlebitis'

On several occasions, Virchow had found blood clots in the arterial system of the lungs without corresponding changes in the vessel wall; also, some clots straddled the site where a pulmonary artery split into different branches. These observations sparked the idea that clots might have originated in veins and had been transported from their site of origin to the pulmonary arterial system. However, it was unclear whether venous blood could actually carry along such chunks and whether passage through the right atrium and ventricle could take place without symptoms.

To test his hypothesis, Virchow performed several experiments in dogs. He exposed the jugular vein on the left side; by applying ligatures, he opened the vessel and, in succession, introduced different kinds of foreign material: at first clots, from cadavers or from venesection, then pieces of wood (elder pith), and finally Indian rubber. Before closing the wound, he pushed the objects downward with a probe, at least as far as the subclavian vein. After a few days, during which time no uncommon symptoms occurred, the animals were sacrificed; invariably he retrieved the objects in the pulmonary arteries.[8]

On studying instances of 'phlebitis' in cadavers, Virchow found that once a clot in a vein had formed, the process of coagulation often did not halt where the vessel joined a larger vein, but extended for some distance into the lumen of the larger vein. In this way, the top of the clot, exposed to a more active flow than at its site of origin, could be detached and carried away by the bloodstream (Figure 7.1).[9]

'Arteritis'

Virchow began by scrutinizing the two arguments underlying the notion that clotting in arteries was secondary to an inflammatory process. The first was the focal redness that was sometimes seen in the intimal layer. Histological examination of the arterial wall made it abundantly clear that nutritive vessels (*vasa vasorum*), if present, were always located at the outside of the vessel, while its inner layers were completely devoid of such nutritive capillaries. As a consequence, he reasoned, inflammatory redness of the intimal layer by capillary hyperaemia is impossible. The second issue was the assumption that a coagulum on the inner surface of an artery was covering an exudate or had merged with it. From a series of experiments on dogs, in which Virchow painted the outer layers of the carotid artery with a variety of corrosive substances, he

[8] Virchow (1846c), Verstopfung der Lungenarterie.
[9] Virchow (1846c), Verstopfung der Lungenarterie; Virchow (1856b), Verstopfung der Lungenarterie, 245.

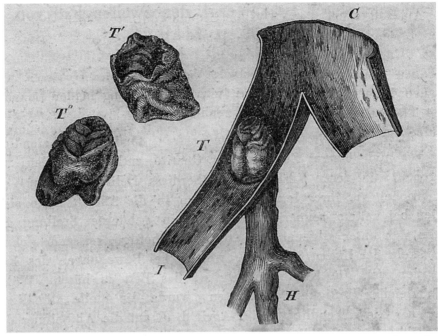

7.1 Venous thrombosis and the manner in which the top of a thrombus can be carried along by the bloodstream. From a 1856 reprint of Virchow (1846), 245. His legend reads, in translation: 'Extension of a thrombus (T) from the *Vena hypogastrica dextra* (H) into the *Vena iliaca* (I). The *Vena cava* (C) is completely free. T′: the [top part of the] thrombus seen from behind and right; T″: the same from the front and left, somewhat enlarged.'

concluded that inflammatory reactions occurred only in the outer layers of a vessel and that exudates never appeared on the inner epithelial layer. If the noxious substances did penetrate the vessel wall as far as the inner covering, the result was necrosis, followed by clotting.[10] All this proved to Virchow that clots found inside arteries represented a primary process, without preceding inflammation.

He cited a case of brain softening as an example of a local clot in an artery that could be directly related to the clinical features. The patient, 46-year-old Friedrich Wichmann, had suddenly been struck by left-sided hemiplegia and a decreased level of consciousness; he died a week later. Dissection showed tortuosity of the arteries at the base of the brain and atheromatous thickening of the right 'artery of the Sylvian fossa', with a thrombus at that same site and extensive softening in the right hemisphere. In the heart, the left ventricle was hypertrophic and the mitral valve thickened at its borders. The descending aorta contained calcifications.[11]

[10] Virchow (1847a), Akute Entzündung der Arterien, 272–312.
[11] Virchow (1847a), Akute Entzündung der Arterien, 323–4.

Virchow added that several analogous cases had been reported in the existing literature. However, he used the findings in this patient only as a starting point, since he wished to draw attention to a special category of arterial occlusions, in which the site of occlusion and the site of origin were not the same:

> In contrast with this kind of a locally occlusive clot, there exists another one. In that kind there are either no essential changes in the vessel wall or its vicinity, or only changes that are evidently of secondary nature. In that case the alterations in the vessel wall have to be regarded as the immediate consequence of the modified shape of its lumen. I feel totally justified in postulating that these clots have never arisen on the very spot, but have been torn off at some distant site of the circulation and were carried with the blood stream, as far as they could.[12]

The directness of Virchow's argumentation is striking. But he had proofs up his sleeve.

Embolism from the Heart

After another experiment in a dog, with a piece of Indian rubber – demanded by his innate rigour, despite the evidence of such transport in veins – Virchow produced seven convincing case reports in humans. In three of them, the brain was involved. Since each of his reports fills several pages, a paraphrase of a single example will have to suffice:

The patient, Franz Kruse, 27 years old, had been feverish for five weeks, when he suddenly started to 'speak nonsense'. The next day he was admitted to the Charité; he could give no information about himself. No important changes occurred until day 13, when he somehow indicated severe pain in his left foot; in the course of the next four days, the pain was unchanged and even moved upwards, as far as halfway up the left thigh. Meanwhile the skin showed blotches of blue-red colour, which became confluent; eventually, parts of the skin came off. On day 33, the patient was 'soporous', and on day 36, he died.

At autopsy, a blood clot emerged from the right carotid artery as it was cut, as part of the procedure to remove the brain; the intracranial part of the artery was patent, but the part from the ophthalmic artery to the bifurcation had an uneven surface. The cortex of the operculum and insula on the right was softened. In the left leg, partly purulent clots had lodged in the popliteal artery, at its bifurcation, and in the femoral artery, where the deep branch went off. On the right, the common iliac artery also contained a plugged clot. In the heart, the left ventricle was hypertrophic; the mitral valve was thickened,

---

[12] Virchow (1847a), Akute Entzündung der Arterien, 327.

especially at its posterior leaflet, and covered with fatty, frayed strands of coagulum.[13]

Even though the findings in this and in six similarly sad case histories almost spoke for themselves, Virchow, one by one, pounded his arguments home:[14]

1. The occluding clots are found where a vessel becomes narrower, or at its bifurcation;
2. Occluding clots can be found in different and distant parts of the arterial tree;
3. The primary coagulum and the distant, occlusive clot are similar in structure;
4. The symptoms caused by the occlusion appear suddenly;
5. At the site of impaction, the clot causes reactive changes, with secondary clotting.

'Embolism' is the term now used for the phenomena Virchow described in 1847; he himself used the term for the first time at a meeting in 1852, more or less in passing; the lecture was published two years later.[15] From then on, he regularly used the term, as if it were a household name. It is uncertain whether Virchow borrowed the expression from an existing source or devised it himself, well versed as he was in classical languages. The word is derived from the ancient Greek word *'embolos'*, for 'something plugged in'. The phenomenon as such was not entirely new in medicine. Wepfer and van Swieten are well-known examples of physicians who entertained the possibility that 'polypous' concretions were ferried along by the bloodstream.[16] Others had reported the simultaneous occurrence of a venous or arterial site where clotting occurred, usually the heart, and occlusion of an artery downstream, but either they had not yet made the connection,[17] or such an event had been suspected but lacked anatomical proof.[18]

VIRCHOW'S 'EMBOLISM' BECOMES KNOWN ELSEWHERE

Given the prominence of Parisian hospitals in the first half of the nineteenth century, medical journals and minutes of scientific societies from that city were well read in other parts of the world. Traffic of new knowledge in the reverse direction was somewhat slower. In the 1850s, Jean-Martin Charcot (1825–1893) (Box 7.2)[19] was one of the first in Paris to follow Virchow's trail. At the time,

[13] Virchow (1847a), Akute Entzündung der Arterien, 338–42.
[14] Virchow (1847a), Akute Entzündung der Arterien, 367–70.
[15] Virchow (1854), Verstopfung der Gekrösarterie, 346.
[16] Wepfer (1658), *Observationes anatomicae*, 196–7; van Swieten (1755–72), *Commentaria*, vol. I, 184.
[17] Buess (1946), Zur Geschichte des Embolie-Begriffs.
[18] Pioch (1847), Un cas de gangrène partielle du pied.
[19] Thuillier (1993), *Monsieur Charcot de la Salpêtrière*; Goetz, et al. (1995), *Charcot: Constructing Neurology*.

Box 7.2 Jean-Martin Charcot (1825–1893).

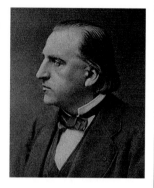

Charcot's father, a carriage-maker and decorator, and his wife Jeanne-Georgette Saussier (almost seventeen at the time of Jean-Martin's birth) were modest, but respectable middle-class citizens. Jean-Martin was their second son; two more boys were to follow; the mother died when Jean-Martin was five years old. He started his medical education in 1843. Formal lectures were only part of the programme, next to walking the wards, dissections, and private courses. Charcot became *externe des hôpitaux* in 1846. All steps of medical careers were highly competitive and often consisted of an examination, both in the medical faculty (thesis, *agrégation*, professorial chair) and in the hospital system. Charcot graduated in 1853 and became a *médecin des hôpitaux* in 1856; his first post was at the central health office, for outpatient triage.

In 1860, he became an *agrégé*, at the second attempt, and two years later chief of service, at the Salpêtrière, together with his friend Alfred Vulpian (1827–1887). Together they undertook a systematic inventory of the thousands of women in the hospice; many had been broadly designated as having 'neuroses'. Meanwhile Charcot had developed an interest in diseases of the nervous system; he attempted to correlate their symptoms with morphological abnormalities at autopsy, including microscopic analysis. In this way, he defined multiple sclerosis, muscular dystrophies, amyotrophic lateral sclerosis, Parkinson's disease (Charcot's term), and locomotor ataxia, called tabes dorsalis by Erb. Also, he encouraged and assisted younger physicians in research on cerebrovascular disease – an undervalued aspect of his work.

In 1872, Charcot obtained a professorship, again at the second attempt in Pathological Anatomy. From the 1870s onwards, Charcot's interest gradually shifted to hysteria. Several factors are responsible for the transition from a clinico-anatomical approach to a functional explanation of disease. To begin with, an administrative decision assigned him a ward with many 'hysterical' patients from the service of a psychiatric colleague. Furthermore, Charcot may well have expected that structural correlations would eventually turn up. Thirdly, while his clinical teaching had always been popular, the demonstrations of hysterical patients, sometimes with the help of hypnotism, had such a dramatic effect that he became caught up in a process of reinforcement by success. In 1882, the government created a special professorial chair of Nervous Diseases for Charcot. The resulting authority and international fame, crowned by his election to the *Académie des sciences* (1883), must have made him impervious to criticism, though there was no lack of it.

Needless to say, Charcot had a large private practice; wherever he travelled, influential patients sought his advice. From 1890, he had attacks of chest pain; three years later, he suddenly died on a brief trip to the countryside. In 1864, he had married Victoire Durvis, a young widow; they had a daughter Jeanne and a son Jean-Baptiste, who trained as a physician but became a celebrated polar explorer.

Source: © *Bibliothèque de l'Académie nationale de médecine*, Paris.

he was only 25 years old and a senior assistant physician (*interne des hôpitaux*); in that function, he still practised general medicine in its broadest sense. All this took place at least a decade before Charcot was to guide Bouchard in his studies of brain haemorrhage and its causes (see Chapter 6).

Charcot Solves a Riddle

In 1851, at a meeting of the *Société de biologie*, Charcot presented the case of a patient he had seen in the Charité, under the supervision of Professor Pierre Adolphe Piorry (1794–1879). A 29-year-old journalist had been admitted with diffuse joint pains. In the course of his illness, he developed fever, delirium, and left-sided hemiplegia; he died after three weeks. At autopsy, the brain showed softening of an area lateral to the right ventricle. The heart was hypertrophic, and the valves thickened, cartilaginous, and ulcerated. The spleen had grown to an enormous size; sectioning revealed many large spots, coloured yellow or dark red. Similar spots were visible in the kidneys and in the small and large bowels; Charcot called them pus-like globules. He had no explanation for the disease and hoped that new observations would resolve the issue.[20]

Four years later, for the same society, Charcot discussed the case history of Marie Fromentin, 86 years old. He had seen her at the end of 1852, during his time as an *interne* at the Salpêtrière. She had already been living for two years in its hospice section when she was admitted to the hospital. By then, she complained of pain in both legs, especially the left, which was also colder than the right leg. On examination, her heart seemed enlarged, with audible bruits; the pulse was irregular. The left leg became progressively gangrenous and the patient died on the eighteenth day after admission. On dissection, the heart was found to be very large; the aortic valve showed some calcified concretions. Clots were found in both femoral arteries and also in the arteries of the left lower leg. The spleen, kidneys, and liver showed one or more yellow-red spots, of varying size, up to 2 centimetres; on microscopical examination, these did not consist of pus, but of fibrin, amorphous or granular, sometimes mixed with elements of blood.[21] In the discussion, Charcot came back on the case history he had presented four years before:

> In the observation we reported in 1851 and recall here, the patient, affected by acute rheumatism of the joints, had died of progressive brain disease, essentially characterised by subdelirium followed by coma, and by paralysis of the entire left half of the body. At autopsy the findings were, apart from multiple fibrinous deposits in the intestines and

---

[20] Charcot (1851), Substance plastique concrète dans plusieurs viscères.
[21] Charcot (1855), Gangrène du pied et de la jambe, 213–16.

numerous haemorrhagic clots, softening of the cerebral substance in the vicinity of the striate body and the optic thalamus, and in the heart fibrinous vegetations on the mitral valves, which had some sort of ulceration at their free borders. At that time, the events that had led to the patient's death were for us inexplicable. [...] Interesting contributions that we owe to foreign physicians, the most important of which are beyond question those of professor Virchow and doctor Kirkes,[22] have in recent times at last thrown some light on this kind of affections, which undoubtedly will be encountered quite often in practice.[23]

This episode illustrates Charcot's habit of reading widely, a characteristic that particularly impressed his superiors, often more so than his responses to direct questions at examinations.[24] On this occasion, however, not everyone was immediately convinced by his interpretation of these two cases.

Hypotheses from 'Beyond the Rhine'

Charcot's audience for his retrospective diagnosis was the membership of the *Société de biologie* he had joined in 1851. This society had been founded in 1848 as a forum where different disciplines could meet, at a time of increasing specialization. The membership included not only physicians, but also chemists, naturalists, anthropologists, anatomists, and physiologists; in these meetings, clinicians could exchange ideas with laboratory scientists, for example François Magendie (1783–1855), Claude Bernard (1813–1878), or Charles-Philippe Robin (1821–1885).[25] A purely clinical society was the *Société médicale des hôpitaux de Paris*, established in 1849 for senior physicians who had gone through the ranks of *interne des hôpitaux* and *chef de clinique* to that of *médecin de l'hôpital*, in other words chief of service. Applicants for membership of the *Société médicale* had to submit a scientific report, which was subsequently examined by a committee of three members.

In 1857, two years after Charcot's above presentation for the *Société de biologie*, Dr Jules Béhier (1813–1876), a future Professor of Medicine, now chairman of an admission committee of the *Société Médicale*, presented and discussed a report submitted by a colleague seeking corresponding membership. The candidate was Dr Bourgeois (n.d.), from the *Hôpital Beaujon* in Étampes, a little south of Paris. Bourgeois invited the opinion of the society on two young patients in whom typhoid fever had been complicated by gangrene of a leg; one case had ended in death (without autopsy), and the other in survival after amputation.[26] Though the committee had doubts about

[22] See below.   [23] Charcot (1855), Gangrène du pied et de la jambe, 217–18.
[24] Goetz, *et al.* (1995), *Charcot: Constructing Neurology*, 24.
[25] Goetz, *et al.* (1995), *Charcot: Constructing Neurology*, 20–3.
[26] Béhier and Bourgeois (1857), Gangrène des membres, 412–16.

the diagnosis of typhoid, Béhier commented, the important question was the cause of the arterial occlusions. The committee members favoured arteritis, a primary inflammatory process at the inner surface of the vessel, as previously described by Guillaume Dupuytren (1777–1835). The theory of 'embolism', proposed by Virchow and taken up by several others, including Charcot,[27] was in their opinion still a hypothesis, lacking rigorous demonstration.[28]

The subsequent discussion was extensive and continued over two subsequent sessions.[29] Several speakers in the audience passionately defended the existence of inflammatory arteritis, though most acknowledged the existence of embolism, for example because it helped to explain 'white softening' of the brain. But Béhier refused to budge:

> Those who, like me, are forced to investigate matters quite closely, see every day that words give a certain weight to the very questionable things they are supposed to signify. I do not wish us to be too easily convinced by those heavy words that have come from beyond the Rhine, like *embolism*, or *uremia*, and which tend to steer ideas in a completely wrong direction. They disguise a serious fact, for they disguise an entirely new and unprecedented pathology, for I see nothing but hypotheses there. It is up to us, us *médecins des hôpitaux*, to proclaim this clearly, in order to protect the minds against these exaggerations.[30]

However, soon afterwards, one of the attendees castigated the provincialism shown by some discussants in another Parisian journal; he extensively cited Virchow.[31] Also in the same year of 1857, Charles Schützenberger (1809–1881), Professor of Medicine at the University of Strasbourg, published a concise treatise in which he confirmed Virchow's findings on every count.[32] Soon the number of publications with similar findings multiplied. In 1860, Bernhard Cohn (1827–1864), a physician in Breslau, published an entire book on blood vessels affected by embolism.[33] One of the chapters dealt with embolism of cerebral vessels.

Brain Softening through Embolism

Cohn's book contained nine histories of patients in whom endocarditis or atherosclerosis of the aortic arch had been the source of embolism to the brain,

---

[27] His presentation had also appeared in a general medical journal (Charcot (1856), *Dépots fibrineux multiples*).
[28] Béhier and Bourgeois (1857), *Gangrène des membres*, 426.
[29] Béhier and Bourgeois (1857), *Gangrène des membres*, 428–32, 488–92, and 501–14.
[30] Béhier and Bourgeois (1857), *Gangrène des membres*, 512.
[31] Sée (1857), *Discussion sur l'artérite*.
[32] Schützenberger (1857), *De l'oblitération subite des Artères*.
[33] Cohn (1860), *Embolischen Gefässkrankheiten*.

with many details. For example, a 66-year-old man became suddenly hemiplegic on the right, which almost completely cleared within days. Six months later, the paralysis recurred, with loss of consciousness and death after five days. Autopsy showed an embolus plugging the common carotid artery, followed by secondary thrombosis with complete occlusion of the internal carotid and part of the Sylvian artery. The corresponding brain area was softened; two large branches contained fresh clots, apparently 'metastatic', broken off from the more proximal site of thrombosis.[34] In seven other patients, the embolus had lodged in the internal carotid artery or the Sylvian artery in its main stem or its branches, and in a ninth patient in the basilar artery. These observations, supplemented by experiments in dogs, led Cohn to conclude that 'brain softening is in its essence nothing else than necrosis, decay of brain tissue'.[35]

Embolism as the Paradigm of Ischaemic Brain Softening

The identification of arterial embolism as a cause of vascular occlusion was important in more than one way. For medicine in general, it allowed an explanation of many morphological and functional abnormalities that had been mysterious until then. But with respect to brain disease, the notion of embolism was crucial in ending the controversy over the question of whether or not arterial occlusion could be the sole cause of cerebral softening. After all, in the 1850s, the pathogenesis of brain softening in general was still heavily controversial. Several schools of physicians still believed that an inflammatory brain lesion preceded the process of clotting – even in patients whose symptoms had appeared suddenly. This is how two Parisian neurologists from the generation after Charcot looked back on this episode in their textbook chapter on brain softening, viewing these old ideas as part of a distant past:

> It is already long ago that this problem provoked so many investigations, so many treatises, so many controversies, all of which have been consigned to oblivion by a brief note of Virchow.[36]

But of course, the medical world had to get used to the new idea. Chance observations such as that of a Parisian patient in whom cerebral softening had occurred as a result of a sarcomatous brain tumour compressing the Sylvian artery also helped to confirm the idea that occlusion of the arterial lumen was the key issue.[37]

---

[34] Cohn (1860), *Embolischen Gefässkrankheiten*, 363–7.
[35] Cohn (1860), *Embolischen Gefässkrankheiten*, 388.
[36] Brissaud and Souques (1904), Maladies de l'encéphale, 193.
[37] Hayem (1869), Oblitération des artères sylviennes. Georges Hayem (1841–1933) became a haematologist.

But in earlier times, before new insights associated brain softening with clots torn loose from heart valves or from atheromatous lesions in the aorta, subsequently becoming wedged downstream in an intracerebral artery, physicians had already found thrombotic lesions in situ, believed to have originated there. Think of Hasse, Carswell, Bouchut, and other authors encountered so far. All these cases had been attributed to 'arteritis' or to local thrombosis; had the causes, in fact, been emboli?

Examples of Local Thrombosis

No, was the emphatic answer of John Syer Bristowe (1827–1895), a pathologist at St Thomas' Hospital in London. In his article of 1859, he referred to the observations of W. Senhouse Kirkes (1822–1864) of a few years earlier, as Charcot had done. Kirkes had written, on account of three patients: '... softening of a portion of the brain, with attendant loss of function, may result from obstruction of a main cerebral artery by the lodgement of a plug of fibrin within its canal, and the foreign substance thus obstructing the vessel is probably not formed there, but is derived directly from warty growths situated on the left valves of the heart.'[38] Kirkes had not mentioned Virchow; his idea may have been original. Despite these associations of arterial occlusion with emboli, Bristowe continued:

> Doctor Kirkes believes that the obstruction of cerebral vessels is mostly due to the transference of accidentally detached cardiac vegetations or clots, which, carried on by the circulating fluid, become impacted in the smaller arteries of the brain. [...] Now, considering the apparently conclusive character of these observations, considering, too, that many confirmatory cases have since been published, it is certainly remarkable that not one of the seven cases which constitute my experience affords a positive instance of doctor Kirkes's law; in five of the number there were no old cardiac clots or vegetations at all; and in the remaining two, although friable excrescences were connected with the valves, it was anything but clear that the plugs in the cerebral arteries were dependent on the conveyance thither, and arrest therein, of fragments of these excrescences.[39]

Indeed, there was little reason to suspect embolism from the heart in Bristowe's seven examples of thrombotic obstruction of the internal carotid artery and its branches (six patients) or the vertebrobasilar system (one patient). This duality of causes – local thrombosis and embolism – raised new questions.

---

[38] Kirkes (1852), Detachment of fibrinous deposits, 300.
[39] Bristowe (1859a), Analysis of seven cases of obstruction of the cerebral arteries.

What kind of occlusion was most common, thrombotic or embolic? Could the two be distinguished during life?

THROMBOSIS OR EMBOLISM?

A First Review

In 1862, Étienne Lancereaux (1829–1910) submitted a doctoral thesis in Paris on thrombosis and embolism in the brain. Later on, he was to discover the relationship between the pancreas and the 'meagre form' of diabetes mellitus.[40] His thesis contained observations from the Parisian hospitals where he had served as *interne des hôpitaux*, supplemented by published cases. Of the 52 patients with occlusion within the carotid system, 40 were probably embolic and 12 thrombotic; though from a variety of sources, these numbers at least showed that cerebral embolism was all but rare.

From his personal observations, amounting to fewer than 10, almost all classified as 'thrombotic arteritis', Lancereaux warned that the aspect of the arterial wall at the site of occlusion did not always allow a distinction between local thrombosis and embolism, at least not with the naked eye, because – as Virchow had warned – embolic material could induce irritative changes in the superficial layers of the vessel. Instead, he suggested that embolic clots are generally less adherent to the wall, tend to be whitish or often heterogeneous, and cartilaginous or calcified inside and fibrinous outside, but always dry and solid.[41]

With regard to brain tissue, Lancereaux regarded the distinction of different kinds of softening according to colour as erroneous,[42] because in his view, it entirely depended on the interval between arterial occlusion and the time of death: red or pink in the first two weeks, yellow thereafter, and white after a couple of months.[43] However, earlier investigators (see Chapter 6) had found white, anaemic tissue in areas of recent softening; contemporary colleagues were soon to correct him on this point.[44] Lancereaux also noted that softening occurred only if the occlusion was located beyond the circle of Willis and that the lesion was often smaller than the area supplied by the artery in question, a difference he attributed to collateral circulation.[45]

---

[40] Wright and McIntyre (2022), Étienne Lancereaux's enduring legacy.
[41] Lancereaux (1862), Thrombose et embolie cérébrales, 17–19.
[42] Rokitansky, in Vienna, had distinguished red, white, and yellow softening as separate categories of disease (Rokitansky (1844), *Handbuch der speciellen pathologischen Anatomie*, vol. 1, 823–31).
[43] Lancereaux (1862), Thrombose et embolie cérébrales, 20–6.
[44] Prévost and Cotard (1866), *Ramollissement cérébral*, 55.
[45] Lancereaux (1862), Thrombose et embolie cérébrales, 27–9.

The clinical features, whether resulting from migratory or from 'autochthonous' clots, are necessarily similar; yet Lancereaux found that premonitory deficits, a gradual onset, and lack of improvement were perhaps more likely with local thrombosis.[46] Much more helpful, he wrote, was circumstantial evidence: if a patient is relatively young, and if there are symptoms or signs suggestive of heart disease, specifically endocarditis, embolism is a much more likely cause.[47]

The Difficulty of Determining the Origin of a Clot

In 1866, a slender treatise on brain softening appeared. It had two authors and was not linked with an academic degree. The first author submitted a formal thesis two years later, on *déviation conjuguée* (conjugate deviation) of the eyes.[48] He was Jean-Louis Prévost (1838–1927), a native of Geneva who had also studied in Zurich, Vienna, and Berlin and who ended his career as Professor of Physiology in his home town. The second author was Jules Cotard (1840–1889);[49] he later graduated with a thesis on 'partial atrophy of the brain', and then became a military surgeon and finally a general practitioner in the suburb of Vanves, developing a special interest in diabetes and mental delusions.

The supervisor of the duo was Jean-Martin Charcot (1825–1893); in that same period, he investigated 'miliary aneurysms' with Bouchard. In the meantime, Charcot had successfully passed the competition to become an *agrégé* and was therefore eligible for an academic career; in 1862, he had returned to the Salpêtrière as *médecin des hôpitaux*, or chief of service. Prévost and Cotard started their study with animal experiments of embolism, in which they injected foreign material into a carotid artery. Initially they used *Lycopodium* spores in rabbits, then tobacco grains in a large series of dogs.

Also, Prévost and Cotard reported post-mortem findings in 11 patients in whom the interval between the onset of symptoms and death had been less than two weeks, mostly less than one week, and in whom a corresponding arterial occlusion had been found. The authors attested to the difficulty of deciding between a local and a more distant origin of the clot by the scarcity of their comments on the issue. Only in the first case history, they came off the fence and favoured a local origin, for want of a possible source of emboli, but in the other ten patients, it is up to the reader to decide.[50] At any rate, this being the Salpêtrière, all women but one were over 50 years of age and six of

---

[46] Lancereaux (1862), Thrombose et embolie cérébrales, 50–1.
[47] Lancereaux (1862), Thrombose et embolie cérébrales, 72–6.
[48] Prévost (1868), Déviation conjuguée des yeux et rotation de la tête.
[49] Walusinski (2011), Jean-Martin Charcot's house officers at La Salpêtrière.
[50] Prévost and Cotard (1866), *Ramollissement cérébral*, 44–64.

them over 80, so that atherosclerotic changes were very common, in the basal arteries of the brain as well as in the aorta.

In two other patients, who had died several months after an apoplectic attack, Prévost and Cotard could still find an occlusion of brain arteries. Of all the 13 patients with verified occlusions, the most common location was the Sylvian artery (10 cases) (Figure 7.2), rarely the internal carotid artery up to its branching site, or the basilar artery.[51]

Interestingly, in five different patients with sudden hemiplegia and brain softening at autopsy, the duo failed to find arterial occlusions, even though in three of them, the interval had been relatively short, around a week.[52] A later presentation from the Salpêtrière reported the same phenomenon, in a patient with brain softening whose leg arteries had been subsequently occluded by blood clots, so there was no doubt about embolism being the cause.[53] In this case, as so often, the heart was the source, in the form of a mitral valve scarred by rheumatic fever; Charcot had provided an illustration of this abnormality in his book on diseases of old age (Figure 7.3).[54]

A Scottish Registrar in Zurich

Eliza Walker (1845–1925) (Box 7.3) deserves to be mentioned with some distinction, not only because of her thesis (1872) on occlusion of brain arteries, but also because she was one of the first women in the UK to qualify and work as a doctor, despite considerable opposition.[55] In order to study medicine, she had emigrated to Zurich, where the medical faculty had, in 1867, decided to admit women.[56] The supervisor of her thesis was Professor Michael Anton Biermer (1827–1892), former student of Virchow in Würzburg; by that time, Biermer had described acute lymphoblastic leukaemia and pernicious anaemia.

Walker tabulated all 121 cases of occluded brain arteries she managed to retrieve, from a variety of European sources; she estimated from these reports that embolism, certain or probable, was about twice as common as local thrombosis.[57] Among the 14 cases she found in the Zurich registry, the preponderance of embolism was even more marked: 10 could be classified as embolism, 3 as primary thrombosis, and in one patient the distinction was not possible.[58]

---

[51] Prévost and Cotard (1866), *Ramollissement cérébral*, 78.
[52] Prévost and Cotard (1866), *Ramollissement cérébral*, 82–6.
[53] Joffroy (1869), Organisation et retraction du caillot embolique.
[54] Charcot and Ball (1868), *Maladies des viellards*, 185 and planche II.
[55] Anonymous (1925a), Eliza Walker, M.D.; Anonymous (1825b), Eliza Walker, M.D. Zürich.
[56] Bonner (1989), Rendezvous in Zurich: a revolution in women's medical education.
[57] Walker (1872), Ueber Verstopfung der Hirnarterien, 22.
[58] Patients II, VIII, and XI; for patient XIV, the records were incomplete; classification in retrospect by JvG, not by Dr Walker.

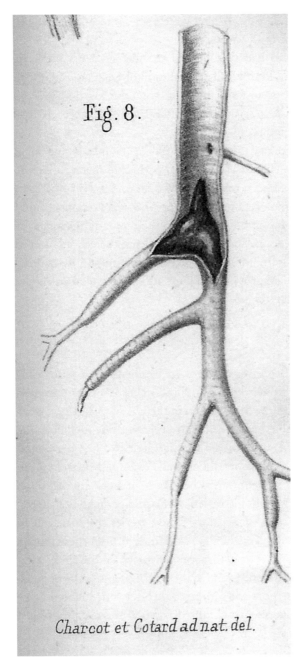

7.2 Sylvian artery obliterated by a thrombus, which extends to its branches (Prévost and Cotard, 1866; original legend, translated). Drawing made by Charcot and Cotard.

The observations of Lancereaux, and especially those of Prévost and Cotard, immediately found their way into new theses and treatises,[59] but also into

[59] Soulier (1867), Ramollissement cérébral; Grenier (1868), Ramollissement sénile du cerveau; De Visscher (1877), Hémorrhagie et ramollissement du cerveau.

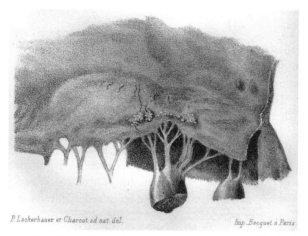

7.3 Alterations of the mitral valve in a case of generalized, chronic rheumatism of the joints (Charcot and Ball, 1868).

textbooks, in different languages. More importantly, their findings helped to ingrain the idea in medical minds, of practitioners and students, that there were two different causes of an apoplectic attack: haemorrhage and, in Charcot's words,[60] *ramollissement apoplectique*. How to tell them apart during life?

SOFTENING VERSUS HAEMORRHAGE

Softening or Haemorrhage – Thermometry?

It soon became clear that preservation of consciousness, a non-progressive course, and survival made softening at least the more likely cause. Yet some physicians, in search of more 'scientific' criteria, judged body temperature to be a suitable candidate. Boerhaave had initiated the measurement of temperature in patients, by means of the mercury thermometer developed in Leiden by Gabriel Fahrenheit (1686–1736). Boerhaave's pupils van Swieten and de Haen had regularly used the method in Vienna; subsequently, suitable instruments were produced elsewhere.[61]

In 1867, Charcot reported in a session of the *Société de biologie* that for the last two years, he had measured the rectal temperature in patients admitted within a few hours after apoplexy, from either haemorrhage or softening. He did not specify how he had made the distinction, but at any rate, the results of his measurements were similar in both groups. In the first few hours, he found a slight decrease, from the normal level of 37.5 degrees Celsius to 37 degrees

[60] Charcot (1873), Discussion, séance du 19 Juillet 1873.
[61] Pearce (2002), History of the clinical thermometer; Astruc (1952), Centenaire de la thermométrie clinique.

Box 7.3 Eliza Walker Dunbar (1845–1925).

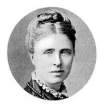 Eliza Louisa Walker was born in Bolarum, Hyderabad, where her father Alexander Walker, a physician from Aberdeenshire, was serving a stint at the Bombay Military Department. She received her secondary education first at the Ladies College in Cheltenham, Gloucestershire, then in Frankfurt am Main, where she became fluent in German. It was her decided wish to become a doctor, like her father and her brother, but unable to enrol in any British medical school, she had to be content with training at St Mary's Dispensary for Women, directed by Elizabeth Garrett (1836–1917). Garrett, her senior by nine years, driven by the same ambition and encountering the same resistance, eventually qualified in Paris. Walker travelled in 1868 to Switzerland, where the University of Zurich had decided to accept female medical students; with six women from other countries, she made up the 'Zurich 7'. Having graduated with distinction in 1872 with a thesis on occlusion of brain arteries, she was an assistant physician in the canton hospital of Zurich, and then spent a year of postgraduate study in Vienna before returning to England in 1873, where she added 'Dunbar' to her surname.

Appointed as a house surgeon at the Royal Hospital for Sick Children in Bristol, but debarred from official registration, her position was marked by controversy and opposition. In the end, she left and set up a private practice in the suburb of Clifton. In 1876, she assisted Miss Read in establishing a Dispensary for Women and Children in Hotwells, Bristol. After the King and Queen's College of Physicians, Ireland, decided to allow the registration of women with foreign degrees, she was officially registered in January 1877. Among a number of other public roles, she founded the Bristol Private Hospital for Women and Children in 1895. Dr Walker Dunbar published on diseases of children and on the role of myxoedema in puerperal eclampsia. Until old age, she remained active as a physician; her death was sudden.

Celsius, or even below, but after 24 hours, the reading was almost always back at 37.5 degrees Celsius, and in the next few days, it generally rose to values of between 37.5 and 38 degrees Celsius. Higher temperatures usually reflected a superimposed, often fatal, inflammation.[62]

A few years later, Charcot's intern Désiré-Magloire Bourneville (1840–1909) (see Box 9.1, p. 295) devoted a thesis to the subject; later on, he combined his medical career with politics and medical journalism, and founded the journal *Le Progrès médical*. Bourneville found a somewhat different pattern of the temperature in patients with brain softening, in that the decrease in the first few hours was more marked – in patients with haemorrhage, it could even be absent – and that, after a stationary phase, the subsequent increase was higher,

[62] Charcot (1867), Température dans l'apoplexie.

up to 39 to 40 degrees Celsius.[63] A later Parisian study failed to confirm the thermometric results of either Charcot or Bourneville.[64]

So it remained the prerogative of the pathologist to make a final distinction between sudden rupture and occlusion of an artery in the brain. Another question that intrigued pathologists was to understand the presence of blood in softened brain tissue.

Infarction

The different shades of white, red, and yellow encountered in softened brain tissue had sometimes spawned ideas about differences in pathogenesis, such as Cruveilhier's notion of *apoplexie capillaire*. Though physicians commonly assumed secondary infiltration by blood, the underlying events remained unclear. The interval between softening and death was not the only factor, if only because some areas of softening remained pale.

The pathologist Julius Cohnheim (1839–1884) investigated the problem systematically in experimental studies, at least for embolism. After some peregrinations, he spent a few years in the pathological institute of Berlin headed by Virchow, to whom he dedicated his monograph. At the time of publication, Cohnheim was Professor of Pathological Anatomy in Kiel; later he exchanged this post for a similar position in Breslau and then Leipzig, until his premature death.[65]

Cohnheim's preferred model for these studies was the tongue of the frog; this organ has a fairly standard pattern of blood vessels. As emboli, he used small particles of wax, blackened with soot, injected via the heart or, mostly, via the common trunk of the lingual and carotid arteries. Meanwhile the tongue had been tacked on in such a way that the events in its blood vessels could be studied with a microscope.[66]

As expected, important changes in the tissue supplied by an occluded artery occurred only if there were no arterial anastomoses distal to the embolus, that is in 'end arteries' – a term coined by Cohnheim.[67] Haemorrhagic transformation, the phenomenon that 'necrobiotic' tissue becomes filled with blood, could be explained by two different phenomena. The first, and sometimes the only, factor was stasis of venous blood, sometimes even engorgement by back flow.[68] Depending on the interval after the occlusion, a second phenomenon

---

[63] Bourneville (1872), Études cliniques et thermométriques.

[64] Hutin (1877), De la température dans l'hémorrhagie cérébrale et le ramollissement.

[65] Borte (1985), Julius Cohnheim. Cohnheim identified diapedesis of leucocytes as the cause of purulent lesions and pioneered the use of frozen tissue sections.

[66] Cohnheim (1872), *Untersuchungen ueber die embolischen Processe*, 4–9.

[67] Cohnheim (1872), *Untersuchungen ueber die embolischen Processe*, 16–18.

[68] Cohnheim (1872), *Untersuchungen ueber die embolischen Processe*, 19–28.

occurred, with extravasation through the walls of small veins and capillaries in the necrotic area – apparently their walls had been damaged by ischaemia, which allowed the passage of colourless fluid, as well as red blood cells (diapedesis), into the necrotic tissue.[69]

In warm-blooded animals, however, the interval after which engorgement and extravasation occurred was much shorter than in the frog; other factors were the position and calibre of the occluded artery – in the brain, occlusion of the main stem of the Sylvian artery could still be followed by white softening.[70] Cohnheim emphasized that the process of haemorrhagic transformation, or 'infarction' (derived from the Latin verb *infarcire*, 'to stuff'), is completely independent from the process of necrobiosis.[71] The irony of terminology has it that in current medical and public parlance, the term 'infarct', *pace* teeth-grinding purists, is used indiscriminately as a synonym for ischaemic necrosis of an organ, especially heart or brain, regardless of whether or not there has been haemorrhagic transformation.

Pathologists gradually learnt to distinguish between primary haemorrhage and haemorrhagic infiltration of softened brain tissue. The explanation of arterial occlusion often remained elusive, as Prévost and Cotard had found out. The association was obvious in young patients with known heart disease, but emboli could also originate elsewhere.

SOURCES OF THROMBO-EMBOLISM

In 1863, Jules Bucquoy (1829–1920) competed for *agrégation* with a thesis on 'sanguineous concretions'. Later, as the chief of service at the *Hôtel-Dieu*, he published a textbook on diseases of the heart that went through several editions. His thesis on blood clotting included a section on embolism of the brain.

The Heart

As a matter of course, this was the first source Bucquoy mentioned in relation to embolism:

> The most common source of arterial embolism one finds in abnormalities of the heart and the large vessels; one can be even more precise and say that in the large majority of cases it is the heart that is the point of departure. One finds here, with regard to blood clots in the heart, the role of endocarditis and especially ulcerative endocarditis; this sometimes

---

[69] Cohnheim (1872), *Untersuchungen ueber die embolischen Processe*, 28–57.
[70] Cohnheim (1872), *Untersuchungen ueber die embolischen Processe*, 58–81.
[71] Cohnheim (1872), *Untersuchungen ueber die embolischen Processe*, 62.

produces ulcerations of the valves, sometimes concretions that are fibrinous, wart-like or calcified. Often one also observes fibrinous clots in the ventricles or the auricles.[72]

However, he also mentioned large vessels:

The next common cause I list consists of changes in the aortic wall, atheroma and ulceration; these can lead to blood clots. Once formed, these [clots] are sometimes propelled into arteries of smaller calibre and produce embolism.

The Aorta

In 1855, the London physician William Gull (1816–1890) reported softening of both hemispheres in a 41-year-old woman in whom fibrous tissue had occluded the origin of both the innominate and the left common carotid artery from the aorta.[73] For Gull, the relationship between softening of the brain and its blood supply was self-explanatory. Since examples of this so-called 'pulseless disease' were uncommon,[74] as they still are, these tended to be published. Most of these unfortunate patients were young; the cause of the fibrotic obstruction was unknown. If progressive obstruction of major vessels caused failure of blood flow to the brain, the symptoms were often non-focal, recurring, or progressive, instead of apoplectic.[75]

Embolism from the aorta was also highly likely in a 50-year-old woman reported by William Markham at St Mary's Hospital in London, in 1854. She had suffered from chest problems since childhood and was eventually struck by hemiplegia shortly before her death; at autopsy, the aortic valve was abnormal and the aortic arch severely atherosclerotic, with aneurysms and thrombi.[76]

A Lemon-Shaped Aortic Aneurysm, Compressing an Extracranial Artery

Fifty years later, a peculiar report of embolism from the aorta to the brain came from Heidelberg, by Wilhelm Heinrich Erb (1840–1921).[77] He contributed much to the knowledge of neuromuscular disease and of tabes dorsalis; moreover, he discovered the medical significance of the knee jerk, at the same

---

[72] Bucquoy (1863), Des concrétions sanguines, 92–3.
[73] Gull (1855), Occlusion of the innominata and left carotid.
[74] Broadbent (1875), Absence of pulsation in both radial arteries.
[75] Yelloly (1823), Preternatural growth in the aorta; Savory (1856), Arteries of extremities and neck obliterated; Kussmaul (1872), Verschliessung grosser Halsarterienstämme; Dejerine and Huet (1888), L'aortite oblitérante; von Weismayr (1894), Stenose der Carotis und Subclavia.
[76] Markham (1857), Aneurysms at the aortic sinuses.   [77] Viets (1970), Heinrich Erb.

time as Karl Friedrich Otto Westphal (1833–1890) in Berlin. The patient Erb reported, a 50-year-old man, had received medical attention four years before; the symptoms at the time were not recorded, but examination had shown an aneurysm of the aorta and absence of pulsations in the left common carotid artery. Six months later, he was struck by hemiplegia on the right side, with aphasia; the deficits were permanent and death followed three and a half years later. Autopsy showed a spherical aortic aneurysm, with the size of a lemon. Its base was small and incorporated the origin of the *arteria anonyma*, while at its other end, it severely narrowed the lumen of the left common carotid artery; this wedged artery was filled by an organized thrombus that extended from the site of compression up to the carotid bifurcation. The left hemisphere of the brain showed cystic softening in the territory of the middle and anterior cerebral arteries. Erb wrote:

> In this case the following interpretation might be the most plausible. In the carotid, compressed by the aneurysm, an autochthonous clot has gradually developed; from this, beyond the complete occlusion of the vessel, some parts have disengaged themselves and have led to embolization in the middle cerebral and anterior cerebral arteries. These emboli have manifested themselves clinically as apoplexy [*Schlaganfall*] and caused the region of softening in the brain.[78]

Many a reader may start wondering about a middle-aged man with a lemon-sized saccular aneurysm of the aortic arch, compressing the nearby left common carotid artery to such an extent that its lumen became obliterated by thrombus. Around the same time, William Gowers (1845–1915) (see Box 12.3, p. 381), commented in his authoritative textbook of neurology that syphilitic disease of arteries was a common cause of brain softening.[79] He mentioned 'growths in the wall' and 'nodular projection on the exterior' as a frequent finding in large brain arteries. Édouard Brissaud (1852–1909) and Alexandre-Achille Souques (1860–1944) even implicated syphilis as the most common cause of arterial brain thrombosis, in their voluminous chapter on brain diseases, as part of a ten-volume '*Traité de médecine*'.[80]

Whether or not the aorta in Erb's patient was indeed infected by spirochaetes is a moot point – it was at least a definite possibility. The comments of Gowers and of his two Parisian colleagues point to an almost forgotten chapter in the history of brain softening. A brief excursion into venerology is indispensable.

---

[78] Erb (1904), Gehirnerweichung bei Obliteration der Carotis communis.
[79] Gowers (1893), *A Manual of Diseases of the Nervous System*, vol. 2, 425–6.
[80] Brissaud and Souques (1904), Maladies de l'encéphale, 211.

SYPHILIS OF THE NERVOUS SYSTEM AND ITS ARTERIES

The Nervous System

Definitive proof that syphilis essentially differs from gonorrhoea dated from 1838;[81] yet it remained still unrecognized that later stages of syphilis involved the nervous system and explained conditions with a separate status: general paralysis of the insane (see Chapter 6) or tabes dorsalis, called *ataxie locomotrice* (locomotor ataxia) west of the Rhine. These two diseases were by no means rare. For example, a physician in Bristol trying a novel treatment for tabes dorsalis could test it on 24 patients in the course of two years,[82] while general paralysis of the insane made up some 15 per cent of the inmates of lunatic asylums.[83] Since a patient's history with respect to venereal disease was notoriously unreliable, the diagnosis largely depended on perceptible manifestations of the disease, such as characteristic skin changes or exostoses, or so-called Argyll Robertson pupils.[84]

It was not until the last third of the nineteenth century that the relation between syphilis and these two serious and common neurological disorders became gradually known. General paralysis of the insane had been recognized as an inflammatory disorder in the 1820s by Antoine Bayle (1799–1858; 'arachnitis') and by Louis-Florentin Calmeil (1798–1895; 'peri-encephalitis'),[85] but it was not until 1857 that Esmarch and Jessen for the first time implicated syphilis as its cause.[86] This is not to say that their three cases instantly convinced the medical community, nor did reports that followed.[87] As late as in 1905, the discussion was still raging.[88]

Tabes dorsalis was named and defined as a clinical syndrome by Romberg in 1846;[89] Duchenne (de Boulogne; 1806–1875) called it locomotor ataxia in 1858.[90] A few years later, Charcot and Vulpian described the corresponding morphological changes in the spinal cord.[91] It was a Parisian dermatologist,

---

[81] Ricord (1838), *Traité pratique des Maladies vénériennes*; Anonymous (1970), Philippe Ricord (1800–1889), syphilographer.

[82] Clarke (1891), Suspension in the treatment of tabes dorsalis. This method to stretch the vertebral column was also recommended by Charcot for some time (Walusinski (2017b), A treatment approach gone astray?).

[83] Davis (2012), General paralysis of the insane and Scottish psychiatry.

[84] Argyll Robertson (1869), Four cases of spinal miosis.

[85] Pearce (2012), Brain disease leading to mental illness.

[86] Esmarch and Jessen (1857), Syphilis und Geistesstörung.

[87] Postel and Postel (1982), La découverte de l'étiologie syphilitique de la paralysie générale.

[88] Martial (1905), L'étiologie de la paralysie générale.

[89] Romberg (1840–6), *Lehrbuch der Nervenkrankheiten des Menschen*, 794–801.

[90] Duchenne (1858–9), De l'ataxie locomotrice progressive.

[91] Charcot and Vulpian (1862), Deux cas de sclérose des cordons postérieurs et de la moelle; Vulpian (1868), Sur l'état des nerfs sensitifs.

Jean Alfred Fournier (1832–1914), who, in 1875, postulated the causal role of syphilis.

More than one authority had reservations about the statistical evidence linking general paralysis to syphilis, for example the psychiatrist Otto Binswanger (1852–1929) and the neurologist Max Nonne (1861–1959).[92] With respect to tabes, it was Charcot who remained unconvinced,[93] perhaps partly because a close friend, the writer Alphonse Daudet, suffered from that painful affliction.[94] To complete this brief review of milestones, in 1905 a 'parasitologist' and a clinician in Berlin detected spirochaetes in genital lesions;[95] eight years later, a similar duo in New York demonstrated the organisms in the brain of patients with general paralysis.[96] Meanwhile, a serological diagnosis had been developed in Berlin.[97] The advent of penicillin in 1943 brought the long-awaited possibility of an effective cure. Back to arteries and brain softening.

Intracerebral Arteries

In 1854, two physicians in Amsterdam described a remarkable disorder in a 25-year-old man. Nine months after a primary genital infection and, after an unknown interval, an exanthematous skin eruption, he was suddenly struck by a left-sided hemiplegia; admitted to hospital, he died after six weeks. Autopsy showed at the base of the brain a yellowish, firm exudate. The right Sylvian artery was occluded by a tight, fibrinous clot; on the same side, the brain tissue was softened in the region of the basal ganglia. The purpose of the publication was to add a new feature to the many pathological manifestations of syphilis. More or less as an aside, the authors seized the opportunity to join the debate about the pathogenesis of brain softening, then at its heyday:

> We find, once more, a confirmation of the relationship that can exist between *emollitio cerebri* and obliteration of an artery, especially in cases that are neither of inflammatory nor of hydrocephalic nature. [...] That it has received the name *gangraena cerebri* is therefore not without justification.[98]

Because of all the stumbling blocks in the recognition of syphilitic arteritis, the diagnosis must often have been missed, or the physician remained uncertain. An example of the former can be found in Rudolf Virchow's epochal

[92] Binswanger (1894), Abgrenzung der progressiven Paralyse; Nonne (1913), Der heutige Standpunkt der Lues-Paralysefrage.
[93] Nitrini (2000), The history of tabes dorsalis.
[94] Thuillier (1993), *Monsieur Charcot de la Salpêtrière*, 166–72 and 195–6.
[95] Schaudinn and Hoffmann (1905), Spirochaeten in syphilitischen Krankheitsprodukten.
[96] Noguchi and Moore (1913), *Treponema pallidum* in general paralysis.
[97] Wassermann, et al. (1906), Eine serodiagnostische Reaktion bei Syphilis.
[98] Gildemeester and Hoyack (1854), Meningitis circumscipta, obturatio art. fossae Sylvii dextrae.

publication in 1847 on 'inflammation of arteries'. One of the patients, a 35-year-old man, had presented with increasing headache and sudden blindness of the left eye; a few days later, he lost a piece of bone through the left nostril. He left the hospital after six weeks, but two months later, he returned in a severely debilitated state and died after only a few days. At autopsy, Virchow found part of the left hemisphere and its membranes invaded by a firm, yellow-white, dry, somewhat friable, cheese-like mass, which had surrounded the terminal part of the left internal carotid artery and the optic nerve. The walls of the artery were abnormally thickened; the narrowed lumen contained clotted blood, extending into the Sylvian artery. There was a small area of softening in the left striate body.[99] At the time, Virchow regarded the lesion as 'tuber-culous', but on republishing this paper with other work in 1856, and having acquired more experience with lesions of syphilis in internal organs,[100] he reclassified the abnormalities as 'syphilitic'.[101]

Three years later, Bristowe still chose to add a question mark to his title 'syphilitic disease' of a paper describing a 34-year-old man with a partial left hemiplegia after a third seizure, probably epileptic in nature, followed by behavioural changes, and finally coma and death two months later. Autopsy had shown, not only two or three tough, hazelnut-sized, opaque-white, fibrinous masses in the right hemisphere, but also on the left side a brownish discoloration and obliteration of the internal carotid artery and its branches by a tough, old coagulum; the blockage corresponded to softening of the left striate body.[102]

As more reports of obstruction of brain arteries by syphilitic changes followed in the latter part of the nineteenth century, it became clear that arterial walls could be affected without simultaneous involvement of the brain parenchyma. In retrospect, Virchow's peremptory dismissal of 'arteritis' was therefore somewhat premature, although he was justified in removing it from the category of inflammations as they were known at the time, with the attendant features of exudate, redness, swelling, warmth, and pain. Another proof of the ubiquity of syphilitic disease of brain arteries is a monograph of 1874 on this subject by Otto Heubner (1843–1926),[103] later a specialist in diseases of children. He cited as many as 44 recorded cases, culled from different European sources.[104] Typically and dramatically, most patients were men in their 20s or 30s. Heubner divided luetic arteritis into three types:[105]

[99] Virchow (1847a), Akute Entzündung der Arterien, 324–6.
[100] Virchow (1858), Constitutionell-syphilitische Affectionen.
[101] Virchow (1856a), *Gesammelte Abhandlungen*, 414–16.
[102] Bristowe (1859b), Syphilitic (?) disease of the brain and liver.
[103] Haroun, *et al.* (2000), Heubner's description of the recurrent artery.
[104] Heubner (1874), *Die luetische Erkrankung der Hirnarterien*, 17–36.
[105] Heubner (1874), *Die luetische Erkrankung der Hirnarterien*, 36–46.

1. Affected arteries enveloped or at least adjoined by lesions of brain tissue, rubbery (*gummata*) or more friable (10 patients). In most of these cases, the lumen of the artery was compressed, with thrombosis. In some, the changes in the vessel wall extended beyond the area of abnormal brain tissue. Brain softening had occurred in all.

2. Lesions in brain tissue coexisted, but at a distance from the affected artery (five patients). All had shown brain softening; a thrombus was detected in all but one.

3. Affected arteries without associated changes of brain tissue (29 cases). However, in five patients of this group, the aspect of the arterial lesions and also the age of the patients were also compatible with atherosclerosis.

Heubner added three clinical observations of his own, in merciless detail, and also, but more concisely, three patients in whom he had performed only the autopsy.[106] Four of these six personal cases corresponded to the third category outlined above, and the other two with the first. Others added histological observations.[107]

Aortitis

Since atherosclerotic disease of the aorta had been implicated as a possible source of embolism to the brain, the same might apply to syphilitic lesions. Ulcerations of the wall of the aorta in young persons had occasionally been observed at autopsy in the previous century, without further comment. But once visceral lesions associated with syphilis were increasingly recognized,[108] the connection was also made for aortitis.[109] At first, separate patients were reported,[110] and later even series. In 1875, Francis H. Welch (1839–1910), a pathologist at the Army Medical School at Netley, alerted, if not upset, his audience at the Royal Medical and Chirurgical Society by claiming a causal relationship between syphilis and atypical aortic lesions, with or without aneurysm, in as many as 117 soldiers who had died – mostly in peacetime, one presumes.[111] Gradually the notion became well known in medical circles. In 1895, Paul Döhle (1855–1928) wrote from Kiel, where he would later occupy the chair of Pathology, before presenting 14 cases, with impressive illustrations (Figure 7.4):

---

[106] Heubner (1874), *Die luetische Erkrankung der Hirnarterien*, 46–123.
[107] Baumgarten (1881), Über gummöse Syphilis des Gehirns; Wendeler (1895), Histologie der syphilitischen Erkrankung der Hirnarterien.
[108] Virchow (1858), Constitutionell-syphilitische Affectionen; Moxon (1868), Visceral syphilis.
[109] Suy (2006), Morphology and aetiology of the arterial aneurysm.
[110] Wilks (1863), Syphilitic affections of internal organs.
[111] Welch (1875), Aortic aneurism in the army.

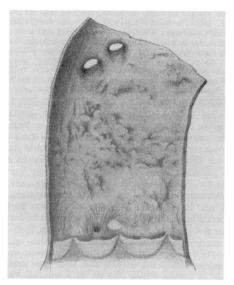

7.4 Syphilitic changes in the ascending aorta (Döhle, 1895). The patient was a 35-year-old man; he collapsed after a party and died the next day. Autopsy showed the lumen of the vena cava superior was entirely occluded and compressed by an external mass, with additional thrombosis of the [left?] jugular vein and the right *vena anonyma*. The wall of the aorta was irregularly thickened. The round, smooth-edged defect was about 4 centimetres from the aortic valve, 1 centimetre deep. On the outside of the artery, this lesion continued as an irregular, yellow-grey mass, 3–4 centimetres wide, partly solid and partly crumbled; it contained thrombus, necrotic parts, and some lung tissue.

> The frequent occurrence of diseases of blood vessels, particularly of the aorta, in patients with syphilis was a well-known fact, confirmed by several, also statistical publications.[112]

Syphilitic inflammation of the aorta or other arteries as a cause of brain softening continued to appear in medical reports until at least the middle of the twentieth century.[113]

Despite all the attention given to the role of embolism from inflamed heart valves or syphilitic aortitis, atherosclerosis remained an important factor. After all, this was the cause of softening Bright, Carswell, and other early pathologists had first implicated. Also, subsequent publications such as those of Prévost and Cotard and of Bristowe had drawn attention to atherothrombosis located more locally, of arteries in or near the brain. But where exactly?

---

[112] Döhle (1895), Aortenerkrankung bei Syphilitischen, 190.
[113] King and Langworthy (1941), Symptoms after occlusion of the carotid artery, 837–41.

AN ASSUMPTION: ATHEROTHROMBOSIS IN BRAIN VESSELS

Intracerebral Arteries?

In 1870, *The Lancet* had a regular column entitled 'Mirror of the Practice of Medicine and Surgery in the London Hospitals'. Dr Charles Kelly (1845–1904),[114] from King's College Hospital, contributed the case history of two women, 60 and 50 years old, with thrombosis of the middle cerebral artery. He criticized the idea, like his colleague Bristowe a decade before, that embolism was the most common cause of arterial occlusion of brain arteries. He therefore presented these two examples as exceptions to this rule:

> For many years the accidental plugging of an artery by a piece of fibrin detached from the valves of the heart has been recognised as a cause of white softening in that part of the brain which was supplied by that vessel. A similar result, too, is obtained when molecular particles are carried from a diseased aorta into the cerebral capillaries. Thrombosis of an artery, or the formation of a clot at the point of obstruction, is a much rarer cause; but of this kind two cases have recently been met with in the hospital. In each case the vessels at the base of the brain were very atheromatous, and at some parts their calibre was greatly impaired. At the spot where the internal carotid artery divides into the anterior and middle cerebral arteries, a firm clot of fibrin was found plugging up the middle cerebral completely. In each case the vessels were much roughened by atheromatous deposit at this point; and the altered surface would thus the more readily allow of fibrin being whipped from the blood as it flowed along. The left side of the heart and the large vessels were quite healthy; and there can be no doubt that the plug of fibrin was formed at the spot, and not carried from a distant point.[115]

The Internal Carotid Artery?

Ever since Wepfer and Willis in the seventeenth century, it was well known that inter-arterial connections safeguarded the integrity of the brain if one, or even more, of its four major arteries were occluded. Reaffirmation of this axiom appeared in *System of Medicine*, a multi-volume handbook commonly used in the second half of the nineteenth century. Under the heading 'softening of the brain', its editor J. Russell Reynolds (1828–1896), writing together with Henry Charlton Bastian (1837–1915), put it thus:

[114] https://history.rcplondon.ac.uk/inspiring-physicians/charles-kelly. [Accessed 21 November 2021]
[115] Kelly (1870), Thrombosis of the middle cerebral artery.

> In almost every case where softening of the brain is associated with
> thrombosis or embolism of the cerebral arteries, it is found that the
> obliteration exists in one of the branches beyond the circle of Willis,
> even though obliteration of the parent trunk also exists at some point
> before it gives off the branches for this anastomosis. Obliteration of the
> trunk of the carotid alone is not sufficient, under ordinary circumstances,
> to produce cerebral softening. [...] Where softening actually did occur,
> this was due either to the extension of a clot upwards, beyond the circle,
> into one of the cerebral arteries, or to some unusual distribution of the
> arteries themselves at the base of the brain, preventing the establishment
> of a collateral circulation, such as ordinarily takes place.[116]

Still, some instances of softening with carotid occlusion failed to fit this theory.
In two middle-aged patients with hemiplegia, reported in 1881 by Franz
Penzoldt (1849–1927) from Erlangen, a thrombus had occluded the contralateral carotid trunk and a proximal part of the internal carotid artery, but in
addition, the middle cerebral artery contained thrombo-embolic material. This
explained the softening and eventual death, but Penzoldt kept wondering
where the embolus had come from.[117] A reverse problem had confronted
the surgeon Norman Chevers (1818–1886) a few decades before. In the course
of an extensive review, in which he questioned the adage that carotid ligation
could always be performed safely, Chevers reported a personal case with
spontaneous occlusion of the common carotid artery in a previously healthy
stonemason with hemiplegia;[118] since the clot did not extend beyond the
carotid bifurcation, he was at a loss to explain the attendant brain softening.

Evasive Textbooks

Still, at the dawn of the twentieth century, something of a consensus seemed to
have been reached in the understanding of brain softening, although (John)
Hughlings Jackson (1835–1911) warned that the term should not be loosely
applied to persons showing a gradual decline of intellectual functions.[119]
Embolism had been well recognized; in cases where this possibility did not
seem to apply, thrombosis seemed to be the obvious explanation, starting in
arterial branches of the brain or at least extending into them. The textbooks of
this period described this process in general terms, with very little evidence.

---

[116] Reynolds and Bastian (1868), Softening of the brain, 455. With regard to anomalies of the
circle of Willis, the authors cited (with errors) a thesis from Paris (Ehrmann (1860), Ligature
de l'artère carotide).
[117] Penzoldt (1881), Thrombose der Carotis.
[118] Chevers (1845), Obliteration of the carotid arteries.
[119] Jackson (1875), A lecture on softening of the brain.

William Gowers, who also drew attention to syphilis as an important cause of softening, summarized the role of atheroma as follows:

> The larger arteries at the base of the brain are very common seats of the thickening of the inner coat, called by Virchow 'endarteritis deformans', which, when fattily degenerated, constitutes 'atheroma'. [...] A similar change may exist in arteries elsewhere, or it may be confined to those of the brain. [...] Alterations in the lining membrane lead to the formation of clot upon it, as on a foreign body. Where the calibre of the vessel is increased the current is retarded, and this also facilitates coagulation. The smaller arteries in the cerebral substance do not suffer in the same degree; but the orifices of branches coming off from an atheromatous vessel are often narrowed or closed, although the main trunk is pervious, and thrombosis may be confined to these. Atheroma is common after middle life, and increases in frequency with age.[120]

One finds a largely similar, but far more extensive, account in the authoritative textbook of 1897 on the pathology of the brain by Constantin von Monakow (1853–1930), head of the Brain Institute in Zurich and of the outpatient department of neurology.[121] In his section 'Thrombosis of Brain Arteries', he stated:

> More often than from embolism the occlusion of brain arteries results from formation of clots locally, at the arterial wall. Such occlusions are mostly secondary to atheromatous changes of the arterial wall. As a rule, the disorder affects the large arteries at the base of the brain. [...] There is no longer any doubt that the first phase consists of aggregation of blood platelets and that the uneven surface is an important factor.[122] Undoubtedly the thrombus formation is facilitated by a host of other factors, for example slowing of the circulation or turbulent flow.[123]

Incidentally, von Monakow did not forget to allot a second place to syphilis as a cause of arterial occlusion, after atherosclerosis.[124]

Lastly, in this round-up of textbooks, the legendary William Osler (1849–1919), at the time Professor of Medicine at Johns Hopkins University in Baltimore, published the first edition of his *Principles and Practice of Medicine* in 1892. His book was destined to become as popular in the first half of the twentieth century as Reynold's book had been in the preceding half century. About thrombosis and the brain, Osler wrote:

[120] Gowers (1893), *A Manual of Diseases of the Nervous System*, vol. 2, 424.
[121] Wiesendanger (2006), Constantin von Monakow.
[122] Schultze described platelets in 1862, and Bizzozero in 1882 identified their role (Brewer (2006), The discovery of the platelet).
[123] von Monakow (1897), *Gehirnpathologie*, 801.
[124] von Monakow (1897), *Gehirnpathologie*, 822.

> Clotting of blood in the cerebral vessels occurs about an embolus, as the result of a lesion of the arterial wall (either endarteritis with or without atheroma or, particularly, the syphilitic arteritis), in aneurysms both coarse and miliary, and very rarely as a result of abnormal conditions of blood. [. . .] The thrombosis is most common in the middle cerebral and basilar arteries.[125]

After Osler had died in Oxford on one of the last days of 1919,[126] his textbook was continued by colleagues. The fifteenth and last edition appeared in 1944; the text on cerebral thrombosis was entirely unchanged.[127]

From Causation to Localization

These textbook authors, though reflecting commonly accepted opinions, were not themselves researchers in the field of vascular brain disease. But even on perusing the minutes of the *Société de biologie* for the last quarter of the nineteenth century, occasions when well-read researchers convened, one finds that discussions on cerebral softening no longer, if ever, involved its *cause*. Sometimes there was dutiful, but transient, attention for the distinction between embolism and thrombosis, but the real focus of attention was shifting to the *consequences* of brain softening, in other words to attempts to find rules establishing the relationships between the site of brain lesions, often neatly demarcated, and the corresponding clinical deficits.

The history of attempts at localizing functions in the brain is a vast subject in itself, but if we leave phrenology aside and acknowledge a few landmarks such as Broca's work on language and the left frontal region,[128] Fritsch and Hitzig's experiments with electrical stimulation of dog brains,[129] and the outcome of debates such as those between Charcot and Brown-Séquard,[130] one can say the principle of localization of at least some brain functions was largely accepted around 1875. Before that time, many physicians had tried to use the presence or absence of convulsions and contractures in order to attain more predictive precision in patients with hemiplegia than the mere fact of whether the right or left hemisphere was affected. From then on, localization was the favourite sport, to put it somewhat ungraciously. Neurologists correlated certain regions of softening with neurological 'syndromes': coherent sets of defects in the motor and sensory systems, or in the patient's capacity to speak, understand, read, and write. As a next step, the process could be reversed: sets of clinical

---

[125] Osler (1892), *The Principles and Practice of Medicine*, 878–9.
[126] Bliss (1999), *William Osler: A Life in Medicine*.
[127] Christian (1944), *Osler's 'The Principles and Practice of Medicine'*, 1271–2.
[128] Broca (1861), Le siège de la faculté du langage articulé.
[129] Fritsch and Hitzig (1870), Über die elektrische Erregbarkeit des Großhirns.
[130] Charcot and Brown-Séquard (1875–6), Discussion (sur les localisations cérébrales).

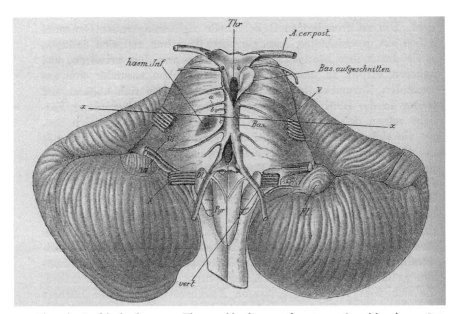

7.5 Thrombosis of the basilar artery. The vessel has been partly cut open (von Monakow, 1897, p. 806).

deficits could be transformed into a mental picture of softened lesions in the brain, the brainstem, or even the spinal cord. In contrast, brain haemorrhages were unpredictable in their extent and their course was progressive. At a further level of sophistication, correlations might include separate brain arteries, or even their branches.

The exact site of arterial thrombosis was no longer a hot topic. The thrombus was thought to have occurred 'somewhere' in the circle of Willis (Figure 7.5), at least beyond the communicating arteries. The World Fair of 1889 in Paris with its Eiffel Tower represented a widely felt impression that technological advances were nearing their peak: electricity, telephones, motor cars, the triumphs in microbiology of Koch and Pasteur – what more could follow?[131] Perhaps medicine, some may well have thought, was also nearing its apogee.

[131] Blom (2008), *The Vertigo Years*, 5–11.

EIGHT

NO MAN'S LAND: THE NECK ARTERIES

SUMMARY

In the late 1880s, Mehnert, performing a systematic study of 'angiosclerosis', found the internal carotid artery commonly affected; a few years later, Chiari identified it as a source of thrombo-embolism to the brain. Yet, throughout the first half of the twentieth century, the role of the extracranial arteries remained underestimated, for two reasons: the presence of communicating arteries and the 'concealed' location of the neck arteries, between the brain arteries and known sources of embolism. Primary atherothrombosis of intracerebral arteries was commonly assumed, even though arteries supplying a softened area could be found patent and intact (Foix and Ley).

In the 1930s and 1940s, X-rays made cerebral angiography possible (Moniz); carotid occlusion was occasionally found. However, these patients had usually manifested progressive symptoms, which had led surgeons to suspect a cerebral tumour; these cases hardly influenced ideas about cerebral softening. Some pathologists re-emphasized the relevance of atherothrombosis near the carotid bifurcation (Dörfler, Dei Poli and Zucha, Hultquist), but their reports contained few clinical details and were not written in English. In the 1950s, Fisher, combining clinical and pathological features, proved the causal relationship between cerebral infarction and stenosis or occlusion of the carotid artery, via arterio-arterial embolism or by associated lesions in other intracerebral arteries. Later studies from Paris confirmed that artery-to-artery embolism was common, especially in the anterior circulation. Carotid dissection as a cause of occlusive disease was first identified in 1944.

As more patients with cerebrovascular disease underwent angiography, surgical treat-
ment of 'carotid insufficiency' increased likewise, despite uncertainty about the balance
between risks and benefits.

The previous chapters revealed a few instances where cerebral softening was associated with thrombotic occlusion of the common or internal carotid artery, even if there was no evidence that the thrombotic process had extended beyond the circle of Willis. This problem is the focal point of the present chapter.

ATHEROSCLEROSIS AT THE CAROTID BIFURCATION

A Thesis about the Distribution of 'Angiosclerosis'

Whereas the story of thrombosis began at the western shore of the Baltic Sea, with Virchow in a pivotal role, the next part of the story starts near its eastern end, in present-day Estonia. First dominated by Polish or Swedish rulers, Estonia formed part of the Russian empire from the beginning of the eighteenth century. Its mixed population included a large German-speaking community. Their cultural centre was Dorpat (now called Tartu), with a flourishing university.

There, Ernst Mehnert (1864–1902) defended in 1888 his doctoral dissertation on the topographical distribution of angiosclerosis. Mehnert was born in St Petersburg; after his doctorate, he became *Prosektor* and Professor Extraordinarius in Halle, where he was to die before reaching the age of 40.[1] Curiously, one of the opponents at his dissertation ceremony was Emil Kraepelin (1856–1926), Professor of Psychiatry; he later taught psychiatry in Heidelberg and Munich, and singled out a category of young patients with psychotic disorders he called *dementia praecox,* now known as schizophrenia.

Though several physicians in the past two centuries had commented on degenerative changes of arteries, now known as atherosclerosis, there had been few, if any, systematic studies. Therefore, Mehnert had carefully studied the frequency and severity of the complete vascular tree in 50 consecutive dissections.[2] Following his teacher Professor Richard Thoma (1847–1923), he distinguished in the arterial system a generalized and a nodular form of 'angiosclerosis'. The generalized form, thickening and stiffness of the intimal layer, could be identified only by means of microscopy, except in severe cases.[3] The nodular form was more easily observable; Mehnert found it was frequent in the carotid artery, in its common part as well as in the internal division, in

[1] Pagel (1901), *Ärzte des neunzehnten Jahrhunderts*, 1114.
[2] Mehnert (1888), Topographische Verbreitung der Angiosclerose, 82–91.
[3] Mehnert (1888), Topographische Verbreitung der Angiosclerose, 37.

56 per cent and 60 per cent, respectively.[4] These proportions cannot be generalized, if only because 18 of the 50 patients were below 40 years of age. Yet it was striking that nodular thickening was much more common in the common and internal carotid artery than in other arteries of similar calibre. The young doctor suggested an explanation for this phenomenon, though only partially:

> The common carotid artery forms an almost direct continuation of the ascending aorta; the peculiar shape of the bifurcation and the acute curves of the internal carotid as it traverses the sphenoid bone undeniably slows down the rush of the blood to the brain, but increases the impulse of the blood in the vascular regions upstream. [...] There is no doubt that this stronger pulsation favours the common occurrence of nodular changes in this vascular region.[5]

Mehnert's dissertation did not remain unnoticed.

An Embolus from the Neck

Hans Chiari (1851–1916) (Box 8.1), Professor of Pathological Anatomy in Prague, reporting a remarkable observation at a meeting in 1905, recalled Mehnert's findings before presenting the following case:[6]

> She was a 45-year-old woman, patient from the department of Prof. Dr Pribram, with the diagnosis 'Right hemiplegia from a brain haemorrhage, 2 days before'. The left cerebral hemisphere showed fresh softening of the posterior third of the frontal lobe, the entire parietal lobe, and the lentiform nucleus with the internal capsule, as a result of an embolic occlusion in the terminal part (1 cm) of the internal carotid artery, [extending into] the initial segment (1 cm) of the Sylvian artery and [also] in a few smaller cortical branches of the latter. All these vessels and all brain arteries were quite smooth.
>
> The search for the source of the embolus was in vain, at least for some time. The heart was normal, except some mottled thickening of the mitral valve and the aortic valve. The aorta showed only in its ascending part and in the arch some lentil-sized spots with thickening of the intima, but otherwise the condition of the walls was smooth. The branches from the arch had the same aspect when cut open for 3–4 cm, according to usual practice. The walls of the limb arteries were equally smooth. Next, we thought of a paradoxical embolus, since the *foramen ovale* was patent in an oblique direction, though only for a standard anatomical probe.

---

[4] Mehnert (1888), Topographische Verbreitung der Angiosclerose, 28.
[5] Mehnert (1888), Topographische Verbreitung der Angiosclerose, 51.
[6] Chiari (1905), Verhalten des Teilungswinkels der Carotis, 326.

Box 8.1 Hans Chiari (1851–1916).

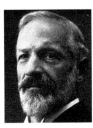 Chiari was born in Vienna; his father was a gynaecologist. Having studied medicine in his home town and subsequently specialized in pathological anatomy, Hans became second assistant to Carl Rokitansky (1804–1878), subsequently first assistant to his successor Richard Heschl (1824–1881). In 1878, after a doctoral thesis on tuberculosis of the thyroid gland, he became *Prosektor* at St Anna Hospital for children in Vienna; there he excelled by his teaching skills and systematic approach. Four years later, he was appointed to the chair of Pathological Anatomy in Prague, where in the meantime his father had been Professor of Gynaecology.

On his arrival in Prague, the university was in the process of splitting into a German-speaking and a Czech-speaking part, after decades of strife between the two factions. Chiari was also the superintendent of the museum for pathological anatomy and saved what he could. Throughout the 24 years of his stay, he kept a tight schedule for himself and his assistants: early in the morning, autopsies were allotted, and at 11, everyone convened for lectures or a discussion of recent publications. Most of his original work dates from this period: descriptions of choriocarcinoma, thrombosis of the hepatic vein (now known as Budd–Chiari syndrome), and malformations of the hind brain, distinguished into three types.

Meanwhile, the agitation and even rioting in Prague had not died down. In 1906, shortly after his paper on the carotid bifurcation as a source of embolism to the brain, he accepted a chair in Strassburg, as the successor of Friedrich von Recklinghausen (1833–1910). His contributions to the pathology of pituitary adenomas date from this period. In 1916, he died from what had started as a throat infection. He had married Emilia Antonia Paulina Anna Schrötter von Kristell in 1878; one of their children also became a pathologist.

But because we detected no thrombus anywhere in the venous system of the body, this idea had to be given up as well.

I then started to investigate the left common carotid artery and its branches more carefully. Very soon it was there that I found the source of the embolus, in the form of a thrombus on the left wall of the common carotid artery in its distal segment (1 cm), extending about 1½ cm into the internal carotid artery. The surface of the thrombus was uneven, as if part of it had been torn off. After removal of the thrombus the aspect of a rather severe *endarteritis chronica deformans* appeared in the bifurcation of the common carotid and the beginning of the internal carotid, partly with atheromatous degeneration. On the right side the *endarteritis chronica deformans* had developed to the same extent, but without thrombosis. On both sides the internal carotid artery was normal in its further course to the skull base, as was the external carotid artery.[7]

[7] Chiari (1905), Verhalten des Teilungswinkels der Carotis, 327.

Alerted by this finding, Chiari paid special attention to the carotid bifurcation in the next 400 dissections he performed in the following five months; 62 of them were newborn babies or less than one year old; all others were at least 12 years of age. Seven times he found thrombosis at the same site, superimposed on what he again called *endarteritis chronica deformans*, in one case bilaterally; five of these seven were women, five aged 70 years or over. The size of the thrombi ranged between that of millet seed and that of a pea. In four of these patients, the thrombus had produced an embolus, followed by brain softening. Thickening of the intimal surface in the region of the carotid bifurcation was generally common, even in four tuberculous patients under 30 years of age. All this justified Chiari's two main conclusions:

> The first is the relative frequency of thrombosis as a result of *endarteritis chronica deformans* in the region of the bifurcation of the common carotid and the initial part of the internal carotid, from which site embolism into the intracranial arteries often occurs. The second is the often early and isolated occurrence of *endarteritis chronica deformans* at the bifurcation of the common carotid and the initial part of the internal carotid.[8]

Since Chiari also diagnosed brain softening in 11 other patients with embolism, from the heart or aorta, he might have added as an extra conclusion that the carotid bifurcation accounted for a sizeable minority of all cases of cerebral softening – 4 out of 15. At that time, valvular heart disease as a sequel of rheumatic fever was quite common.

Feeling the Carotid Artery

James Ramsay Hunt (1872–1937), who had settled as a neurologist in New York after an extensive European tour, alerted the North American medical community in 1914 to the possible role of obstructed neck arteries in the pathogenesis of brain softening, despite the general emphasis on primary occlusion of intracranial vessels:

> Hemiplegia from occlusion of the intracranial branches of the internal carotid is one of the most frequent clinical pictures met with in medical practice, and yet one of the rarest from obstruction of the main arterial pathway in the neck. However, when one considers that these vessels are frequently ignored both in clinical and pathological studies, it is not unlikely that many such conditions are overlooked.
> The reason for our neglect in this aspect is obvious, and springs from the assumption that the circle of Willis is sufficient to carry the blood into an obstructed vascular area when such obstruction is situated below the

[8] Chiari (1905), Verhalten des Teilungswinkels der Carotis, 327.

level of the communicating arteries. [...] On the other hand, in those individuals with disease and weakened hearts and sclerotic vessels, the necessary compensatory changes for the establishment of the collateral circulation may not develop. [...]

We also know that, entirely apart from a weakened heart and arterio-sclerotic vessels, obstruction of a carotid may produce permanent hemiplegia because of inadequate arteries of communication in the circle of Willis or other vascular anomalies.[9]

Hunt did not provide proofs for his hypothesis of failing collateral pathways, or mention the problem that such explanations might fail. The cases from his own practice were all associated with neck trauma, while the other patients with spontaneous carotid occlusion he cited had manifested only headache or visual symptoms, or also had aortic disease. Chiari's work had apparently not reached him.

Instead, Hunt proposed diminished pulsation as circumstantial evidence:

[...] I would call attention to the occurrence of diminished pulsation of the carotid artery in the neck on the side of the softening in cases presenting the symptoms of thrombotic hemiplegia. Among a series of twenty cases of hemiplegia occurring in advanced life, which I examined for this symptom in the neurological service of the Montefiore Home for Chronic Invalids, it was possible to demonstrate its presence in four cases, all of which presented the clinical picture of an extensive lesion of the hemisphere: hemiplegia with contractures, hemisensory disturbance and mental deterioration. The optic nerves were normal on both sides in all four cases.[10]

Oblivion

Chiari's article, having appeared in the transactions of the German Society for Pathology, failed to attract wide interest. A single case report in 1928 by Gerhard Wüllenweber (1894–1942) from Cologne documented the case of a 62-year-old man who had suddenly become unconscious and died three days later. Both internal carotid arteries in the neck showed atherosclerosis and occlusion by grey-red thrombus, from the bifurcation to their intracranial divisions. The left hemisphere showed mild scars of softening, corresponding to mild deficits of language and movement that had occurred one and a half years before death. On the right side, the middle cerebral artery (MCA) contained a loose-lying, fresh thrombus, and extensive, recent softening.[11]

---

[9] Hunt (1914), The role of the carotid arteries in vascular lesions of the brain, 704–5.
[10] Hunt (1914), The role of the carotid arteries in vascular lesions of the brain, 711.
[11] Wüllenweber (1928), Doppelseitiger Verschluß der Aa. Carotides internae.

The point the author wished to make was not so much the possible origin of the recent thrombus, but rather the peculiarity of a patient who had lived on for a considerable time, given the aspect of the thrombi, despite both internal carotids being occluded.

Textbooks in the German language might sometimes refer to extracranial arteries in their listing of possible sources of embolism,[12] or even specifically to the carotid bifurcation,[13] but not all did.[14] Elsewhere, the role of neck arteries entirely failed to make its way into popular textbooks in other parts of Europe,[15] or in the United States.[16] The explanation is not just a matter of language: no matter how important Chiari's observations may seem in later eyes, they had very little impact on the thoughts and actions of clinicians in the early twentieth century; these colleagues were first of all faced with the task of distinguishing between haemorrhage and softening in patients with acute and spontaneous lesions of the brain, while treatment remained speculative in either case.

Given the well-known collateral pathways in the arterial system of the human brain, what explanation for apoplectic softening was more plausible than primary obstruction of branches beyond the circle of Willis, either by local thrombosis or by embolism from the heart or aorta?

THE PERSISTENT PARADIGM OF INTRACRANIAL THROMBOSIS

A Thrombus that Escaped Attention?

Often the idea of intracranial thrombosis as the common cause of acute brain ischaemia was so ingrained, at least if embolism from the heart or aorta was unlikely, that physicians, on failing to find such a thrombus, concluded their search had not been exhaustive enough. An example is a 1933 article by Herbert H. Hyland (1900–1977) at the Toronto General Hospital. The purpose of the paper was to draw attention to sites of arterial occlusion other than the MCA. One of his cases was a 58-year-old man who had died 10 days after a sudden left hemiplegia, with blindness of the right eye. A thrombus was found in the intracranial part of the right internal carotid artery (ICA), beginning in the carotid canal and ending before its terminal division; however, there was a separate clot in the right MCA. The heart and aorta were essentially normal. The pathologist who studied microscopic sections of the intracranial part of the

[12] Strümpell and Seyfarth (1926), *Pathologie und Therapie der inneren Krankheiten*, 737.
[13] Hirsch (1909), Die Zirkulationsstörungen des Gehirns, 607.
[14] Oppenheim (1913), *Lehrbuch der Nervenkrankheiten*, 1063.
[15] Brissaud and Souques (1904), Maladies de l'encéphale, 195, 211; Turner and Stuart (1910), *Textbook of Nervous Diseases*, 193; van Gehuchten (1920), *Les Maladies nerveuses*, 456.
[16] Jelliffe and White (1923), *Diseases of the Nervous System*, 701.

ICA found very few changes in its wall and concluded: 'It is probable that the sections did not pass through the point of origin of the thrombus.' In his comment, Hyland wrote:

> The internal carotid artery is not commonly the site of primary thrombosis, and the reason for the occurrence of a thrombus in it in this case was not clear. The thrombosed artery and the other cerebral arteries examined showed less atheromatous change than might be expected considering the patient's age.[17]

The solution may well have been in the neck. But Hyland was not a pathologist like Hans Chiari, who did not give up until he had found the origin of a thrombus that had become stuck in an intact artery. Nonetheless, Hyland was an innovative neurologist;[18] the above story has been chosen merely as an example to illustrate the track neurologists' thoughts commonly followed at the time.

Missing Occlusions

As far back as in the 1860s, when the vascular form of cerebral softening was being defined, the lumen of a major cerebral artery had sometimes been found patent despite necrotic changes in its corresponding territory.[19] In those instances, thoughts sometimes wandered to obstruction more distally in the vascular tree, to small arterial branches or capillaries.[20]

Much later, in the 1920s, a new study from Paris reported on arterial lesions in cerebral softening. The senior author Charles Foix (1882–1927) tragically died before the study was fully completed, presumably from appendicitis. The junior author Jacques Ley (1900–1983) from Brussels, who was to continue his career as a psychiatrist, continued as well as he could and published the final results in a journal of his home country, after a preliminary presentation in Paris.[21] Foix and Ley had investigated 63 arteries corresponding to a defined area of softening; they found a complete occlusion in only 19 of these arteries, a subtotal occlusion in 14, a partial occlusion in 27, and no obstruction of the lumen at all in three.[22] The interval between disease onset and death had no appreciable effect on this distribution. Ley concluded (the italics are his):

---

[17] Hyland (1933), Thrombosis of intracranial arteries, 356.
[18] JCR (1978), Herbert Hylton Hyland.
[19] Prévost and Cotard (1866), *Ramollissement cérébral*, 82–6.
[20] Lancereaux (1862), Thrombose et embolie cérébrales, 95–106; Proust (1866), Ramollissement du cerveau, 39–46.
[21] Foix, *et al.* (1927), Importance relative des oblitérations artérielles.
[22] Foix and Ley (1927b), État anatomique des artères du territoire nécrosé, 669.

> The result of our numbers is that *a person with cerebral softening is in only a limited proportion of cases (complete embolism or thrombosis) a patient who suddenly plugs an artery.* As a rule, it is, in contrast, *someone who, presenting diseased arteries, but not more diseased on the day of the attack than on the previous day or the day before that, yet is suddenly hit by necrosis of an insufficiently irrigated territory.*
>
> From this, it follows that there must necessarily exist an *occasional* or *accessory* cause for cerebral softening.[23]

In other words, the course of events must be more complicated than local thrombosis and subsequent occlusion. In London, Kinnier Wilson (1878–1937) commented as follows on the findings of Foix and Ley, in his textbook appearing a few years after his death: 'I have remarked on several occasions how the affected artery has not been so conspicuously diseased as others in the same brain.'[24] Few clinicians cited the article of Foix and Ley or reported similar experiences.

Meanwhile, a new diagnostic technique with invisible rays had drawn some attention to the ICA, though rather inadvertently. It is appropriate to go back a few decades and follow this new development from its onset.

X-RAYS

Röntgen

Near the end of 1895, Wilhelm Röntgen (1845–1923) discovered in his physics laboratory in Würzburg that some cathode rays could penetrate soft tissues, whereas they were absorbed by bone and metals (Figure 8.1); he christened them X-rays.[25] On 28 December of that same year, Röntgen submitted a handwritten article to the local physico-medical society; the members of the editorial board decided to include it in the *Transactions* of that same year, although no meetings had been scheduled for the Christmas break. In the first few days of 1896, Röntgen sent offprints to some colleagues. That the technique promised important applications in medicine was obvious: the news spread across the world with uncommon rapidity. In that same month of January 1896, X-rays of the hands were produced in Paris, London, and New York.[26] Soon hospitals were fitted with X-ray machines, and in the First World War, wounded soldiers in the tragic battlefields of Flanders and Northern France could be investigated by a fleet of mobile X-ray units; some

[23] Foix and Ley (1927b), État anatomique des artères du territoire nécrosé, 670.
[24] Wilson and Bruce (1940), *Neurology*, 1087.
[25] Röntgen (1895), Ueber eine neue Art von Strahlen.
[26] Glasser (1959), *Die Geschichte der Röntgenstrahlen*, 16–30.

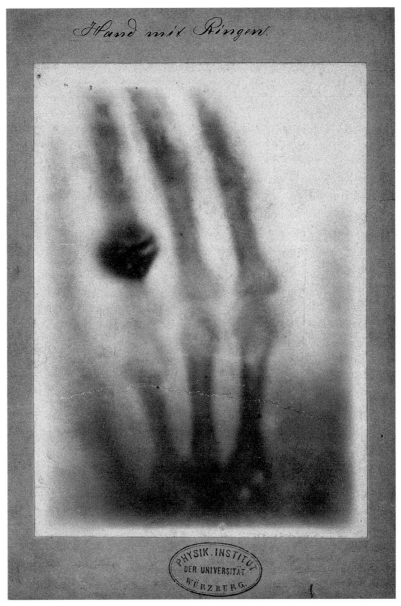

8.1 Radiograph of the hand of Conrad Röntgen's wife, made on 22 December 1895. *Source:* Courtesy of Welcome collection.

were organized or even manned by Marie Curie-Sklodowska (1867–1934) and her young daughter Irene.[27]

Contrast agents as a method for outlining contours of body spaces not shown on plain X-ray pictures were soon applied, but for the nervous system, such techniques become relevant only after the First World War.

[27] Giroud (1991), *Une femme honorable, Marie Curie*, 137–41.

Spaces in and around the Nervous System

For the brain cavities, Walter Dandy (1886–1946) devised ventriculography, by introducing air into the ventricles, through direct puncture.[28]

Visualization of the spaces around the spinal cord for the detection of tumours or cysts was first achieved in 1921 by Jean Sicard (1872–1929) and Jacques Forestier (1890–1978); they injected a compound of iodine, opaque to X-rays, mixed with ethyl esters of poppyseed oil (Lipiodol®).[29] They used a hollow needle to access the spinal fluid space, between the two processes of the lower lumbar spine. The first person to carry out this 'lumbar puncture' had been Heinrich Quincke (1842–1922), Professor of Internal Medicine at the University of Kiel, in 1891;[30] initially he used it only as a therapeutic procedure, to relieve increased pressure in the skull, particularly in hydrocephalic children.[31]

Egas Moniz and Cerebral Angiography

Egas Moniz (1874–1955) (Box 8.2), a neurologist in Lisbon,[32] applied his innovative spirit to medicine only after the end of his political career, when he was around 50 years of age. Trying to achieve for brain tumours what Sicard had done for spinal tumours, without the invasiveness and perceived risks of ventriculography,[33] he figured that the shape of the arterial system in the brain was fairly constant, so that most tumours would betray their location by displacement of arterial branches, especially in the carotid territory. With his collaborators, he tried a variety of contrast agents and concentrations, first in the carotid artery of dogs, then in human cadavers.[34]

After unsuccessful attempts with a percutaneous approach, Moniz and his team reverted to surgical exposure of the ICA; this method also facilitated the application of a temporary ligature during the injection of contrast agent, initially strontium bromide. However, of the first few patients, one showed transient neurological deficits and the next, a 48-year-old woman with severe post-encephalitic parkinsonism, died a few hours later. This accident prompted the use of a safer contrast agent, sodium iodide. Moniz reported his preliminary results in a session of the *Société de neurologie* in Paris, in 1927.[35]

[28] Dandy (1918), Ventriculography following the injection of air.
[29] Sicard and Forestier (1921), Méthode radiographique d'exploration de la cavité épidurale.
[30] Quincke (1891), Die Lumbalpunktion des Hydrocephalus.
[31] Frederiks and Koehler (1997), The first lumbar puncture.
[32] De Barahona Fernandes (1956), Egas Moniz; Walker (1970), Egas Moniz.
[33] Moniz (1927), L'encéphalographie artérielle, 72–7.
[34] Moniz (1927), L'encéphalographie artérielle, 77–83.
[35] Moniz (1927), L'encéphalographie artérielle, 83–9.

Box 8.2 Egas Moniz (1874–1955).

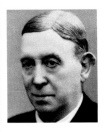

Moniz was born as António Caetano de Abreu Freire de Resende, but at some stage, the family changed the surname 'de Resende' to that of 'Moniz', to indicate the link with a noble medieval forefather. As a medical student at the University of Coimbra, Egas developed a taste for literature and also became a republican activist, for which he was jailed twice. Meanwhile, he had developed an interest in neurology and psychiatry; after graduation in 1899, he submitted a doctoral dissertation on sexuality (1901), became a staff neurologist in Coimbra, and married Elvira de Macedo Dias (1902). From 1903, he served as deputy in the national parliament. He spent some time in Bordeaux and Paris, where he struck up a friendship with Joseph Babinski (1857–1932).

In 1910, the First Republic was established; Moniz became Professor of Neurology but was chiefly engaged in politics, as the leader of a centrist party, as ambassador to Madrid, and – briefly – as minister of foreign affairs. After having represented Portugal at the peace conference at Versailles in 1919, he gave all his attention to medicine and pioneered cerebral angiography in the mid-1920s.

In the next decade, Moniz started thinking about psychosurgery, in order to alleviate suffering from chronic psychosis, depression, or compulsive disorders. He experimented with lesions of the frontal lobe, given the absence of effective drugs. Since a few observations had shown that lesions of the frontal lobe could change behaviour without gross neurological deficits, he developed 'leukotomy' – slicing through the frontal lobes with a pointed instrument. A proportion of the patients improved. It was his young colleague Pedro Almeida Lima (1903–1985) who carried out the procedures, because Moniz suffered from severe gout. The method was controversial from the start, but in modified form it became widely applied, especially in North America; in 1949, Moniz received the Nobel Prize for Medicine for this work.

He retired at the age of 70; five years before, he had been severely wounded by an ex-patient.

Even the first successful image, of a hypophyseal tumour displacing several intracranial arteries, was not easy to interpret. New adaptations followed. One was the switch, in 1931, to a new contrast agent, a suspension of thorium dioxide (Thorotrast®); the associated risks of radiation exposure were not yet known. Side effects were no longer a problem, Moniz reported. Also, this new agent allowed visualization of the venous system, a few seconds after the arterial phase; arteriography had become angiography.[36] Another modification was to inject the fluid in the common carotid artery instead of in the internal division, and so to include its cervical segment in the radiograph.

---

[36] Moniz (1934), *L'angiographie cérébrale*, 16–18.

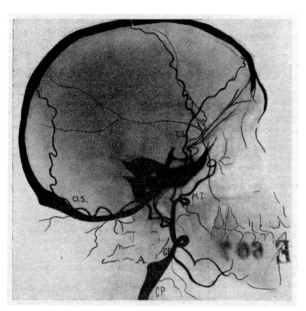

8.2 Occlusion of the left internal carotid artery (Moniz *et al.*, 1937). The patient was a 43-year-old man with gradually progressive weakness of the right limbs and aphasia. The angiogram of the right carotid artery was completely normal; both pericallosal arteries were filled, but no other arteries on the left side. CP, common carotid artery; A, the site where the internal carotid artery was occluded at its origin; CE, external carotid artery; MI, internal maxillary artery; OS, superficial occipital artery; TS, superficial temporal artery.

Carotid Occlusion on Angiograms

By 1937, when Moniz had performed a total of 537 angiographies, he had come across four patients with an occlusion of the ICA (Figure 8.2).[37] Three of them had presented with a gradually progressive hemiparesis, with or without symptoms of aphasia; it was the suspicion of a tumour that had led to the angiogram.[38] In these cases, Moniz supposed that the collateral circulation had failed, perhaps because of spasm. In the fourth patient, the clinical picture was complicated by tabes dorsalis and a bullet wound in the neck.

Following Moniz's article, a flurry of other papers reported the occurrence of carotid occlusion, mostly in combination with neurological deficits. The diagnosis was always made by angiography, and in one case by operative inspection.[39] Although a percutaneous technique, instead of surgical dissection, was soon reported,[40] its adoption took time; at any rate, the procedure

---

[37] Ferro (1988), Egas Moniz and internal carotid occlusion; Oliveira (2018), History of carotid occlusions.

[38] Moniz, *et al.* (1937), Hémiplégies par thrombose de la carotide interne.

[39] Webster, *et al.* (1950), Spontaneous thrombosis of the carotid arteries in the neck.

[40] Loman and Myerson (1936), Visualisation of cerebral vessels by direct intracarotid injection; Shimidzu (1937), Arteriographie des Gehirns – einfache percutane Methode.

remained firmly in surgical hands. The main indications for angiography were, according to neurosurgeons from Baltimore, 'patients suspected of having a brain tumor, aneurysm, or cerebral vascular anomaly'.[41] Finding a brain tumour was not entirely a fruitless exercise. Neurosurgery was still in its infancy, but several abnormal growths could be safely operated; the first successful removal of a meningioma had taken place in 1879, by William Macewen.[42] Angiography soon proved helpful in detecting and localizing acoustic neuromas, meningiomas, gliomas, hypophyseal tumours, tuberculomas, and subdural haematomas.[43]

As long as cerebral angiography was restricted to patients whose symptoms suggested a condition for which an operation was feasible, the finding of carotid occlusion was almost invariably unexpected. Such chance events created, at least for some time, an incomplete and distorted picture of the symptoms and causes of carotid occlusion. The simple explanation is that most patients with carotid occlusion who were struck by 'common apoplexy', with sudden-onset and full-blown deficits, did not end up on the surgical ward of a hospital, but in an institution for chronic care.

Surgeons and Carotid Occlusion: Particular Symptoms, Particular Causes?

Two surgeons from Birmingham, for example, presented six such cases in 1949, reviewed previous reports, and wrote in the discussion section:

> Symptoms arising from thrombosis of the internal carotid artery contrast with those due to ligation of the artery. In the case of internal carotid ligation there is usually no disturbance at all, or there may be slight hemiparesis from which the patient often recovers with no further incident. In some patients, however, rapid and complete hemiplegia develops within a few minutes of the ligation of the artery. Thrombosis of the carotid artery, on the other hand, is characterised by repeated minor pareses or attacks of dysphasia during the early stages. [...]
>
> The first symptom is often some transient weakness of one of the extremities, usually on the right side, associated sometimes with a minor disturbance of speech. Partial recovery usually takes place, and there ensue several recurrent exacerbations of weakness and disturbance of speech culminating in a dramatic incident with increased weakness, aphasia, loss of consciousness, or visual defect, leading the patient to come for treatment.[44]

[41] Johnson and Walker (1951), Spontaneous thrombosis of the carotid arteries, 631.
[42] Macmillan (2005), William Macewen's early brain surgery.
[43] Shimidzu (1937), Arteriographie des Gehirns – einfache percutane Methode.
[44] Ameli and Ashby (1949), Non-traumatic thrombosis of the carotid artery.

This perception was not unique. Between 1936 and 1951, the year in which a landmark paper on carotid occlusion was to appear, 95 patients with carotid occlusion and relevant neurological deficits were reported in 29 papers; these have been conveniently tabulated elsewhere.[45] Apart from premonitory symptoms, in about half of these articles a gradual or stuttering onset of focal symptoms – almost invariably involving hemiparesis – was thought characteristic of carotid occlusion, as had happened early on in the patients of Moniz. The preponderance of right-sided hemiparesis was another common feature in most series. Undoubtedly this represents another example of referral bias, given that unilateral weakness is more likely to attract medical attention when accompanied by defects of speech and comprehension.

Age was also a misleading factor. Since especially young patients were suitable candidates for angiography, they formed a sizeable proportion of reported patients with carotid occlusion. Of the total of 95 patients with carotid occlusion mentioned above, 29 were less than 40 years of age and 61 were aged between 40 and 60. One author even highlighted the juvenile factor by separately republishing four patients under 40 in his series.[46] The young age of some patients with carotid occlusion did not fail to inspire alternative explanations: retrograde thrombosis from an intracranial aneurysm,[47] of course syphilis, and repeatedly a cerebral form of thrombo-angiitis obliterans.[48] Though thrombo-angiitis obliterans was known to occur in peripheral arteries, the criteria for a cerebral variant remained fuzzy, despite lengthy articles;[49] ultimately, its very existence has been called into question.[50]

Why Does the Collateral Circulation Fail?

Without exception, authors reporting occlusion of the common or internal carotid artery on angiography did not sufficiently explain contralateral weakness or other deficits. George Marinesco (1863–1938), a neurologist in Bucharest who had received most of his training in Paris, used arteriography post-mortem to demonstrate once more how the vertebral arteries sustained the cerebral circulation after occlusion of both common carotid arteries.[51]

[45] Johnson and Walker (1951), Spontaneous thrombosis of the carotid arteries.
[46] Sorgo (1939), Art. carotis interna-Verschluß bei jüngeren Personen.
[47] James (1949), Thrombosis of the internal carotid artery.
[48] Sorgo (1939), Verschluss der Art. carotis interna; Andrell (1943), Thrombosis of the internal carotid artery; Krayenbühl and Weber (1944), Thrombose der Arteria carotis interna; Frøvig (1946), Thrombose der Arteria carotis interna; Wolfe (1948), Unexplained thrombosis of the left internal carotid artery.
[49] Lindenberg and Spatz (1939), Thromboendarteriitis der Hirngefäße.
[50] Fisher (1957b), Cerebral thromboangiitis obliterans.
[51] Marinesco and Kreindler (1936), Oblitération des deux carotides primitives.

The explanation remained elusive. Moniz and several others implied a structural anomaly or additional atherosclerosis elsewhere in the circle of Willis. Others assumed a functional disturbance: spastic narrowing of the arteries in the vicinity, resulting from hyperactivity of sympathetic nerves or 'carotid hypersensitivity'. This theory was based on the work of René Leriche (1879–1955), a surgeon in Lyon, later in Strasbourg and Paris, with special expertise in disorders of blood vessels. From his experiments, he concluded that 'an obliterated artery ceases to be an artery and becomes a diseased sympathetic nerve'.[52] Suiting the action to his words, Leriche resected thrombosed arterial segments, seemingly with favourable results.[53] Colleagues followed Leriche and removed a segment of the occluded ICA, sometimes also of the common and external carotid; others performed only sympathectomy by excision of the superior cervical ganglion, or combined both procedures.[54]

The association of carotid occlusion with 'spasm' in the first half of the twentieth century was less common in the medical world at large, since angiography solidly belonged to the surgical domain. Though an activist surgeon wrote 'where angiography is not yet available patients with carotid occlusion are diagnosed as "hemiplegia" and are left to their fate',[55] physicians who took care of elderly patients with apoplexy were fully aware of the lack of therapeutic implications. To begin with, they were uncertain whether the brain lesion was haemorrhagic or ischaemic, even though softening proved more than three times as common as massive bleeding, at least in deceased patients.[56]

Research in neurology was almost exclusively pathological research of the nervous system in isolation. Post-mortem study of blood vessels remained restricted to what was 'on the table' of the neuropathologist. Despite recurring inconsistencies, ideas about brain softening continued to revolve around thrombosis of intracranial vessels, as attested by popular textbooks of the 1960s.[57] Occlusion of the carotid artery remained an angiographic curiosity, until a few young physicians took this up again.

---

[52] Leriche (1931), Arterectomy in the treatment of localized arterial obstructions, 56.
[53] Leriche, et al. (1937), Arterectomy – with follow-up studies on seventy-eight operations.
[54] Riechert (1938), Verschluß der Carotis interna; Chao, et al. (1938), Thrombosis of the left carotid artery; Galdston, et al. (1941), Thrombosis of the carotid arteries; Krayenbühl (1945), Zerebrale Erscheinungen bei der Endangiitis obiliterans; Barré, et al. (1947), Thrombose de la carotide interne; Wolfe (1948), Unexplained thrombosis of the left internal carotid artery.
[55] Sponer (1941), Verschluß der Arteria carotis interna, 481.
[56] Foix and Ley (1927), État anatomique des artères du territoire nécrosé.
[57] Brain (1962), *Diseases of the Nervous System*, 362–6; Biemond (1961), *Hersenziekten*, 453–5.

THE CAROTID ARTERY REVISITED

Atherosclerosis of the Carotid Artery in Unselected Autopsies

Mehnert's observation of 1888 about the common occurrence of 'angiosclerosis' at the carotid bifurcation was confirmed in the 1920s and 1930s by two British pathologists. These findings were hardly cited before the 1950s, because they had no obvious connection with cerebrovascular disease: one, by D.R. Dow (1887–1979), was a purely anatomical inventory,[58] and the other hypothesized that hypertension was the effect of carotid atherosclerosis rather than its cause.[59]

A pathologist in Munich, Joseph Dörfler (n.d.), writing in 1935, was especially struck by atheromatous lesions in the tortuous part of the ICA, in the cavernous sinus.[60] Five years later, Hans Anders (1886–1953), a pathologist at a municipal hospital in Berlin,[61] hosted the young pathologists Dei Poli and Zucha, from Padua and Bratislava, respectively. Together they undertook an inventory of atherosclerotic lesions, comparable to Mehnert's work half a century before, in a consecutive series of 40 post-mortem dissections; only three were aged under 50 years. In all 40 patients, the duo found atherosclerotic lesions in the ICA, in variable degrees of severity. However, the lesions were unevenly distributed over the long course of the artery. Predilection sites were the carotid sinus in the neck, and the cavernous curved part,[62] dubbed 'carotid siphon' by Moniz.[63] Atherosclerotic changes occurred far less often in other segments of the artery.

The two papers from Munich and Berlin received very little attention in the anglophone and francophone literature, if at all. The Second World War was not the only reason; both papers were published in rather inconspicuous journals, aimed at psychiatrists and neurosurgeons, respectively. A third study, written in German from a neutral country, reached a wider circle of physicians. Its strong point of interest was that the patients had all died of ischaemic brain disease.

Carotid Atherothrombosis in Patients with Brain Softening

In 1942, the pathologist Gösta Hultquist (1910–1993) followed Chiari's lead and obtained his doctoral title in Stockholm by submitting a study of thrombo-embolism in the territory of the carotid artery. Over a period of four years, he

---

[58] Dow (1925), Incidence of arterio-sclerosis in arteries.
[59] Keele (1933), Pathological changes in the carotid sinus.
[60] Dörfler (1935), Arteriosklerose der Arteria carotis interna.
[61] In 1933, the Nazi regime removed Anders from his post.
[62] Dei Poli and Zucha (1940), Erkrankungen der Arteria carotis interna.
[63] Moniz (1934), L'angiographie cérébrale, 19.

had investigated the common and internal carotid arteries in all 1300-odd cases of dissection in St Erik's hospital, at least the extracranial parts. In cases of cerebral softening, he also studied their intracranial course.[64]

Of the different regions in the carotid artery, Hultquist found the carotid sinus was most commonly affected by atherosclerosis and subsequent thrombosis; also ulceration of lesions at that location occurred more often than elsewhere. Most relevant was the subset of patients with cerebral softening in whom Hultquist found 'primary' atherothrombosis in either the extracranial (25 patients) or the cerebral part (7 patients) of the ICA.[65] In several cases, such an intracranial thrombosis coexisted with a thrombotic lesion in the carotid sinus, with a stagnation thrombus in between. In some instances of separate thrombi in the same artery, Hultquist regarded the intracerebral thrombus as the initial occlusion, in view of morphological features on microscopic study, especially the cohesion between the sclerotic vessel wall and the overlying thrombus. Other criteria were a lamellar structure and the consistency and colour of the clot: he attributed redness to stagnation of erythrocytes, and a greyish colour to deposition of leucocytes by a still active bloodstream.[66] Clinical information was generally scarce and unhelpful, apart from the presence and the side of limb weakness and the interval between the onset of symptoms and death – almost invariably less than one week.

Despite application of these criteria, it was often difficult to exclude embolization from the carotid sinus to the intracerebral part of the artery.[67] It is not inconceivable that other pathologists might have come to different conclusions in cases where Hultquist regarded the distal thrombosis as an independent lesion (Figure 8.3). At any rate, in five patients, aged between 54 and 80 years, Hultquist found atherothrombotic lesions in the cerebral part of the carotid artery alone, whereas the area of the carotid sinus was free of thrombus and no source of embolism appeared in the heart or aorta (Figure 8.4).[68]

Carotid Occlusion in Patients with Brain Softening and a Clinical History

C. Miller Fisher (1913–2012) (Box 8.3) appeared in Chapter 5, on account of his work on the pathology of small arterioles in the 1960s. In the late 1940s, Fisher was still based in Montreal, apart from a stint in Boston. Building on the

---

[64] Hultquist (1942), *Thrombose und Embolie der Arteria carotis*, 11–16.
[65] Hultquist (1942), *Thrombose und Embolie der Arteria carotis*, 48.
[66] Hultquist (1942), *Thrombose und Embolie der Arteria carotis*, 51.
[67] Hultquist (1942), *Thrombose und Embolie der Arteria carotis*, 85–9.
[68] Hultquist (1942), *Thrombose und Embolie der Arteria carotis*, 48.

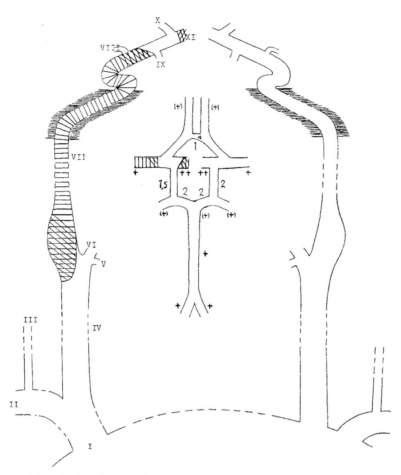

8.3 Thrombosis in the carotid system; case 34 of G. Hultquist (1942); the patient was a 77-year-old man. The arteries in the neck and the skull are indicated by Roman numerals: VII, (right) common carotid artery; VIII, ophthalmic artery; IX, posterior communicating artery; X, anterior cerebral artery; XI, middle cerebral artery. The numbers near the segments of the circle of Willis indicate the width in millimetres; the symbols (+), +, and ++ indicate the degree of atherosclerosis. The dense striation represents the intra-osseous segment of the internal carotid artery. In the arterial lumen, single stripes signify red thrombus, and double stripes grey or mixed thrombus. Hultquist's legend reads: 'In both sinuses atherosclerotic changes of the wall, most marked on the right side. [...] The thrombus extends peripherally with a secondary red thrombus, which in its intracerebral part again contains more fibrin and leukocytes (but not to the extent that it gives the impression of having originated locally); it ends just before the posterior communicating artery. [...] Separately from this clot there is a thrombus in the middle cerebral artery, which also has the character of a local thrombus, with marked changes in the wall and a clear relation between its layers and the wall. [...].'

work of Chiari and Hultquist – having mastered the German language as a prisoner of war – he published, in 1951, an article in English, entitled *Occlusion of the Internal Carotid Artery*. This paper had a much greater impact than the publications mentioned in the previous paragraphs. He began by pointing out why the neck arteries had been overlooked for so long:

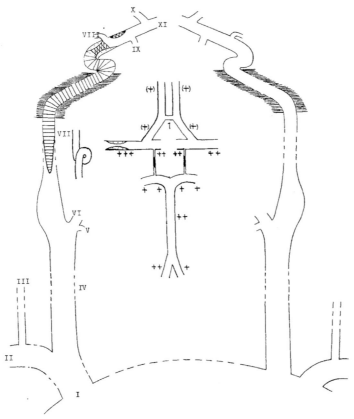

8.4 Thrombosis in the carotid system; case 39 of G. Hultquist (1942), a 67-year-old man. For explanation of symbols, see Figure 8.3. The legend reads: 'In both carotid sinuses marked atherosclerotic changes in the vessel wall, especially on the right. In the intracranial part of the internal carotid artery is a thrombotic mass, which on microscopic examination has the character of autochthonous thrombosis; it has probably arisen as a result of the extensive atherosclerotic changes of the walls. In the distal part of this arterial segment there is an isolated patch of thrombosis. No source of embolism has been found. The occluding thrombus extends downwards towards the carotid sinus, in the form of a secondary red thrombus. [...] The occluding thrombus abruptly stops at the origin of the ophthalmic artery. More peripherally the vessel lumen is free, except for the isolated patch. The middle cerebral artery shows a tight stenosis in its distal part.'

Clinicians and pathologists have heretofore failed to appreciate this condition, because the cervical portion of the carotid artery lies in a 'no man's land' between general pathology and neuropathology, its examination at autopsy being therefore neglected.[69]

He went on to recount the conundrum with which he had grappled during his fellowship in Boston, as others had before him, in failing to find the occlusions of the main intracerebral arteries that had been predicted from the clinical

[69] Fisher (1951), Occlusion of the internal carotid artery, 346.

Box 8.3 C. Miller Fisher (1913–2012).

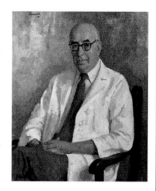

(Charles) Miller Fisher was born in Waterloo, Ontario, third of nine children of Frieda Kaufman and George Middleton Fisher, a traveling insurance salesman. His mother died after childbirth when he was 11 years old. At that time, the family already called him 'the doctor'. Indeed, he matriculated at the Toronto Medical School in 1931. After graduation, he obtained a one-year internship at the Henry Ford Hospital in Detroit, not far across the border. In 1939, he married Doris Stiefelmeyer, his girlfriend from high school. After a brief period of training in internal medicine in Montreal, war broke out and in 1940, he joined the Canadian Navy as a surgeon-lieutenant. A year later, his ship was sunk in the South Atlantic; Fisher was among those captured and ended up in prisoner-of-war camps near Bremen, where he 'learned not to complain'.

After repatriation, he was anxious to make up for the lost years and started retraining in Montreal. During his rotation at the Neurological Institute, Wilder Penfield (1891–1976) encouraged him to pursue neurology. For experience abroad, Fisher chose the Boston City Hospital (1949–50), attracted by the neurologist Derek Denny-Brown (1901–1981) and the neurologist–neuropathologist Raymond D. Adams (1911–2008). Back in Montreal, Fisher divided his time between clinical work and the laboratory for pathology. He had developed a special interest in the pathogenesis of stroke.

In 1954, he moved to the Massachusetts General Hospital, where Adams had been appointed Chief of Neurology. It was there that he did most of his research, especially in the field of cerebrovascular disease, but not exclusively; he also described a variant of the Guillain–Barré syndrome, now named after him. Fisher was not just methodical, but also, as his biographer Louis Caplan noted, 'never in a hurry and completely oblivious to the time of day or night'. As a person, he was uncommonly kind. The year 1980 marked his official retirement, but this hardly changed his routines: he kept his office at the hospital, to where his wife Doris would drive him each morning for the next 25 years, until her health failed. Doris died in 2008 and Fisher moved to Albany, where one of their three children lived. He died at the age of 98.

Source: © Massachusetts General Hospital.

---

features. More or less at the same time, an article by two pathologists from Boston, Samuel P. Hicks (d. 1996) and Shields Warren (1898–1980), concluded that: '... in 60 of the hundred cases of infarction there was no mechanical occlusion of cerebral vessels by thrombosis, embolism or arteriosclerosis';[70] in their eyes, the only possible explanation left was vasospasm.

---

[70] Hicks and Warren (1951), Infarction of the brain without thrombosis.

Fisher, however, did not give up his attempts to find a less far-fetched interpretation of brain infarction without apparent cause:

> My interest in this subject was aroused while working at the Mallory Institute of Pathology, under the directorship of Raymond D. Adams. There, in case after case, neuropathological examination failed to confirm the clinical impression of disease of the middle cerebral artery. During a period of nine months, in which the brains in 200 cases of cerebrovascular disease were examined, not a single case of thrombosis of the middle cerebral artery was found, although the diagnosis had often been made clinically. [. . .] Moreover, during our study of brain embolism, in many cases no source for the embolus could be found in the conventional locations – the pulmonary veins, the left auricle, the left ventricle or the ascending aorta. The neglected area, again, seemed to lie in the carotid system [. . .][71]

So, once back in Montreal, Fisher undertook a methodical search for lesions of the carotid artery, including its extracranial part. A practical hitch was that by removing the carotid bifurcation at autopsy, he created a difficulty for the morticians; they used the external carotid artery as an access for perfusing the face of the deceased, a procedure allowing relatives to view an open casket. Fisher solved the problem by leaving a rubber tube in the external branch.[72] In his 1951 report, he presented details about eight patients with hemiplegia.

These eight patients with a fatal stroke and carotid occlusion were all men; predominance of males over females had been a constant feature in all previous reports of atherothrombosis and would remain so. Also, they were older, on average, than patients in whom carotid occlusion had been detected after angiography. Several of them had reported fleeting symptoms days, weeks, or months before; such premonitory attacks are the subject of a separate chapter; here the question is why the collateral circulation failed in the major attack.

Fisher's first four patients are most informative, because in them, pathological examination of the brain, as well as of blood vessels, was possible. In each of these four, the ICA was occluded at the level of the carotid sinus, but proved completely unaffected in its further course. In two, a sudden hemiplegia had occurred several years before death; in one of these two patients, the stroke had been precipitated by severe iatrogenic hypotension (vasodilator drugs as treatment for gangrene of a foot), and in the other, with a subtotal occlusion, the anterior communicating artery was abnormal, being trabeculated into three or four smaller vessels. The two other patients died within a few days of the corresponding event; one had become hypotensive during an operation in the neck to remove metastases of a nasopharyngeal carcinoma

---

[71] Fisher (1951), Occlusion of the internal carotid artery, 346.
[72] Feindel and Leblanc (2016), *The Wounded Brain Healed*, 184.

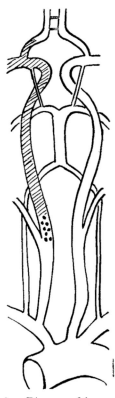

8.5 Diagram of the cerebral arteries in patient 3 of Fisher's publication of 1951. The patient was a 67-year-old man with nasopharyngeal carcinoma, operated for resection of lymph node metastases in the right cervical region. During the operation, the systolic blood pressure fell to about 70 millimetres for one and a half hour. The patient died 72 hours later from massive infarction of the left hemisphere. The corresponding text reads: 'The circle of Willis showed a very small anterior communicating artery, and the posterior communicating vessels were small in comparison with the posterior cerebral arteries. The right internal carotid artery was tightly packed, with a dark red clot extending distally into the middle and anterior cerebral arteries and proximally to the region of the carotid sinus. At the sinus, the right internal carotid artery was narrowed by a white, firm atherosclerotic deposition, so that the diameter of the lumen was at one place no greater than 0.5 mm'. *Source:* © Archives of Neurology and Psychiatry.

(Figure 8.5); in the other, with a subtotal carotid occlusion on one side, it appeared that concomitant occlusion of the basilar artery and one vertebral artery had caused subsequent sudden loss of consciousness and death.

So far, the evidence seemed to suggest that the pathophysiology of brain softening after carotid occlusion or extreme narrowing was determined by failure of the collateral supply, either by a fall in blood pressure or by associated abnormalities of other intracranial vessels. Fisher did not profess to such a general 'haemodynamic explanation' in so many words, but seemed to imply it:

> [...] the extent of damage to the brain following spontaneous occlusion
> of the internal carotid arteries is a function of the adequacy of the

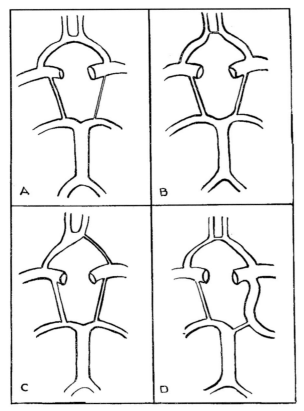

8.6 Diagram of common variations in the circle of Willis (from Fisher, 1951). *Source:* © *Archives of Neurology and Psychiatry.*

collateral circulation. It is usually possible to explain most of the pathological picture by studying the vascular pattern and the patency of its vessels. But the pattern of the circle of Willis must be studied in its entirety.

He continued by underlining the importance of the arrangement of the collateral pathways in individual patients, partly exemplified by findings in his own series (Figure 8.6):

For example, it is not sufficient to examine the anterior communicating artery and, finding it large, conclude that failure of collateral circulation cannot be used to explain the pathological picture. The size of the involved anterior cerebral artery must be considered too, for it may be small and inadequate when the anterior communicating artery is ample. A large posterior communicating artery may be a liability, rather than an asset, if the proximal posterior cerebral artery is small. If the anterior communicating and posterior communicating arteries are small, the territory of the middle and anterior cerebral arteries will be infarcted. If

the anterior communicating artery is small and the posterior communicating artery is large, the entire hemisphere will usually be softened.[73]

Notwithstanding this emphasis on the relative width of arterial connections,
Fisher was well aware of Chiari's case, in which the carotid sinus had been a
source of embolus:

> I have so far been unable to corroborate Chiari's observations in detail
> but have not infrequently noted thrombus material on the wall of the
> carotid sinus. Emboli can thus be expected to complicate the picture of
> internal carotid artery disease [...][74]

Fisher did not leave it at that. Continuing in the dual roles as a neurologist and
a pathologist in two hospitals in Montreal, he went on studying the arterial
system in the brain, as well as in the neck, in deceased patients.

EMBOLISM FROM THE CAROTID SINUS

Carotid Occlusions Can Have Different Effects

In 1954, Fisher published additional observations in 45 cases of carotid atherothrombosis from 432 consecutive autopsies. He found much variety, both in the
arterial lesions, as Hultquist had recognized, and in the clinical manifestations.
Still, some patterns emerged. Sometimes carotid occlusion was asymptomatic
or it accompanied other brain diseases, but in most, it had caused sudden
unilateral hemiplegia, aphasia, hemianopia, or combinations of these symptoms.
With few exceptions, patients were aged 55 or over and atherosclerotic lesions
had been followed by thrombotic occlusion or, in about one-third, tight
stenosis. The location of the primary lesion was almost invariably the carotid
sinus, and in only a few the common carotid artery or the intracranial segment
of the ICA. The corresponding area of softening did not always correspond
to a particular artery or branch, but was sometimes located between different
territories ('watershed area'),[75] a phenomenon previously noticed.[76]

Chiari Vindicated

In 9 of his 45 patients, Fisher found what one might call 'Chiari's pair': an
embolus in an intracranial artery, together with a mural thrombus in an

---

[73] Fisher (1951), Occlusion of the internal carotid artery, 372.
[74] Fisher (1951), Occlusion of the internal carotid artery, 376.
[75] Fisher (1954), Occlusion of the carotid arteries: further experiences, 192.
[76] Sorgo (1939), Verschluss der Art. carotis interna, 169. In World War II, Wolfram Sorgo
(1908–1983) carried out criminal operations (Czech (2017), Vienna School of Medicine,
1939–1945, 146–7).

occluded or extremely narrowed carotid sinus. The following case history
is exemplary:

> The patient, aged 81, had a left-sided stroke two years previously. She
> was admitted finally because of a fracture of the neck of the femur
> following a fall. The hip was pinned, with the patient under anesthesia
> after which she remained comatose until she died, five days later.
> Pathological examination showed an extensive softening of the right
> cerebral hemisphere and a transtentorial herniation of the temporal lobe.
> The right carotid sinus was narrowed to a hole 0.5 mm or less by a large
> atherosclerotic plaque. More distally, an embolus (confirmed microscop-
> ically) was found tightly occluding the right anterior cerebral artery
> opposite the mouth of the anterior communicating artery. It was con-
> cluded that such a large embolus could not have passed through the
> remaining lumen of the carotid sinus and therefore must have arisen
> distally. The embolus probably arrested the blood flow reaching the right
> hemisphere via the anterior communicating artery.[77]

From these and similar findings, Fisher warned:

> This possibility is of great importance, for it no doubt is one of the
> mechanisms by which an incompletely occluded carotid vessel can pro-
> duce a hemiplegia. In such cases examination months later will show no
> vessel occlusion intracranially, for the embolus, as a rule, will have long
> since disintegrated and disappeared.[78]

He concluded:

> [...] [in the past] there remained a substantial residue of unexplained
> cases. In my experience, routine examination of the cervical portion of
> the carotid arteries reduces this residuum to less than 5% of cases.[79]

Like Ramsay Hunt 40 years before, Fisher also advocated palpation of the
carotid artery on both sides, despite the possible negative and positive errors
with this procedure. A few years later, he added that in a minority of patients
with carotid occlusion, a bruit could be heard over the eyeball on the other
side, that is the side of the patent artery.[80]

Two Possible Explanations

In a few years' time, Fisher's proofs of the importance of atherothrombotic
lesions in extracerebral arteries, especially the carotid artery, became widely

---

[77] Fisher (1954), Occlusion of the carotid arteries: further experiences, 202.
[78] Fisher (1954), Occlusion of the carotid arteries: further experiences, 191.
[79] Fisher (1954), Occlusion of the carotid arteries: further experiences, 203.
[80] Fisher (1957a), Cranial bruit associated with occlusion of the internal carotid artery.

accepted. The medical community increasingly abandoned the somewhat vague, but convenient, notion of 'cerebral thrombosis' for large ischaemic strokes that could not be explained differently. A steady stream of supporting publications appeared. To cite them all would make dull reading; some offered more statistics than insight. Still, some questions remained to be answered.

To begin with, if cerebral infarction was associated with atheromatous lesions at the carotid bifurcation, far proximal to the circle of Willis, had, in all these cases, a distal embolus been fragmented and carried downstream? After all, previously Fisher had also implicated associated anomalies in communicating or other intracranial arteries. Which explanation was the most common? And: was the pathogenesis the same for the posterior circulation?

MOSTLY ARTERIO-ARTERIAL EMBOLISM, OR FAILING COLLATERALS?

Pathologists and neurologists approached these problems in a variety of ways. Some tabulated the distribution of atherosclerotic lesions in all extracranial arteries, in unselected post-mortem procedures, or only in patients with ischaemic brain disease. Others tried to reconstruct the course of events by comparing the site of atherothrombotic lesions with the location and extent of brain softening. Also, angiography was increasingly performed, but it was less helpful than autopsy in understanding the extent of thrombo-atheromatous disease.

Frequency of Atherosclerosis in Carotid or Vertebral Arteries

Of the entire meandering course of the ICA, Fisher's studies in the 1950s had not included the segments in the skull base and in the cavernous sinus; Hultquist, who had, found little evidence of atherothrombosis there. K. C. Samuel (n.d.), on study leave from Jaipur, India, studied the entire trail of the carotid artery in 82 consecutive autopsies of adults at Hammersmith Hospital. Indeed the carotid sinus was the most common site of atherosclerotic and superimposed thrombotic lesions, but the next most common site in his sample was the intracavernous part, followed by the intracerebral and petrous portions; the cervical part above the sinus was the least often affected.[81] A pathological study of the carotid siphon, with Fisher – now in Boston – as first author, found calcification there in 74 of 99 unselected specimens, with a tendency towards an inverse relationship between the degree of calcification and the severity of atheroma.[82]

---

[81] Samuel (1956), Atherosclerosis and occlusion of the internal carotid artery.
[82] Fisher, *et al.* (1965), Calcification of the carotid siphon.

Atherosclerosis of the vertebrobasilar, as well as carotid, arteries was the subject matter in a study of 93 unselected autopsies by C. J. Schwartz (n.d.) and the neurologist Tony Mitchell (1928–1991), in Oxford. The distribution of atheromatous lesions over the carotid trajectory was grossly similar to that in Samuel's study.[83] Somewhat surprisingly, they found that atheroma in the vertebral artery (VA) was even more frequent than in the carotid sinus; it was most often located near the origin from the subclavian artery. Since the calibre of VAs was generally smaller than that of the carotids, relatively modest degrees of atherosclerosis could lead to severe vertebral stenosis. A sample of similar size from the Mayo Clinic in Rochester, Minnesota, showed comparable results.[84]

Overall, the new studies of atherosclerotic lesions in extracranial arteries were in agreement with the findings of Mehnert and Dow at the beginning of the century. Though such statistical observations helped to re-establish the VAs as additional predilection sites of atherosclerosis, in individual cases the question remained how superimposed thrombosis caused occlusion of major cerebral arteries: via arterio-arterial embolism or by local thrombosis, at single or several locations.

The Role of the Posterior Circulation in Cerebral Infarction

In the late 1950s, a duo from Manchester Royal Infirmary, the neurologist Edward Charles Hutchinson (1921–2002),[85] collaborating with the pathologist P. O. Yates (1921–2001), pointed out that the role of atheromatous lesions in the neck section of the VA had been as much neglected as in the case of the carotid artery before Fisher. In a first study, they scrutinized the entire course of the neck arteries in 48 patients who had died of 'a variety of cerebrovascular disease'; the emphasis was on the VA, which was stenotic or occluded in 19 patients. The VA lesions occurred most often at or near the origin of the VA from the subclavian artery, as in the Oxford study; elsewhere they were scattered, without predilection, even for the tortuous trajectory around the atlas and axis.[86]

Since the presence of vertebral atherosclerosis tended to parallel that in the carotid artery, the same duo performed a further study in which they recorded intra- and extracerebral occlusions in 22 patients with recent cerebral infarction. They drew special attention to a group of eight patients with combined stenosis of the carotid and vertebral arteries, on one or both sides, for which they proposed the term 'carotico-vertebral stenosis'. All showed infarction in

---

[83] Schwartz and Mitchell (1961), Atheroma of the carotid and vertebral arterial systems.
[84] Martin, *et al.* (1960), Occlusive vascular disease in the extracranial cerebral circulation.
[85] Aber and Hutchinson (2002), Edward Charles Hutchinson.
[86] Hutchinson and Yates (1956), The cervical portion of the vertebral artery.

several parts of the brain or cerebellum. The extent of the infarcts, often in the territory of the MCA, was mostly incomplete and patchy; the authors interpreted this as 'an expression of the inadequacy, in the final stages, of the collateral blood-supply'.[87] A few years later, the same authors confirmed these conclusions in a larger series of patients,[88] as did physicians from Philadelphia General Hospital (41 autopsied patients with supratentorial infarction).[89] The Manchester group added that especially the combination of stenosed neck vessels and string-like narrowing of one posterior communicating artery was associated with infarction.[90]

In the early 1970s, atherothrombotic changes in the posterior circulation were meticulously compared with associated areas of infarction by a group from the Salpêtrière with Paul Castaigne (1916–1988) as first author.[91] The location of the primary occlusion of the VA (15 patients with 17 occlusions) differed from that reported by the Oxford and Manchester groups: the terminal part of the artery in 12, the first section in only four instances, and the middle part in one patient. In 10 of these 15 patients, with or without associated occlusion of the posterior inferior cerebellar artery, infarction had occurred beyond the site of vertebral occlusion: in the upper brainstem, the occipital lobe, or both. Most occipital lobe infarcts could be attributed to emboli from the occluded VA, but haemodynamic failure may well have contributed to at least some of the supratentorial ischaemic lesions, given the frequent association with atherosclerosis in the carotid system.

Arterio-arterial Embolism from the Carotid Sinus

Further Parisian studies of the carotid system in the early 1970s provided rather decisive evidence that in the anterior circulation arterio-arterial embolism was more common than 'misery perfusion', at least in their series.

Castaigne's group studied the brains of 27 patients in whom cerebral infarction was associated with carotid occlusion, mostly in or near the carotid sinus, otherwise in the carotid siphon.[92] In one-quarter, antegrade thrombosis had extended beyond the intracranial bifurcation of the ICA; in this subgroup, infarction tended to be extensive, often involving the territory of both the middle and anterior cerebral arteries. In the remaining three-quarters of patients, they often found emboli to the main or smaller branches of the ICA, single or multiple; these emboli were mostly associated with restricted

[87] Hutchinson and Yates (1957), Carotico-vertebral stenosis.
[88] Yates and Hutchinson (1961), *Cerebral Infarction*.
[89] Wiener, *et al.* (1964), Intracranial circulation in carotid occlusion.
[90] Battacharji, *et al.* (1967), Developmental abnormalities in normal and infarcted brains.
[91] Castaigne, *et al.* (1973), Arterial occlusions in the vertebro-basilar system.
[92] Castaigne, *et al.* (1970), Internal carotid artery occlusion.

areas of infarction. Some old emboli could be related to past episodes in which angiography had shown ICA stenosis, so that the disruption of the thrombus and arterio-arterial embolism should have taken place before total occlusion occurred.[93]

Another approach was to collect instances of infarction in the territory of the MCA and to try and detect its source. This was done by the same group at the Salpêtrière, now led by François Lhermitte (1921–1998).[94] In the important subgroup where both the ICA and the MCA had been occluded, embolism by a thrombus that had been torn loose was more common than antegrade thrombosis extending beyond the intracranial ICA bifurcation. In addition, non-occlusive stenosis of the ICA had sometimes led to thrombo-embolism downstream. These conclusions were compatible with an earlier, somewhat less detailed study from London, by William Blackwood (1910–1990) and others.[95] In both series, primary atherosclerotic occlusion of the MCA was distinctly rare, in keeping with the earlier results of Foix and Ley, Hicks and Warren, and Fisher.

Embolism is also a likely explanation for the dramatic complication that manipulation of the carotid artery is followed by permanent contralateral hemiplegia,[96] previously attributed to arterial spasm.[97] More compelling evidence for the importance of arterio-arterial embolism in the pathogenesis of cerebral infarction, at least in the anterior circulation, was to emerge from observations in patients with transient attacks, as Chapter 10 will attest. As a final note, embolism from the heart still accounted for a sizeable minority of some studies in the 1960s;[98] this may well reflect the high incidence of rheumatic fever at the time when these patients had been young.

Increase in Angiographic Studies

Carotid angiography, initially restricted to patients with clinical features suggesting either a cerebral tumour or a ruptured basal aneurysm, became gradually performed more often, but not in elderly patients with a massive stroke, given the lack of therapeutic implications. So when physicians reported a 'striking variability of the clinical picture and prognosis in individual patients

[93] Castaigne, *et al.* (1970), Internal carotid artery occlusion, 251.
[94] Lhermitte, *et al.* (1970), Occlusions of the middle cerebral artery.
[95] Blackwood, *et al.* (1969), The carotid arterial system and embolism from the heart.
[96] Calverley and Millikan (1961), Complications of carotid manipulation.
[97] Askey (1946), Hemiplegia following carotid sinus stimulation.
[98] Blackwood, *et al.* (1969), The carotid arterial system and embolism from the heart; Lhermitte, *et al.* (1970), Occlusions of the middle cerebral artery, 84–5.

with carotid occlusive disease',[99] they were actually just telling the reader the characteristics of patients they selected for angiography.

A centre in Detroit, less restrictive, had performed 800 cerebral angiograms by 1961 and found 42 brain tumours, 30 aneurysms or arteriovenous malformations, and eight subdural haematomas, next to hundreds of arterial occlusions. Complications of the procedure were not rare,[100] not even in the 1970s.[101] Although Sven Ivar Seldinger in Stockholm had developed a catheter technique in the 1950s,[102] it took a few decades before his method was generally adopted. Indeed, as authors from National Hospital in London mused in 1960, 'At present it is impossible to strike a balance between gain and loss when using angiography in the management of acute strokes.'[103]

In terms of understanding the pathophysiology of cerebral ischaemia, angiography was still less informative than autopsy. Only if unilateral carotid occlusion occurred together with non-filling of the ophthalmic artery from the contralateral side, the inference was justified that thrombosis had extended beyond the bifurcation of the ICA.[104] On the other hand, angiography proved extremely helpful in diagnosing a new and non-atheromatous cause of carotid occlusion.

Carotid Dissection

The first recorded patient with carotid dissection was associated with neck trauma, as in most later reports. The accident happened during the Second World War, in the Arabian Peninsula; in the wording of the authors, the neurosurgeon Captain George Bernard Northcroft (1911–1996) and Captain A. D. Morgan (n.d.):

> On the morning of Aug. 19, 1942, the patient, a signalman aged 31, was walking along a military road, accompanied by a friend, when they were overtaken from behind by a lorry travelling in the same direction. According to the statement of his friend, a piece of loose rope hanging from the side of the lorry wound itself round the patient's neck, threw him to the ground, and then unwound itself without dragging him along. He picked himself up, and, though he felt faint and was suffering from a superficial laceration in the right parietal region, he was able to accompany his friend on foot to the Unit Medical Officer.

[99] Hurwitz, et al. (1959), Carotid artery occlusive syndrome.
[100] Broadbridge and Leslie (1958), Cerebral angiographic contrast media.
[101] Matthews (1972), The investigation of cerebrovascular disease.
[102] Seldinger (1953), Catheter replacement of the needle in percutaneous arteriography.
[103] Bull, et al. (1960), Cerebral angiography in the diagnosis of the acute stroke.
[104] Castaigne, et al. (1970), Internal carotid artery occlusion.

After the scalp wound had been stitched with a single suture, the patient was referred to the nearest hospital, where he was detained overnight because of mild amnesia. On the following morning he was alert and rational; there were some superficial abrasions on the throat, especially on the left. But, when a nurse was dressing the scalp wound, the soldier suddenly failed to respond; twenty minutes later he had flopped over in bed and after another fifteen minutes the medical officer found him unconscious, with a complete right flaccid hemiplegia. An exploratory burr hole in the left temporal region failed to show an extradural haematoma; the patient died 48 hours after the accident. At autopsy, the neck region was most important:

The first 1½ in. of the left internal carotid artery were transformed into a hard bluish, spindle-shaped swelling as a result of traumatic thrombosis. [...] On cutting the thrombosed internal carotid artery longitudinally, the mechanism of the thrombosis was revealed. The main thrombus lay just above the origin of the internal carotid artery, extending upwards for 1½ in. The original lesion was presumably a tearing of the intima and media, with extravasation of blood into the media, raising both intima and media from the outer layers of the vessel wall. As the haemorrhage increased in size, the lumen of the vessel became narrowed, until finally the rucked-up intima and media completely blocked the lumen in the form of an inverted valve, with the thrombosed blood below it. Following total occlusion, more recent thrombosis occurred above the level of injury, spreading upwards into the petrous and cavernous portions of the vessel to continue into the left middle cerebral artery, resulting in massive infarction of the left cerebral hemisphere.[105]

In other cases of relatively mild trauma followed by hemiplegia, one can recognize, or at least suspect, similar events, such as in a boy who, in 1908, sustained not only unilateral paralysis, but also, a few weeks later, blindness on the other side.[106]

Subsequent reports of carotid dissection also included 'spontaneous' cases – that is, the history did not uncover blows, strangling, or other accidents involving the neck; of course, normal life is full of unremembered 'mini-injuries'. The first instance of this kind committed to the medical literature concerned a man of 41 years who had presented with hemiplegia of the right body half and aphasia at National Hospital in London; angiography showed a configuration that was to prove typical in subsequent cases: narrowing of the contrast column, starting closely above the origin and gradually tapering to occlusion or near-occlusion (Figure 8.7).[107] Also in this patient, massive infarction led to a fatal outcome within less than three days; autopsy

---

[105] Northcroft and Morgan (1944), A fatal case of traumatic thrombosis of the internal carotid artery.
[106] Guthrie and Mayou (1908), Right hemiplegia and atrophy of left optic nerve.
[107] Anderson and Schechter (1959), A case of spontaneous dissecting aneurysm of the internal carotid artery.

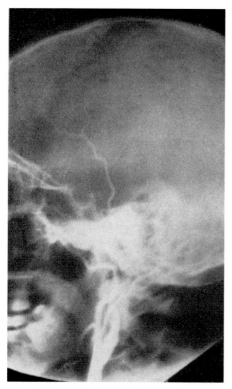

8.7 Carotid angiogram showing arterial dissection in a patient without a history of trauma (from Anderson and Schechter, 1959). The original legend reads: 'The needle point, which is not shown, must be proximal to the end of the common carotid artery. The external carotid artery and its branches are outlined. The internal carotid artery tapers 3 cm above its origin (A film taken 1.5 seconds later showed some delayed filling of more distal parts of the internal carotid artery).' *Source:* By permission of the *Journal of Neurology, Neurosurgery, and Psychiatry.*

completely confirmed the diagnosis. In 1972, Ojemann and Fisher, describing another patient with spontaneous carotid dissection complicated by hemiplegia, cited 10 others up to that time. Their patient underwent surgical removal of the thrombus, survived, and gradually improved.

It is a sobering fact that angiography by means of direct puncture of the artery could not only show, but also cause carotid dissection.[108] The danger of iatrogenic complications also looms heavily over the subject of therapeutic attempts: the wish to prevent brain ischaemia, or at least worsening of existing lesions, by means of surgical intervention.

THE SURGEON AND THE CAROTID ARTERY

The history of carotid surgery began in the 1930s and 1940s, as recounted above, with resection of the occluded arterial segment, the superior cervical

---

[108] Fleming and Park (1959), Dissecting aneurysms of the carotid artery following arteriography.

ganglion, or both; these interventions depended on hypotheses about vaso-spasm, secondary to occlusive disease. Others supposed, given the known relationship between the vagus nerve and the carotid sinus, that atherosclerotic tissue not only narrowed the lumen, but also induced sympathetic hyperactiv-ity and hypertension.[109]

In the 1950s, after Fisher's work had focused the attention of the medical world on thrombotic processes in or near the carotid sinus, surgeons became interested in the possibility of restoring the blood supply to the brain, in line with the surgical treatment of chronic leg ischaemia.[110] This activist stance reverberates in the term 'cerebral arterial insufficiency',[111] and even more in the unrestrained optimism emanated by some:

> To realize the full potential of this new and encouraging form of treatment, a much more aggressive approach must be taken toward the problem of cerebral arterial insufficiency. In our opinion, all patients with cerebrovascular occlusive disease should be suspected of having a poten-tially curable lesion.[112]

The first carotid endarterectomy may well have been performed in China, Argentina, or, as some claimed, in Houston, Texas, but the event that gener-ated by far the most intense publicity, through a report in *The Lancet*, was the resection and reconstruction of a stenosed carotid artery at St Mary's Hospital in London, in 1954.[113] The patient, a 66-year-old housewife, had experienced more than 30 attacks 'lasting from ten minutes to half an hour, in all of which there was loss of vision in the left eye, right hemiparesis and aphasia, preceded by this heavy feeling in the chest, associated with rapid palpitation of the heart'. The attacks of paroxysmal tachycardia continued after the operation, but they were no longer followed by manifestations of focal brain ischaemia. More sobering is an early report of 27 operated patients.[114] Of the 16 patients with complete occlusion, the flow was restored in only four; of the 11 patients with stenosis, one woke up with hemiplegia, and in the entire series of 27 patients, three died fairly soon afterwards, from vascular diseases other than ischaemic stroke.

Modified techniques for restoring blood flow to the brain were introduced: arterial homografts,[115] vein grafts,[116] and nylon bypass grafts;[117] yet thrombendarterectomy

---

[109] Keele (1933), Pathological changes in the carotid sinus.
[110] Ellis (2019), The story of peripheral vascular surgery.
[111] Corday, *et al.* (1953), Cerebral vascular insufficiency.
[112] Fields, *et al.* (1958), Surgical considerations in cerebral arterial insufficiency.
[113] Eastcott, *et al.* (1954), Reconstruction of internal carotid artery.
[114] Rob and Wheeler (1957), Thrombosis of internal carotid artery treated by arterial surgery.
[115] Denman, *et al.* (1955), Insidious occlusion of carotid arteries, treated by arterial graft.
[116] Lin, *et al.* (1956), Carotid artery occlusion treated by primary resection and vein graft.
[117] Lyons and Galbraith (1957), Surgical treatment of atherosclerotic occlusion of the internal carotid artery.

remained the mainstay. The actual problem remained the lack of proof that, on average, the gains exceeded the losses. Publication of uncontrolled studies plummeted, especially in the United States. In 1974, precisely at the point in time when the story in this book comes to a halt, the closing sentence in an editorial on carotid surgery in the *British Medical Journal* was as ambiguous as it was optimistic: 'Operative risks can never be completely eliminated but there is no longer any doubt about the value of successful surgery.'[118] Successful for whom, was the question.

Meanwhile, transient attacks of brain ischaemia were increasingly often recognized. In such patients, the question of whether or not to advise angiography with a view to surgical treatment with its associated risks was even more difficult. A first randomized trial of carotid surgery in the United States claimed benefit in patients with transient attacks,[119] but apart from the pitfalls of subgroup analysis, the assessment of outcome was unmasked and the numbers were small. Admittedly, the benefits of medical treatment were equally unknown at the time, but the potential downsides were definitely less.

What exactly are 'transient attacks of cerebral ischaemia'? A British neurologist muttered somewhat facetiously in 1972: 'There are some towns where it is unwise to complain of dizziness for fear of being subjected to direct puncture vertebral angiography.'[120] The subject deserves a separate chapter; but first an excursion to small, deep infarcts.

---

[118] Editorial (1974), Internal carotid stenosis.
[119] Fields, *et al.* (1970), Surgery or nonsurgical treatment for transient cerebral ischemic attacks.
[120] Matthews (1972), The investigation of cerebrovascular disease.

NINE

LACUNES

SUMMARY

In the middle of the nineteenth century, small holes in deep regions in the brain were recognized as widened perivascular spaces (Durand-Fardel: 'état criblé'). Later researchers (Laborde, Proust, Campbell) reported in these areas some larger cavities with ragged borders, presumably damaged brain tissue ('lacunes'); these authors did not correlate such lesions with symptoms, and their pathogenesis remained unclear.

Hemisensory disorders were the first symptoms attributed to lacunar lesions (Türck, Bourneville). In the early twentieth century, lesions causing hemiparesis followed; these were studied more systematically (Marie, Ferrand; Foix and Hillemand). In the 1960s, Fisher not only confirmed the relationship with hypertension that had previously been suggested (Hughes), but also defined several 'lacunar syndromes': pure motor hemiplegia (internal capsule or pons), pure sensory stroke (internal capsule, probably thalamus), ataxic hemiparesis (pons), and 'dysarthria–clumsy hand syndrome' (pons).

Fisher also studied the arterial lesions, which had long remained elusive. Small lacunes (below approximately 1 centimetre) almost invariably resulted from occlusion of terminal twigs through thickened walls, infiltrated by fatty material ('lipohyalinosis'); symptomatic lacunes tended to be larger and associated with thrombotic occlusion of an arteriolar branch from a major artery.

Small, deep cavities in the brain were first distinguished in the course of the nineteenth century. They are of historical interest firstly because some, as it turned out, are ischaemic in origin but others are not. Also, the pathogenesis of small ischaemic lesions is somewhat different from that of large artery disease.

Most, if not all, articles about historical aspects of lacunar stroke begin with an explanation of the term 'lacune'. This seems strange but is appropriate, since physicians first used it for cavities unrelated to ischaemia.

THE TERM

A Small Lake

'Lacuna' is a Latin word, often with a poetical ring, for a small pit or hole where water collects; it is a diminutive of *lacus*, for 'lake'. It goes almost without saying that the term has been used for a host of things, such as a missing verse in transcripts of ancient poems.

Medicine has also used the word in various senses. An example is Dechambre, whose paper of 1838 is always dutifully cited; however, his article had nothing to do with small brain lesions. Dechambre wanted to prove that lesions of brain softening could heal, while the corresponding symptoms also improved. He used the term, in a very casual fashion, to indicate the loculated structure in large areas of softening in the brain ('a stack of lacunes').[1]

État Criblé *(Perivascular Spaces)*

Another 'usual suspect' is Maxime Durand-Fardel (1815–1899), an ardent proponent of inflammation as the primary cause of brain softening in the history of *ramollissement*. Indeed, he identified small holes in the brain, but these were unrelated to softening. In 1842, the year before his book on brain softening appeared, he published an article on a 'peculiar alteration' in the substance of the brain. He began by reminding readers of the well-known small area on either side of the optic chiasm where many small holes allowed blood vessels to perforate deep regions of the brain. After injection of fluid into the parent vessels in a human cadaver, these small penetrating vessels became much wider, he explained, whereas normally they did not entirely fill their small canals. And he continued:

> But what has not yet been noticed, as far as I know, is the presence, inside the brain, deep in the white matter of the hemispheres, of vascular channels that form, on the surface of the customary brain cuts, a perforated aspect, similar to that on the outside of the brain. [. . .] This alteration

---

[1] Dechambre (1838), Curabilité du ramollissement, 309: *une foule de petites lacunes.*

I will designate, because of the aspect it presents, with the name *état criblé* [sieve-like state] of the brain.[2]

Durand-Fardel found that these holes were widely distributed across the white matter of the cerebral hemispheres and that they were abnormally large in some patients. He then presented several case reports to make the point that widening of these perivascular spaces was a sign of cerebral congestion. He also implied that this congestion had contributed to the symptoms before death. For example, it was the only detectable abnormality in a patient with general paralysis and dementia, and in a patient with 'simple dementia'; seven other patients had a variety of concomitant brain lesions. In some of them, softening of the brain had occurred, but in large and remote areas.

A year later, when Durand-Fardel published the voluminous book in which he championed inflammation as the explanation for acute, as well as chronic, brain softening, he briefly described a few cases with 'vacuoles' in the region of the basal ganglia. Yet these holes were multiple and, importantly, there was no relationship with cerebral dysfunction; once he used the word 'lacunes' for such aggregated lesions, but only in passing.[3]

All said and done, Durand-Fardel described small, perivascular holes in the brain, but not lacunes – at least not in the sense of tissue damage with corresponding acute loss of function. Other reports mentioned holes in the brain that looked more like lesions and were also somewhat larger, but purely in the sense of morphological phenomena, unrelated to symptoms.

THE LESIONS, NOT THE SYMPTOMS

Pea-Sized Lacunes, with Ragged Borders

At the Parisian Bicêtre, Jean-Baptiste Vincent Laborde (1830–1903) mentioned 'pea-sized lacunes' in his 1866 book on *ramollissement*, in which, parenthetically, he muddled the subject rather than clarified it, by conflating all different kinds of cerebral softening, including the lesions of dementia paralytica. More or less in passing, he wrote:

> *Pea-sized lacunes.* [...] Their cavity is not entirely empty, for in their centre some *ragged filaments* are floating, where one sees fragments of fibrillary elements or tiny capillaries. They clearly result from a partial and progressive disorganisation.[4]

---

[2] Durand-Fardel (1842), Altération particulière de la substance cérébrale, 23. Other possible translations of '*criblé*' are 'perforated' or 'buckshot'.

[3] Durand-Fardel (1843), *Traité du Ramollissement du Cerveau*, 291.

[4] Laborde (1866), *Le Ramollissement et Congestion du Cerveau*, 94: *lacunes pisiformes, foyers pisiformes*.

Later that year, Adrien Achille Proust (1834–1903) – the father of the novelist, mentioned on p. 221 – wrote in his thesis on brain softening:

> Perhaps changes of capillaries should also be implicated as the cause of *lacunes*, small cavities with the size of a pea, which are commonly found in the striate bodies and to us often seem very small areas of softening.[5]

And he continued, in a chapter about scars resulting from circulatory disturbances:

> One often finds, in sections including the corpus striatum, the thalami or, more rarely, the pons, small, pea-sized cavities, sometimes tortuous, and with ragged borders. [...] These small cavities, which have received the name of *lacunes*, and in which one finds granular bodies, show a variable dimension, but in general they do not exceed the size of a lentil or a small pea; in some cases, they are numerous and give the striate body a sieve-like appearance, which has led Mr. Durand-Fardel to describe them with the name *état criblé*. This author regarded them as the result of widening of vessels, secondary to repeated congestion. Authors are not in agreement about the interpretation one has to apply to these lacunes; but it is probable that sometimes they arise from a small area of haemorrhage or a small area of softening.[6]

Proust overinterpreted Durand-Fardel here, in conflating the other's smooth, round, pinpoint openings attributed to perivascular dilatation with the somewhat larger, pea-sized vacuoles with frayed borders he had seen himself.

A Minute Rupture?

Almost three decades later, in 1894, Alfred W. Campbell (1868–1937) also described small lesions in the region of the basal ganglia. He did not call them lacunes and did not correlate them with symptoms. Campbell was born in New South Wales and had studied medicine in Edinburgh; in 1905, he returned to Sydney.[7] During his time as a pathologist in the Lancashire County Asylum at Rainhill, he studied the brains of old and demented patients. He phrased his findings in general terms, for example the comment that several aged patients with the diagnosis of 'insanity' failed to show the pathological characteristics of 'general paralysis of the insane'. He confirmed Durand-Fardel's observation of an *état criblé*, but added that some small lesions required a different explanation:

> Examining a microscopical section of one of the basal nuclei which is disorganized by perivascular dilatation in the manner which I have

---

[5] Proust (1866), Ramollissement du cerveau.

[6] Proust (1866), Ramollissement du cerveau, 74.   [7] von Bonin (1970), Walter Campbell.

described, one notices that one has to deal not only with a perivascular dilatation pure and simple, but that an actual irregular-shaped small cystic cavity has formed round the vessel and occasioned the destruction of a considerable amount of nervous tissue. This cavity contains fibro-cellular material, blood crystals, leukocytes, compound granule cells, and debris. The diseased blood vessel can be seen lying near its centre.

Campbell thought leakage of blood was responsible for the small area of tissue destruction:

> What actually occurs primarily to set up this condition is this – a minute rupture of the vessel wall takes place, through this blood is infused into and further distends the already dilated perivascular space and this effusion mainly by pressure destroys the immediately surrounding tissues.[8]

For the true beginning of the story of 'lacunar strokes', one has to go further back in the nineteenth century, to isolated case reports of patients with sudden neurological deficits that, after autopsy, seemed to correspond to small lesions in the brain.

THE LESIONS AND THEIR SYMPTOMS

Lacunar Softening

In the third quarter of the nineteenth century, two articles correlated small, deep lesions with clinical deficits. The symptoms were actually the main point of interest, since both papers described patients with persistent hemianaesthesia after the accompanying motor deficits had cleared; the aim was to localize the sensory fibres ascending from deep regions of the brain to the cortex. One author was Ludwig Türck (1810–1868),[9] a neuropathologist and laryngologist in Vienna,[10] and the other Désiré-Magloire Bourneville (1840–1909) (Box 9.1),[11] Charcot's younger colleague who had tried to distinguish haemorrhagic apoplexy from softening by thermometry.

A difficulty in these attempts at localizing sensation was that their patients had more than one lesion. Yet, most lesions they identified were small enough, with the largest measuring 2×1 centimetres, and the smallest 5×2 millimetres, to correspond to 'lacunes' in the sense that the term was to acquire later, at least in some of Türck's four patients and in Bourneville's only patient, a 64-year-old woman known only as *Hortense*, who was admitted to the service of Charcot.

---

[8] Campbell (1894), Morbid changes in the nervous system of the aged insane, 642–3.
[9] Türck (1859), Die Beziehung gewisser Krankheitsherde des grossen Gehirnes zur Anästhesie.
[10] Schmahmann, *et al.* (1992), The mysterious relocation of the bundle of Türck.
[11] Benda (1970), Désiré Magloire Bourneville; Zarranz (2015), Bourneville: a neurologist in action; Brigo, *et al.* (2018), First descriptions of tuberous sclerosis.

Box 9.1 Bourneville (1840–1909).

Champion of social justice and *égalité*, Bourneville chose to use only his surname, without the ponderous first names 'Desiré-Magloire'. He was the eldest of three sons in a family of modest landholders in Normandy. During his time as a medical student in Paris, he helped to combat a severe epidemic of cholera in Amiens. He also voluntarily assisted Louis Delasiauve (1804–1893), who took care of the psychiatric patients at the Salpêtrière and was Editor of the *Journal de médecine mentale*. 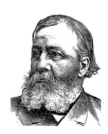 Bourneville spent the last year of his internship with Delasiauve and with Charcot, who supervised his graduation thesis on thermometry in patients with apoplexy. In 1870, an administrative move made Charcot responsible for patients with 'hystero-epilepsy' who had until then belonged to the service of Delasiauve. Bourneville edited the first clinical lessons on hysteria for Charcot, who was not familiar with this category of patients; he also co-authored the three volumes of the *Iconographie photographique de la Salpêtrière* (1877–80). Meanwhile Bourneville had founded the journal *Le Progrès médical* (1873); it was to continue for 110 years. In 1879, he obtained the position of *chef de service* for psychiatric patients at the Bicêtre, where he would remain until his retirement in 1905. His wife died a year later, and their son Marcel in 1914.

Maintaining his radical and anticlerical political ambitions, Bourneville was elected to the municipal council of Paris in 1876 as deputy for one of the poorer districts, and to membership of the National Assembly in 1883. His proposals with regard to public health included purification of the water supply, improved facilities for the mentally ill, and training of nurses. In his own hospital, he reorganized the care for children with physical or mental handicaps. Bourneville was a tireless debater, writer, and editor, not afraid of making enemies.

At the age of 46, he had married Maria Breugnon, with whom he had a son; she predeceased him by three years.

What is more, Bourneville used the term 'lacunes'; yet he did not intend to define a new clinico-anatomical category of brain lesions, as others were to claim later for themselves, but he merely used the word to describe the smallness of the lesions:

> In this case we see that the hemianesthesia, which ends precisely at the midline, involves the entire right half of the body, the face as well as the limbs and the trunk. [. . .] The lesions the autopsy allowed to recognise were located in the central area of the left hemisphere of the brain; these consist in multiple foci of softening belonging to an anatomical variety commonly designated with the name of *lacunar softening*.[12]

The italics were put in by Bourneville himself, but in the same sentence, it transpires that 'lacune' was already a household name (*forme anatomique désignee*

---

[12] Bourneville (1873), De l'hémianesthésie liée à une lésion d'un hémisphère du cerveau, 245.

d'ordinaire . . .), at least in the laboratory of the Salpêtrière, as in the descriptions of Proust and Laborde. What followed in both papers were the exact anatomical descriptions of the lesions in the five patients, in or near the corona radiata and the basal ganglia. Neither Bourneville nor Türck was concerned with the pathogenesis of the small areas of softening; they seemed to assume, without further explanation, that the small areas of softening (*Erweichung, ramollissement*) in patients with sudden neurological deficits were analogous to larger and more common lesions.

It was not until the beginning of the twentieth century that lacunar brain lesions were regarded as a separate pathophysiological category of disease.

'Lacunes of Disintegration'

Pierre Marie (1853–1940) (Box 9.2),[13] the chief of service at the hospital of the Bicêtre, the Parisian asylum for old men, wrote in 1901:

> Having for several years been at the head of an important [health] service for the aged, in whom hemiplegia is a frequent event, I have been struck by the relatively small number with haemorrhage or softening of the brain at the autopsy of my hemiplegic patients. In the largest number of these, one finds one or more lacunes, situated in or near the central grey nuclei or in the pons. [. . .] It is strange that despite the frequency of this lesion, and despite its importance from the point of view of the clinic as well as of pathological anatomy, authors pass it over in silence or at least give only a summary description.[14]

Marie found these 'lacunar foci of disintegration' as isolated lesions, but also in multiple form, up to 10 or more, and in both hemispheres. They occurred especially in the lenticular nucleus, sometimes involving the internal capsule (Figure 9.1), and also regularly in the thalamus or the pons; they occurred less often in the head of the caudate nucleus, the semi-oval centre of white matter, or in the thalamus. These structures were best visualized with, in Marie's words, 'Flechsig's horizontal cut': this plane of section started at the front end of the corpus callosum and was angled upward towards the Sylvian fissure. The size of these lacunes was that of millet seed, hemp seed, or peas, rarely like small beans. Typically, their borders were irregular. Marie described the lesions as well as the symptoms of his 50 patients only in general terms, without details or even histories of individual patients. On microscopy, the borders showed infiltration of tissue debris by granular bodies and sometimes red blood cells, at least in the acute stage; in a later phase, they became contracted and sclerotic. It follows from this description, Marie went on:

[13] Goetz (2003), Pierre Marie; Teive, *et al.* (2020), Duels of Pierre Marie and Jules Dejerine.
[14] Marie (1901), Foyers lacunaires de désintégration, 281.

Box 9.2 Pierre Marie (1853–1940).

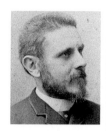

Marie grew up in a comfortable Parisian milieu and was initially destined for a career in law. Yet he soon switched to medicine, in which he excelled. After internships with Paul Broca and Charles Bouchard, he moved to the Salpêtrière as a disciple of Jean-Martin Charcot, who imbued him with the clinico-anatomical method. Among the studies Marie performed with Charcot's help are those on acromegaly and its relationship to pituitary tumours, on familial forms of polyneuropathy, later known as Charcot–Marie–Tooth disease, and on hereditary forms of ataxia. He became a *médecin des hôpitaux* in 1888 and an *agrégé* a year later. The intrigues after Charcot's death in 1893 caused him to move to the hospital of the Bicêtre, where diseases of the nervous system had received no special attention. In this period, Marie published on lacunes, on ankylosing spondylitis, and on what is now called the 'carpal tunnel syndrome'.

His temperament often failed to endear him to his colleagues. This reached a climax through Marie's criticisms of cerebral localization, especially in relation to aphasia. His chief opponent in these skirmishes, starting in print in 1906 and culminating two years later in an open debate, was Jules Dejerine (1849–1917); a duel with pistols was narrowly avoided. Dejerine, raised in Geneva, worked after his move to Paris with Vulpian and did not belong to the 'clan' of Charcot; yet Dejerine was appointed to Charcot's 'sacrosanct' chair of Neurology, after the 'neutral' successor Fulgence Raymond (1844–1910). It was not until 1907, after the death of Dejerine, with Paris being ravaged by war, that Marie, aged 66, was voted into Charcot's chair and could return to the Salpêtrière. On his retirement, six years later, he moved south and died at the onset of the next World War, having lost his wife and two children earlier on.

Source: Portrait courtesy of Wellcome Collection.

> [...] that its aspect is precisely that of a 'microscopic softening'. We have
> to take proper account of this fact when we seek to perceive the nature of
> this lesion and it seems indeed clear it is in blood vessels that one has to
> look for the cause of lacunes.[15]

The small blood vessels in or near the lacunes appeared pale, in all three layers. Similar changes of colour occurred in lenticulostriate arteries of larger calibre. It seems, Marie concluded, that arteriosclerosis, in its widest sense, is the primary cause of the lesion.[16] But how? Obliteration of the lumen was probably a factor, although the tiny vessels in the lesions were almost always permeable. Rupture of a small vessel was another possibility; in support of this idea, he added that of the 50 patients with lacunar lesions he had observed, almost half (23) had died after cerebral haemorrhage, against seven with

---

[15] Marie (1901), Foyers lacunaires de désintégration, 284.
[16] Marie (1901), Foyers lacunaires de désintégration, 286.

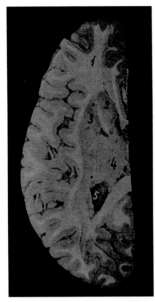

softening of the brain. He summarized this ambiguous interpretation as follows:

> One might thus imagine the anatomo-pathological events in the development of lacunes as follows: under the influence of the general causes responsible for atherosclerosis, the vessels carrying out the irrigation of the brain undergo change, the nutrition of the brain decays, its different parts undergo atrophy, which contributes to dilatation of ventricles and perivascular spaces; when the vascular changes continue, a progressive course, rupture or obliteration occurs in one or more of the small branches, resulting in the development of one or more lacunes, for it is known that in the deep parts of the brain the arrangement of vessels is *terminal*, in other words that there are no or very few anastomoses [...][17]

9.1 Lacunes (Marie, 1901). His legend is as follows: 'Horizontal cut of the left hemisphere; 1, frontal lobe; 2, head of the caudate nucleus; 3, lenticular nucleus; 4, lenticular nucleus; 5, occipital horn of the ventricle. One will note the existence of a lacune (small black triangle), situated precisely at the knee of the internal capsule; this lacune had given rise to a very distinct hemiplegia.'

Apart from the issue of haemorrhage versus occlusion, it is clear that Marie amalgamated the development of lacunes with other changes of old age in the brain. This even applied to the meninges: he found the dura mater was often adherent to the skull, and the pia mater thickened over the anterior two-thirds of one or both hemispheres.

The clinical features of lacunes consisted almost invariably of hemiplegia, according to Marie. Typically, the weakness was not accompanied by loss of consciousness; also, the weakness tended to improve in the course of weeks or months. Sometimes the hemiplegia was incomplete, but Marie did not correlate separate limbs with segments of the internal capsule; he did not believe in such a refinement of localization, he explained in a later paper.[18] At any rate, aphasia never accompanied hemiplegia in these patients, he emphasized, but dysarthria could be present; rare accompaniments were conjugate deviation of the eyes or hemianaesthesia. He regarded incontinence and an increased tendency to laughing or crying as mental phenomena.

If lacunes were multiple, one might see a shuffling gait (*marche à petits pas*) or features of a pseudo-bulbar syndrome such as dysphagia;[19] shortly before, Albert Comte (1868–1944), who assisted Dejerine at the Salpêtrière, had shown that the pseudo-bulbar syndrome corresponded to bilateral lesions of

[17] Marie (1901), Foyers lacunaires de désintégration, 286–7.
[18] Marie and Guillain (1902), Existe-t-il en clinique des localisations dans la capsule interne?
[19] Marie (1901), Foyers lacunaires de désintégration, 288–90.

the fibres from the motor cortex to the nuclei of the facial, lingual, and laryngeal muscles;[20] others had found also that an increased tendency to crying or laughing was part of the pseudo-bulbar syndrome.[21]

Finally, Marie distinguished lacunes from other cavities, such as *état criblé* or other dilatations of perivascular spaces. Apart from morphological differences, such other vacuoles were not associated with any symptoms.

A Nosological Entity in the Aged, with Patent Small Blood Vessels

A young collaborator of Pierre Marie, Jean-Baptiste Ferrand (1873–1957), expanded on his master's findings. In a thesis submitted in 1902, he included more patients and more technical details, such as injecting formalin in the subdural space soon after the patient's death. He echoed Marie's view of the lacunar lesions as part of a larger constellation of pathological changes – a syndrome of old age. In addition, Ferrand claimed that lacunes causing hemiplegia were almost never found below the age of 55.[22] This was a bold statement, given that the Bicêtre was almost exclusively populated by elderly males. Ferrand made no bones of his wish to secure a separate place for lacunar disintegration in the nosological firmament:

> We also have to consider the diverse alterations of the nervous system coming close to it and with which [other] observers have surely confused it, in order to show that it indeed constitutes a separate lesion, which justifies our efforts to elevate it to the rank of an anatomical entity and to provide it with a place of its own among softening, haemorrhage, and encephalitis.[23]

In discussing these three main groups of brain disorders from which 'lacunar disease of the aged' should be distinguished, Ferrand dealt first with haemorrhage. He invariably represented the lacune as surrounding a blood vessel, whereas Marie had left this open. Ferrand did not follow up on Marie's suggestion that rupture of the central vessel might underlie the development of lacunes. Such haemorrhages were usually extensive, he argued, and if minor haemorrhages from smaller vessels did occur, they left a different type of scar. Also, miliary aneurysms were never found in or near lacunes. With regard to softening, Ferrand agreed with Marie that the changes in nerve tissue were indistinguishable, but the problem was that he always found a patent central

[20] Comte (1900), Des paralysies pseudo-bulbaires.
[21] Dupré and Devaux (1901b), Rire et pleurer spasmodiques.
[22] Ferrand (1902), Les lacunes de désintégration cérébrale, 99.
[23] Ferrand (1902), Les lacunes de désintégration cérébrale, 106.

arteriole; occlusion might have been occasionally missed in sections of a single specimen, he argued, but not in all of them.[24]

The last category was encephalitis. Ferrand had to admit that inflammation should always be secondary to something, for example to microbes; the great triumphs of Koch and Pasteur had occurred some 20 years before. Yet, he briefly played with the idea of a chronic, but limited, inflammatory condition in the perivascular sheath, a kind of 'destructive vaginalitis', at which Marie had hinted in a footnote to his article. But in the end, Ferrand still regarded changes of the central end artery as the primary cause – not occlusion, but narrowing, with slow starvation of nerve tissue, in keeping with the often gradual or stuttering onset of symptoms, and with their tendency to ameliorate.[25]

Another disciple of Marie who discoursed on the chief's 'new disease' was Giunio Catola (1875–?) from Florence; soon afterwards he was to return home and teach neuropathology there. Catola's article, in the same journal in which Marie had launched the 'lacunes of disintegration' three years before, covered largely the same ground.[26] A new element was his list of no fewer than 19 authors who had failed to find a corresponding brain lesion in patients with sudden hemiplegia, implying that they had overlooked lacunes. With regard to pathogenesis, he remained close to Marie's idea of disintegration secondary to a lesion of the central arteriole, but added the hypothesis that atherosclerosis was accompanied by something else, such as syphilis, alcohol abuse, or uraemia.

The work of Marie and his pupils prompted quite a few new publications. Several of these applied the term 'lacune' to a variety of holes in the brain without any relationship to symptoms with sudden onset. Since the present book is about stroke, there is little place for purely morphological descriptions such as putaminal lacunes in parkinsonism,[27] or perivascular demyelination in chronic mental disease.[28] Also, it is no more than marginally relevant that some subdivided 'lacunes' into subtypes according to size,[29] or into 'proper disintegration', 'microscopical softening', and 'punctate haemorrhages'.[30] Similarly, the proposal of a new name for atherosclerosis of small brain arteries, 'cerebrosclerosis',[31] was not accompanied by new insights.

[24] Ferrand (1902), Les lacunes de désintégration cérébrale, 46–7.
[25] Ferrand (1902), Les lacunes de désintégration cérébrale, 110–32.
[26] Catola (1904), Lacunes de désintégration cérébrale.
[27] Vogt and Vogt (1920), Erkrankungen des striären Systems, 808–10.
[28] Barbé and Lévy-Valensi (1908), Lacunes de désintégration cellulaire; Moore (1954), Perivascular encephalolysis.
[29] Dupré and Devaux (1901a), Foyers lacunaires de désintégration cérébrale.
[30] Foix and Nicolescu (1923), Grands syndromes de désintégration sénile.
[31] Grasset (1904), La cérébrosclérose lacunaire.

Minimal Lesions of Softening, Unilateral or Bilateral

Charles Foix (1882–1927), a former pupil of Pierre Marie,[32] published in his brief life on ischaemic lesions in the region of the pons, together with Pierre Hillemand (1895–1980), a future gastroenterologist. They confirmed Marie's observations of 'lacunes' in that area, with the proviso that the smallest lesions were related to paramedian twigs from the basilar artery and were often bilateral, resulting in a pseudo-bulbar syndrome. In an extensive study of brain softening in the Sylvian area and the corresponding symptoms that Foix published a year later with Maurice Lévy (n.d.), 'lacunar' lesions as the cause of hemiplegia were implied rather than explicitly described:

> There is a predilection site where partial deep softening gives rise to a marked hemiplegia through a lesion minimal in size, even more so at the time it is detected. This predilection site [in the white matter] is located, with a [horizontal] cut according to Flechsig, at the level of middle of the putamen. [...] There are absolutely no sensory symptoms, and of course no hemianopia.[33]

Foix and Lévy went on to add that not only the pseudo-bulbar syndrome, but also the *marche à petits pas* occurred if the small lesions of softening were bilateral. It is striking that they attributed the small lesions to *ramollissement*, without paying special attention to small arterioles or venturing any comments about their pathogenesis. The main purpose of their study was to establish clinico-pathological correlations; the circumstance that Marie was still alive might have been at the back of their minds.

A Pause

After the publications of Marie and his pupils, the first half of the twentieth century saw but little new knowledge about small brain lesions in relation to stroke. The two disastrous World Wars and the attendant disruption of scientific institutes may be part of the explanation. Another factor was the gradual fragmentation of medicine into separate specialties, which took off at around the turn of the century. Clinical duties of neurologists increased as the scope of the discipline expanded, often complicated by an ambiguous relation-ship with psychiatry. Since most research efforts were focused on the anatomy, pathology, and physiology of the nervous system, laboratory scientists acquired key roles; in other words, 'the field was being taken over by basic scientists',[34] who had only a limited interest in clinical aspects of disease. As neurology drifted away from general medicine, interest in blood vessels waned for some

---

[32] Caplan (1990), Charles Foix – the first modern stroke neurologist.
[33] Foix and Lévy (1927), Les ramollissements sylviens, 20.   [34] Casper (2014), *The Neurologists*.

time; even in the twenty-first century, health authorities in some countries do not regard the care for patients with stroke as part of neurology.

At any rate, in 1954, William Hughes (1904–1981), a geriatrician in Bristol, was struck by the occurrence of small foci of softening in the region of the corpus striatum and thalamus; he did not refer to foreign publications. The message of his paper was that these lesions were especially found in hypertensive patients and corresponded to a history of 'small strokes'. He suggested their pathogenesis might be haemodynamic failure, given the perpendicular origin of the penetrating arteries.[35]

REVIVAL

The Role of Hypertension

It was not until 1965 that the pathogenesis of lacunar lesions regained a place in the limelight. The initiative came from C. Miller Fisher (see Box 8.3, p. 275), who also took centre stage in Chapters 5 and 8. Fisher marked his position in the opening sentences of his article:

> Lacunes may be defined as ischemic infarcts of restricted size in the deeper parts of the brain. Absent from the cerebral and cerebellar cortex, they are best known in the chronic healed stage when they form irregular cavities, 0.5 to 15 mm in diameter, principally in the basal ganglia and basis pontis.[36]

The words 'ischaemic infarct' may sound as a pleonasm, but at that time, 'infarct' presumably still had the ring of a lesion sogged with blood, for pathologists at any rate. Fisher had but little documentation about the symptoms of the patients whose brains he had examined; clinico-pathological correlations were therefore limited. After a full review of previous studies, broadly similar in scope to the text above, he presented his own findings.

In contrast to the Parisian authors of half a century before, Fisher preferred brain sections in the coronal plane (Figure 9.2). He found lacunes in 11 per cent of the brains of more than 1000 individuals, on average three per brain; the lenticular nucleus was most often affected. He listed a variety of details: number, position, laterality, colour, and shape (walls irregular in the grey matter, and more rounded in the white matter). About size, he wrote:

> About 17% of the lacunes measured 10 mm. or more in diameter. The size that an infarct may attain and yet qualify for the term lacune has not been set down, and it may seem pointless to do so. Preferably, the nature

---

[35] Hughes, *et al.* (1954), Chronic cerebral hypertensive disease.
[36] Fisher (1965a), Lacunes: small, deep cerebral infarcts, 772.

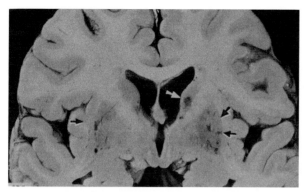

9.2 Lacunar infarcts (Fisher, 1965a). The author's legend was: 'Section showing lacunes in putamen and head of caudate nucleus'. *Source:* By permission of *Neurology*.

and site of the lesion rather than its size should be the chief criterion. It is suggested, however, that, in order to emphasize the unusual size of the larger lacunes, those 10 mm. or more in diameter be designated as giant.[37]

Two issues remained to be resolved. The first was the pathogenesis of lacunes. Hypertension had been documented in all but three patients in Fisher's series of 114 patients. Atheromatous changes in the basal brain arteries, from mild to severe, were ubiquitous; in 50 per cent, such plaques extended into the small surface vessels over the cerebral and cerebellar cortex, against none in 100 control subjects. This strongly suggested a circulatory problem and Fisher had therefore no hesitation in naming the small lesions 'infarcts'. Yet he did not find the expected occlusions, at least not where the mouths of arterioles branched off from a parent artery. Ferrand had assured that each lacune contained a central arteriole, but without demonstrable occlusion. Yet it was in only a few instances that Fisher could identify a vessel within the lacune, at least as could be made out from the surface of the brain slice.[38] For the time, the solution remained up in the air: 'The essential vascular change underlying lacunar formation remains at present undisclosed.'[39]

The second remaining task was the clinico-pathological correlation. Could specific lesions indeed be regarded as the morphological counterpart of specific stroke-like episodes such as hemiplegia? Marie, Ferrand, and later Foix and Hillemand had clearly suggested this in a general sense, but had never shown examples of a stroke-like episode 'X' as corresponding to lacune 'Y'. Fisher addressed this problem as well.

[37] Fisher (1965a), Lacunes: small, deep cerebral infarcts, 780.
[38] Fisher (1965a), Lacunes: small, deep cerebral infarcts, 779.
[39] Fisher (1965a), Lacunes: small, deep cerebral infarcts, 783.

The Symptoms

In 1965, the same year in which he drew renewed attention to lacunes and emphasized the role of hypertension, Fisher published three more papers, each of which described a different clinical syndrome related to a particular small ischaemic lesion.

First of all, with the help of Hiram B. Curry (1927–1989), he studied lesions associated with 'pure motor hemiplegia', the most common clinical manifestation of lacunar lesions. They examined 50 patients in whom unilateral weakness of the face, arm, and leg had appeared more or less suddenly, without other neurological deficits.[40] In nine of them, post-mortem examination of the brain had been possible – already an indication that the outcome was generally less bleak than with larger lesions. In six of these nine patients, the corresponding lesion was located wholly or partly in the posterior limb of the internal capsule. The paper contained clinical and pathological details about three of the six patients; one lesion, 7 × 10 millimetres, could be called a lacune, while the other two exceeded 1 centimetre in one or more dimensions, as did probably some of the unrecorded three cases. Three other patients had unilateral lesions in the pons; in two of them, the size of the lesions also seemed to correspond to the description of a 'giant lacune' – the third was not documented. In no case was the arterial lesion identified, although in the vicinity of one of the pontine lesions, a penetrating artery was thin and whitish as it branched off from the basilar artery. Old haemorrhagic lesions were not identified.

An almost complementary lacunar syndrome was 'pure sensory stroke'.[41] Fisher saw 26 patients of this type within 'a few years'. Fixed sensory deficits had occurred in 13 patients, and transient symptoms in eight others; five had symptoms that were atypical or affected only part of the body. In one patient with transient symptoms, the brain could be examined.

> The patient, a 72-year-old man, jumped out of bed one morning and developed tingling in the right fingers. A few minutes later it appeared in the right upper and lower lips, the right side of the tongue, and the two medial toes of the right foot. The attack reached its peak in fifteen minutes and then subsided. One-half hour later there was a recurrence of greater severity. Several further attacks occurred in the next five hours. There were no associated symptoms or signs. Examination showed slightly decreased pin-prick sensation in the right fingers. [...]. At autopsy three years after the ictus there was a single lesion in the brain, a lacune 7 mm in diameter situated in the postero-ventral (sensory) nucleus of the thalamus on the appropriate [left] side.

---

[40] Fisher and Curry (1965), Pure motor hemiplegia of vascular origin.
[41] Fisher (1965c), Pure sensory stroke.

Fisher commented that other patients might have lesions at different locations in the sensory system. Indeed, one can think not only of the 'thalamic syndrome' Dejerine and Roussy described,[42] but also of the earlier cases of Türck and Bourneville. He also emphasized the rarity of major strokes after isolated episodes of sensory loss.

The third 'lacunar syndrome' Fisher proposed in 1965, this time in collaboration with Monroe Cole (1933–2008), was that of unilateral weakness with pyramidal signs, in combination with cerebellar-like ataxia.[43] The only patient whose brain became available for study, three years after Fisher and Cole examined him, had several small lesions in the appropriate hemisphere; more than a decade later, in three new observations in patients with the same syndrome, now named 'ataxic hemiparesis', Fisher found isolated small cavities of infarction in the base of the pons, contralateral to the side of the symptoms, at most $8 \times 8 \times 6$ millimetres in size.[44]

Two years after the 'triad', Fisher reported another combination of symptoms he had seen in no fewer than 20 patients, the so-called 'dysarthria–clumsy hand syndrome'. In one patient, he was able to retrieve the lesion – again in the base of the pons on one side, but this time in the upper, rather than the lower, part. The cardinal clinical features were:

> [. . .] moderate to severe dysarthria; central weakness of one side of the face; deviation of the tongue on protrusion; impairment of la-la-la; a trace of dysphagia; clumsiness, awkwardness, and slowness of fine manipulations of the affected hand; questionable weakness of the hand; difficulty in writing; a wavering ataxia on the finger-nose test not clearly cerebellar in type; mild imbalance on walking; possibly enhanced tendon reflexes on the affected side: a Babinski sign; and reduced arm swing.[45]

OCCLUSIONS

Blocked Arterioles

It was again Fisher who developed, over the course of several years, 'by trial and error',[46] a method for the systematic study of arterioles corresponding to lacunar infarcts. After a preliminary communication,[47] the full article appeared in 1969.

---

[42] Dejerine and Roussy (1906), Le syndrome thalamique.
[43] Fisher and Cole (1965), Homolateral ataxia and crural paresis.
[44] Fisher (1978), Ataxic hemiparesis. A pathologic study.
[45] Fisher (1967a), A lacunar stroke. The dysarthria–clumsy hand syndrome.
[46] Fisher (1995), Lacunar infarction – a personal view, 16.
[47] Fisher (1965b), The vascular lesion in lacunae.

He had examined, in serial microscopic sections, entire uncut blocks of the basal ganglia and pons from the brain of patients with a history of arterial hypertension, in the expectation that lacunes would be found. Indeed, lacunes occurred in six of the nine blocks, from four patients who had manifested complete or partial hemiparesis, pseudo-bulbar syndrome, or other motor deficits, but it was not possible to attribute any of these symptoms to a particular lacune. The paper contained the description of the first 50 lacunes he encountered; 36 of these were from a single patient. The entire research project entailed the examination of some 18,000 microscopic sections. For each lacune, Fisher tried to find the corresponding artery:

> In each of the 50 lacunes the tiny arterial tree supplying the region of the infarct was identified with reasonable certainty and in most instances beyond the question. The finest vascular twigs were traced from the walls of the infarct cavity and usually from one or more of its fibrous trabeculations. While some lacunes contained a prominent central vessel, this was not the rule. The affected artery was almost always followed proximally until it became a normal blood-containing vessel. [...] Gray matter contained many more small vessels (60–200 microns in diameter) than white matter and the frequency of branching was most impressive, e.g. in some regions a vessel 40 microns in diameter gave rise to a small branch every 35 microns.[48]

He then described the changes seen in the wall of these small arteries:

> In 45 of the 50 lacunes an arterial occlusion was identified which accounted anatomically for the infarction. The commonest vascular lesion took the form of an advanced 'segmental arterial disorganization' often with *local* enlargement of the vessel and evidence of a focal *haemorrhagic extravasation* through the wall. This type of lesion accounted for 40 lacunes. Of the other five with totally occluded vessels, in two recent thrombosis had occurred within a microaneurysm, in two, subintimal foam-cell accumulations obliterated the lumen and in one a mass of homogeneous pink-staining material lay within a thin partially disorganized wall.[49]

Four of the five remaining arteries showed other abnormalities: partial occlusion (three) or compression by a nearby micro-aneurysm (one); the fiftieth artery was entirely patent.

---

[48] Fisher (1969), The arterial lesions underlying lacunes, 3.
[49] Fisher (1969), The arterial lesions underlying lacunes, 3. The italics are Fisher's. In line 2, the original text reads '*look* the form', no doubt a typesetting error.

Lipohyalinosis, Encroaching upon the Lumen

These findings were surprising, since many had assumed an analogy with larger infarcts, in that the occlusive process was thought to take place primarily through local clotting or, at any rate, by accumulation of blood elements. Several authors had specifically assumed thrombosis of micro-aneurysms as the cause of small areas of softening, mainly in studies of patients with hypertension, with or without intracerebral haemorrhage.[50] At any rate, small aneurysms proved to be uncommon in patients with lacunes.

Instead, the pathogenesis could be reconstructed as follows. High blood pressure, strongly related to atherosclerosis in large and middle-sized arteries, gives rise to a different kind of changes in arterioles measuring less than 175–200 microns in diameter, changes in the form of focal deposition of fibrinoid material below the intimal layer. Fisher called these alterations 'lipohyalinosis'; they had been previously described in studies of hypertensive patients,[51] even in detail,[52] with terms such as 'hyalinosis', 'angionecrosis', 'arteriolosclerosis', 'fibrinoid necrosis', or 'plasmatic infiltration'. The material readily took up stains for fat, techniques Fisher had not applied. As a next stage, as Fisher reconstructed the sequence in the process of degeneration, the elastic and middle layers can no longer be distinguished ('disorganization'); fatty macrophages (foam cells) are seen between the collagenous strands. The vessel wall starts to bulge outwards and inwards, in a more or less circular or an irregular fashion. As a result, the lumen becomes occluded and on the outside the vessel dilates to two or three times its regular size, over a more or less similar distance (Figure 9.3). The occlusion causes retrograde thrombosis, until the vessel reaches the subarachnoid space and joins other vessels (Figure 9.4). In most cases, blood elements leak through the wall to the perivascular space, also in wall segments that are not dilated. In the final stage, the fibrinoid matter may become replaced by an onion-like fibrous ball.[53]

It is a bit ironic and perhaps confusing that Fisher's term 'disorganization' resembles Marie's 'disintegration', but it should be kept in mind that Marie was applying the term to brain tissue, whereas Fisher was describing the walls of arterioles.

[50] Green (1930), Miliary aneurysms; Beitzke (1936), Kleine Aneurysmen; Ross Russell (1963), Intracerebral aneurysms.
[51] Mehnert (1888), Topographische Verbreitung der Angiosclerose, 37; Rühl (1927), Apoplektische Gehirnblutung; Wolff (1937), Apoplektische Hirnblutung, 591–602; Scholz and Nieto (1938), Pathologie der Hirngefässe; Anders and Eicke (1939), Gehirngefässen bei Hypertonie; Anders and Eicke (1940), Gehirngefässe beim Hochdruck, 13–24.
[52] Arab (1959), Hyalinose artériolaire cérébrale.
[53] Fisher (1969), The arterial lesions underlying lacunes, 4–15.

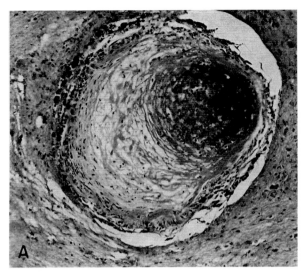

9.3 Segmental disorganization (angionecrosis), with local enlargement of the artery to three times the normal diameter of 130 microns (Fisher, 1969). *Source:* By permission of *Acta Neuropathologica*.

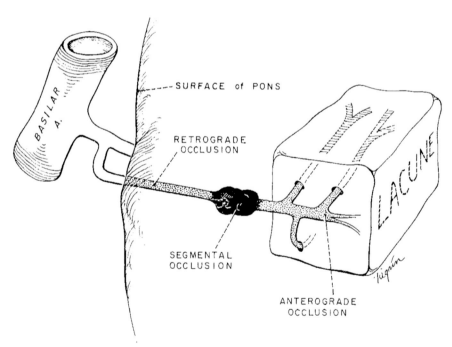

9.4 Diagram of the pons showing the relation of a larger lacune to the vascular lesion (Fisher, 1969). *Source:* By permission of *Acta Neuropathologica*.

Atheroma of Perforating Branches

Still, occlusion of end arterioles by lipohyalinosis applied only to lacunes without known symptoms. Did it also explain symptomatic lacunar infarction? In the paper about 'pure motor hemiplegia', Fisher and Curry had guessed that

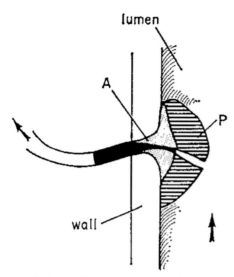

9.5 'Diagram illustrating the basilar branch arterial supply to the infarct in the lower pons and the intramural lesion. A = atheroma and P = plaque' (Fisher and Caplan, 1971; original legend). *Source:* By permission of *Neurology*.

the somewhat larger lacunes of this type might be 'the product of small vessel thrombosis in the region of the internal capsule or basis pontis'.[54] A few years later, Fisher could confirm this in another pathological study, assisted by Louis R. Caplan (1936–). They described two patients with a pontine infarct, in both cases associated with hemiparesis.[55] In one patient, a 67-year-old woman in whom the lesion measured 10 × 10 × 6 millimetres, the unilateral weakness was of the 'pure' type; in the second, an 86-year-old man, there had also been temporary disturbances of horizontal eye movement.[56]

The arterial lesion, in both patients, consisted of occlusion of a branch of about 0.5 millimetres in diameter, near the point where it took off at right angle from the basilar artery before penetrating the surface of the pons. In the first, female patient, the vascular abnormality was not found in the branch itself, but in the parent vessel. At the site where the branch took off, it traversed a clump of macrophages that formed part of an atherosclerotic plaque; the lumen of the arteriole was obstructed by a mixture of large macrophages, fibroblasts, collagenous connective tissue, and some red blood cells (Figure 9.5). In the second patient, the atheromatous plaque in the wall of the basilar artery continued along the wall of the arteriolar branch. The branch lumen was narrowest as it passed the muscular layer of the basilar wall (Figure 9.6). As the plaque extended outside the wall of the basilar artery for

---

[54] Fisher and Curry (1965), Pure motor hemiplegia of vascular origin, 41.

[55] Fisher and Caplan (1971), Basilar artery branch occlusion.

[56] The so-called 'one-and-a-half syndrome' (Fisher (1967c), Some neuro-ophthalmological observations).

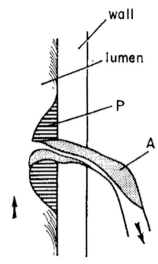

wall

lumen

P

A

9.6 'Diagram illustrating the arterial supply to the infarct in the lower pons and the vascular lesion. A = atheroma and P = plaque' (Fisher and Caplan, 1971; original legend). *Source:* By permission of *Neurology.*

about 2 millimetres, 'the lumen was narrowed to 50 microns and irregularly divided into compartments, suggesting a very small local mural dissection'.

Brain Softening in General: Two Types of Occlusion, Three Levels

By the mid-1970s, the notion of the existence of small ischaemic lesions had been fully ingrained in the minds of neurologists, in terms of clinical syndromes and morphological changes. But what about their pathogenesis? Had Pierre Marie's ambition come true that the small scars of brain tissue responsible for 'lacunar hemiplegia' and related syndromes represented a separate category of vascular disease?

Basically, almost all brain infarcts, from massive lesions to the smallest deep ischaemic cysts, share a common underlying pathological process: atherosclerosis. Also, the final process is identical: death of nerve tissue for want of nutrition. Yet between these two extremes, there is a dichotomy in the process of occlusion, according to the size of the affected artery. In large brain arteries of patients with devastating infarction, one finds fibrinous plugs made up of blood elements, through local thrombosis or embolism. At the other end of the spectrum, the brains of hypertensive patients show the smallest types of lacunar infarction, with or without corresponding symptoms, where the arteriolar lumen has become blocked by its own walls, distended by hyaline deposits.

Which of the two occlusive processes is most common in strokes of the lacunar type, with sudden unilateral weakness as the predominant feature? As a rule, these lesions, though also deeply situated, in the region of the basal ganglia and internal capsule, or in the pons of Varolio, are somewhat larger than those found in Fisher's first study: 'giant lacunes'. In this type of lesion, the arterial occlusion has rarely been identified with certainty; as Fisher and Caplan wrote: 'generalizing from two cases is hardly warranted'.[57] So the conclusion might be, at least for the time being, that clinically manifest episodes of lacunar infarction are associated with thrombotic or atherosclerotic occlusion of penetrating arteries of approximately 0.5 millimetres in diameter.

Though this is the end, at least for some time, of the story of lacunes, it does not yet end the narrative of the brain lesion that has been designated, in the

---

[57] Fisher and Caplan (1971), Basilar artery branch occlusion, 905.

course of time, as *ramollissement*, 'softening', 'encephalomalacia', 'ischaemic necrosis', or 'infarction'. An intriguing aspect, fully discussed in Chapter 10, is the occurrence of 'stroke warnings' in patients who later experienced a definitive attack. Such preliminary symptoms also occur in patients with 'lacunar attacks', especially in the form of transient hemisensory loss,[58] or transient hemiparesis.[59]

[58] Fisher (1965c), Pure sensory stroke, 77.
[59] Fisher and Curry (1965), Pure motor hemiplegia of vascular origin, 31 and 32.

TEN

STROKE WARNINGS

SUMMARY

Around the mid-nineteenth century, it became commonly known that the deficits of brain softening had sometimes been preceded by temporary attacks of the same kind (hemiplegia, disorders of language). In the middle of the twentieth century, Fisher recognized that episodes of monocular blindness, identified in 1898 as embolic (Knapp), were also potential harbingers of cerebral ischaemia. Studies addressing the risk of stroke after such warnings, conducted in the 1960s and early 1970s, were sparse and difficult to interpret.

Explanations of transient cerebral ischaemia initially included arterial spasm and relative hypotension. In the second half of the twentieth century, artery-to-artery embolism became the dominant explanation, at least in the carotid territory; white material moving through retinal arteries proved to consist of aggregated blood platelets; transient loss of vision in one eye could, in turn, be related to the same extracerebral atherothrombotic lesions that caused cerebral ischaemia (Fisher, Ross Russell). By 1975, studies of medical or surgical treatment to prevent stroke in patients with episodes of cerebral ischaemia were largely inconclusive.

In the course of the centuries, several physicians who tried to understand apoplexy noted that sometimes transient symptoms had preceded a severe, definitive attack. Up to the mid-twentieth century, such preliminary symptoms were diverse and mostly non-specific, thought with hindsight to represent impending 'fullness of the head'. Conversely, a wide range of phenomena could be interpreted as 'warning symptoms'. Only recently the definition of preliminary spells became stricter; the more the transient symptoms resembled the characteristics of permanent stroke, the greater the danger they signified.

TRANSIENT PHENOMENA – STROKE-LIKE OR OTHER

Non-specific Spells

For example, Thomas Willis distinguished apoplexy into two kinds: one was unexpected, 'accidental', and the other 'habitual', in susceptible patients:

> However, in addition we have observed that this *disease* is sometimes *habitual*, that is, in some persons there resides a *permanent diathesis*, through which they are at first bothered by skirmishes of a rather mild sort; later more serious attacks seize them, with shorter intervals. In the end most die of them.[1]

Willis did not specify these preliminary 'skirmishes', nor would many later authors. A wide range of temporary sensations were regarded as potential portents of apoplectic mischief, for example by William Heberden (1710–1801),[2] and – more specifically associated with brain softening – by Léon Rostan in the early nineteenth century, and even in the middle of the twentieth century, by Kinnier Wilson (1878–1937):

> Premonitory signs, lacking in embolism, are often conspicuous in thrombotic cases (more so than in haemorrhagic); days or weeks beforehand they may give the observer an inkling of what is likely to occur. Here are comprised headache (not infrequently on the same side as the commencing damage), vertigo, defective memory, transient confusion of thought; and, more specifically, heaviness or momentary weakness, numbed feeling or other paraesthesia, in the limb or limbs on the verge of becoming involved. Whether such symptoms constitute minor antecedent attacks or merely indicate general vascular trouble is immaterial; they are straws which show how the intracranial wind is blowing.[3]

Some others, however, noted the similarity between particular preliminary symptoms and the definitive attack.

Transient Hemiplegia

An early example is Conrad Heinrich Fuchs (1803–1855), at the time Professor of Medicine in Würzburg. The chapter on *ramollissement* relates, with a brief

---

[1] Willis (1672), *De Anima Brutorum*, 269.
[2] Heberden (1802), *Commentarii de Morborum Historia et Curatione*, 288–9.
[3] Wilson and Bruce (1940), *Neurology*, 1088.

biography (see Box 6.2, p. 199), his support of Rostan's view that brain softening was a separate and non-inflammatory disorder, but without reproducing his inclusive array of premonitory symptoms. In his book on encephalomalacia, published in 1838, Fuchs wrote:

> Instead, I found in three of my cases a very characteristic precursor symptom of which Rostan does not make mention. For from time to time, during a walk, the limbs on one side would suddenly stop functioning; the patients had to sit down or they collapsed on the floor, without losing consciousness. In two patients these warning attacks had started to occur already a few weeks before the actual, permanent onslaught of hemiplegia and increased in frequency as time passed; in the third one they appeared only on the day before the next stage. The weakness in the limbs always lasted only a few hours or minutes; as a rule, they could get up from their fallen position without assistance and continue their journey. The limbs only retained for some time a sense of numbness and heaviness.[4]

Fuchs emphasized that such prophetic symptoms never preceded brain haemorrhage.[5] A few years later, Karl Ewald Hasse (1810–1902) from Zurich recounted how temporary hemiplegia had preceded a definitive and ultimately fatal attack.[6]

Subsequent publications mentioned a mix of fleeting attacks, specific and non-specific. J. Ramsay Hunt (1872–1937) wrote in 1914 that more attention should be paid to the carotid artery, though most of his examples were traumatic in origin:

> Unilateral headaches and vertigo, especially in assuming the upright posture, epileptiform attacks, failing memory, attacks of threatened hemiplegia, intermittent cerebral claudication, are some of the vascular symptoms which should suggest the possibility of carotid obstruction.[7]

Hunt did not specify the observations that had induced him to suppose these diverse relationships. He probably supposed, as Rostan did at a time when localization of certain brain functions was still on the horizon, that temporary interruptions of local blood flow ought to affect not only specific, but also more general brain functions.

Transient Dysphasia

A personal experience of temporary 'loss of words' was recorded in the 1780s in Paris, a few years before the Revolution. It was not written as a medical

---

[4] Fuchs (1838), *Beobachtungen über Gehirnerweichung*, 96.
[5] Fuchs (1838), *Beobachtungen über Gehirnerweichung*, 123.
[6] Hasse (1846), Verschliessung der Hirnarterien und Hirnerweichung, 96.
[7] Hunt (1914), The role of the carotid arteries in vascular lesions of the brain, 712.

report, but as a scientific curiosity; it never influenced medical thinking until it was discovered by twentieth-century neurologists with an interest in disorders of language.[8] The author-patient was Jean-Paul Grandjean de Fouchy (1707–1788), a keen astronomer. As the long-term secretary of the *Académie royale des sciences*, he submitted his own story to the records of the *Académie*. An intriguing detail is that on the day before the episode, de Fouchy, then 77 years old, had tripped over an uneven pavement, fallen, and hurt his nose – he used the anatomical term *vomer* – and also the right orbit; the pain radiated to the left eye. Once at home, he had dressed the superficial wounds and slept well. The next day, he was healthy until dinner time:

> Near the end of the dinner, I felt a mild increase of the pain above the left eye and at the same instant I lost the ability to pronounce the words I had in mind. I heard what was said, and I knew what I ought to respond. Yet I pronounced other words than those needed to express my thought; or, if I began them, I did not finish them, or put other words in their place. Nevertheless, I could make all movements as freely as usual; I did not drop my fork or the piece of bread I was holding. I saw all objects with sharpness, I clearly heard what was said, and the organs contributing to thought were, as it seemed to me, functioning normally.
>
> This kind of paroxysm lasted about one minute, during which time I was sufficiently alert to reflect on the particular arrangement in the sensorium of the soul, in which only a single of its faculties was affected while the other ones showed not even the least derangement.[9]

Transient impairment of language functions was increasingly recognized in the twentieth century,[10] especially after the introduction of angiography;[11] it was often accompanied by right-sided weakness. However, the relationship with arterial disease was almost always made in retrospect, and not 'hot off the fire'. This included the examples of transient dysphasia in three of the eight case histories in Miller Fisher's seminal 1951 paper on carotid occlusion (see Chapter 8); yet what stood out was that Fisher, a keen neuropathologist, but also a perceptive neurologist, had recorded these preceding events *in extenso*. Especially illustrative was his first patient, though some of the symptoms indicated ischaemia in areas other than the dominant hemisphere:

---

[8] Benton and Joynt (1960), Early descriptions of aphasia.
[9] Grandjean de Fouchy (1787), Observation anatomique.
[10] Pickering (1948), Transient cerebral paralysis in hypertension.
[11] Siegert (1938), Verkalkung oder Thrombose der Carotis interna, 802; Chao, *et al.* (1938), Thrombosis of the left carotid artery, 102; Andrell (1943), Thrombosis of the internal carotid artery, 345; Krayenbühl and Weber (1944), Thrombose der Arteria carotis interna, 303; Govons and Grant (1946), Angiographic visualisation of cerebrovascular lesions, 615; Ameli and Ashby (1949), Non-traumatic thrombosis of the carotid artery, 1097; Budínová-Smelá, *et al.* (1949), Thrombosis arteriae carotis internae, 96 and 98; Sugar, *et al.* (1950), Spontaneous thrombosis of the carotid arteries, 824.

A man aged 64 complained of transient attacks characterized by dizziness, inability to speak and paralysis and numbness of the right hand. He said he had had at least 100 attacks in eight months. His family confirmed this statement, although he had tended not to acquaint them with his complaints. All the attacks were similar but varied in duration and severity. They usually began with a severe pounding sensation behind the left ear. Next there appeared a steady headache over the left eye. Then severe rotatory dizziness (clockwise) began, causing him to sweat and become nauseated, sometimes to the point of vomiting. During the vertigo, diplopia occurred, one image lying directly above the other. At the same time, the right hand became numb and paralyzed, and he was unable to speak a word, although he knew what he wanted to say. He retained complete awareness. A short attack lasted 15 minutes; a 'long one' would take 40 minutes to clear.[12]

Sadly, the patient died in hospital from a massive stroke; autopsy showed recent occlusion of the basilar artery, together with near-occlusion of the left internal carotid artery.

Transient Blindness

Temporary loss of vision has always been a well-known phenomenon for ophthalmologists. The term *amaurosis fugax* was introduced in 1869 by Richard Foerster (1825–1902), an ophthalmologist in Breslau and the inventor of the perimeter;[13] he used it to map his own flashing scotomas.[14] Foerster's attacks occurred in both visual fields, but in the course of time, the term *amaurosis fugax* has come to mean – rather imprecisely – temporary blindness of a single eye.[15]

Attacks of blindness in one eye. These were observed not only in middle-aged or older persons, but also in young men. The ophthalmologist Arthur Benson (1852–1912) in Dublin provided an early example of 'temporary visual obscurations' in one eye. The patient was a mariner, 32 years of age when he was first seen in 1894.

In 1890, four years ago, when in Alaska on board a man-of-war, he for the first time noticed a sudden complete obscuration of the left eye, without any cause that he could assign. He was in good health at the time and was exposed to no unusual circumstances. After about a couple of minutes the blindness cleared away, and the sight was as good as ever.

From that time forward till the present he has suffered at intervals from similar transient obscurations of sight, sometimes affecting the whole of

[12] Fisher (1951), Occlusion of the internal carotid artery, 348.
[13] Grzybowski and Sobolewska (2015), Richard Foerster (1825–1902).
[14] Foerster (1869), Amaurosis partialis fugax. In 1835, the ophthalmologist Richard Middlemore (1804–1891) used the term 'periodical amaurosis', also referring to both eyes (Middlemore (1835), *Diseases of the Eye*).
[15] Fisher (1989), 'Transient monocular blindness' versus 'amaurosis fugax'.

the field of vision, but most frequently implicating only one section of the field. These obscurations at first occurred only once a month or so, but have since, by degrees, increased in frequency, until latterly he sometimes has two in a day.[16]

Benson found central scotomas in both eyes, so several causes were probably involved; the past history included three bouts of 'rheumatic fever' and the patient was a heavy smoker.

Attacks of monocular blindness with brain dysfunction on the same side. In older patients, an association with atherosclerosis would seem more likely, particularly if the same patient also had one or more attacks of weakness in the opposite half of the body. In 1868, (Jacob) Hermann Knapp (1832–1911) (Box 10.1),[17] Professor of Ophthalmology in Heidelberg and about to move to New York City, published case histories of patients with occlusions of retinal or ciliary vessels. One of these is highly relevant:

> Heinrich Weiss, a 46-year-old farmer from Waldmichelbach, came to the Eye Clinic because of visual loss in the right eye. He is a staunch person and is said to have been healthy until three months before the visual loss. From that time onwards he was often troubled by headache, dizziness and numbness, especially on the left side of the head; at the same time he felt distracted, dim-witted and inattentive. These phenomena occurred episodically but later more continuously and were accompanied by an unpleasant sensation of ants crawling and itching at the skin of the left arm and leg; on that same side he perceived some weakness of muscle power, which for some time made him unable to walk. Together with the weakness there was loss of skin sensation. What most worried the patient was the loss of vision in the right eye; it had occurred overnight without any other trouble. Also at some time in the past this eye had suddenly become dark, to the extent that he could make out only large objects. That disturbance had lasted a few days and had then completely disappeared. This time he could only distinguish light from dark, and it did not improve.[18]

The aspect of the retina and its vessels, Knapp wrote, was typical for embolism of the central retinal artery. He viewed it indirectly, with the aid of a lens, as well as directly with the ophthalmoscope, invented in 1850 by Hermann von Helmholtz (1821–1894).[19] Furthermore, he proved to be an inquisitive and, one might even say, holistic physician:

> Now, in order to determine the source of embolism, I examined the heart, but I could not find even the slightest abnormality. I then

---

[16] Benson (1894), Recurrent temporary visual obscurations, 83.

[17] https://en.wikisource.org/wiki/American_Medical_Biographies/Knapp,_Jacob_Hermann.

[18] Knapp (1868), Verstopfung der Blutgefässe des Auges, 212–13.

[19] Helmholtz (1851), *Beschreibung eines Augen-Spiegels*.

Box 10.1 Hermann Jakob Knapp (1832–1911).

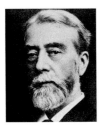

Knapp was born into a wealthy family, in Dauborn (Hessen-Nassau). He studied medicine at the universities of Munich, Würzburg, Berlin, Leipzig, Zürich, and finally Giessen, where he graduated in 1854. He then decided to apply himself to ophthalmology, working with Franciscus Donders in Utrecht, William Bowman in London, Albrecht von Graefe in Berlin, and Hermann von Helmholz in Heidelberg. In 1860, Knapp qualified as *Privatdozent* for ophthalmology in Heidelberg, and five years later, he was appointed Professor of Ophthalmology.

In 1868, at the age of 36, he moved with his family to New York City, where he founded a private clinic for diseases of the eye and ear, soon incorporated into the Ophthalmic and Aural Institute, open to the rich and poor alike. One year after his emigration, he collaborated with the otologist Salomon Moos (1831–1895) to found *Archives of Ophthalmology and Otology* (*Archiv für Augen-und Ohrenheilkunde*), a monthly international scientific journal published both in Wiesbaden and in New York. A decade later, the periodical split into two independent journals, one for ophthalmology and one for otology. In 1882, Knapp became Professor of Ophthalmology at the Medical Department of the University of the City of New York; six years later, he accepted a similar chair at the College of Physicians and Surgeons, which was the medical department of Columbia University.

Knapp developed several instruments and appliances, for example improved lid forceps, which permitted bloodless operations on the lid, roller forceps for the treatment of trachoma, and a needle-knife for the resection of secondary cataract. His character has been described as gruff and short-spoken, but extremely generous and completely free of envy. His bibliography contains hundreds of titles.

Source: Portrait courtesy of U.S. National Library of Medicine.

---

examined the large vessels in the neck and found at the bifurcation of the right common carotid artery a hissing sound, like one hears with aneurysms; on the other side one heard the carotid sounds quite normally. On the side where the bruit was heard, one also felt a circumscribed, dough-like swelling.

Again, this was 1868! Until 1951, when Fisher's paper alerted the neurological world to the role of atherosclerosis at the carotid bifurcation, a few more observations appeared in print about patients in whom temporary loss of vision in one eye coexisted with a brain lesion on the same side, but failed to attract much attention. In Baltimore, Frank B. Walsh (1895–1978), in his seminal textbook of neuro-ophthalmology of 1947, mentioned a woman with right hemiparesis, followed by transitory episodes of blindness in the left eye;[20] two

---

[20] Walsh (1947), *Clinical Neuro-ophthalmology*, 935.

papers with other reports were atypical in the sense that the patients were under 40 years and factors other than atherosclerosis were possible: an old neck wound and possibly a carotid aneurysm on the side of the affected eye,[21] or coexisting pulmonary tuberculosis, while heart disease and syphilis were not ruled out.[22]

In his 1951 paper, Miller Fisher noted, more or less parenthetically, that some of the eight patients he reported, all with carotid occlusion complicated by cerebral infarction, had experienced transient episodes of blindness in the eye on the side of the occluded artery, 'as a sort of warning that disaster threatened'. Having made the same observation a few times afterwards, the next year, he published a separate paper with seven patients who all showed this striking combination of symptoms.[23] His new article also contained a long historical section for the ophthalmological readership, citing as many as 150 previous observations of transient monocular blindness. Yet, the vast majority of those patients were younger, or the attacks were associated with explanations other than carotid atherothrombosis, such as heart disease or migraine.

TRANSIENT ATTACKS ATTRIBUTED TO THE POSTERIOR CIRCULATION

Given the large number of brain functions depending on an intact brainstem, permanent ischaemia of structures in the posterior fossa became associated with a great variety of symptoms. In an early series from Boston of 22 patients (18 fatal), in whom thrombosis or embolism had resulted in occlusion of the basilar artery, Charles S. Kubik (1891–1982) and Raymond D. Adams (1911–2008) wrote:

> The first symptom is usually headache, 'dizziness,' confusion or coma. Difficulty in speaking and unilateral paraesthesias occur in a large proportion of the cases. Common findings are pupillary abnormalities, disorder of ocular movements, facial palsy, hemiplegia, and/or quadriplegia, and bilateral extensor plantar reflexes. Cranial nerve palsies and contralateral hemiplegia may be combined.[24]

Later articles confirmed this wide spectrum of symptoms.[25] But, in the context of early warnings, was it possible to reverse the relationship and correctly

[21] Foerster and Guttman (1933), Cerebrale Complicationen bei Thrombangiitis obliterans, 510–14.
[22] Sie-Boen-Lian (1948), Spasm of macular arteries.
[23] Fisher (1952), Transient monocular blindness associated with hemiplegia.
[24] Kubik and Adams (1946), Occlusion of the basilar artery, 109–10.
[25] Biemond (1951), Thrombosis of the basilar artery; Silversides (1954), Basilar artery stenosis and thrombosis.

interpret transient phenomena as ischaemia of the posterior circulation? Only on rare occasions could survivors be interviewed about attacks in the preceding days, weeks, or months; vertigo and visual field disorders topped the list.[26] The interpretation of such studies is problematic: if enquiry is made once a stroke has occurred, recollections may be dominated by unrelated and harmless symptoms, to say nothing about bias of recall and interpretation.

Denis (John) Williams (1908–1990), with a large outpatient practice in London,[27] had in the course of two years seen as many as 65 patients with 'minor attacks' resembling the early phenomena in patients with confirmed basilar artery thrombosis. In the paper he wrote with T. Grahame Wilson (1916–1983), the most common symptoms were, in order of decreasing frequency: vertigo, disorders of consciousness, hallucinations, visceral sensations, ataxia, drop attacks, and diplopia. Visual field defects, mentioned more than once in reports of fatal basilar artery occlusion, were less often mentioned as a transient phenomenon.[28] The authors were careful enough not to base their diagnosis on any of these phenomena in isolation. Neurologists at the time were well aware of the difference between rotatory vertigo and non-specific dizziness;[29] also, it did not take long before perceptive physicians identified an innocuous, though sometimes distressing, form of drop attacks in middle-aged women.[30]

Whatever the type of possible transient ischaemic attack of the brain, the only reliable method for assessing the risk of stroke was to wait and see. For example, it is well known that some episodes of myocardial infarction are preceded by episodes of pain in the chest, but it has turned out that the large majority of chest pains do not signify an impending heart attack. The question remained: how great is the risk of stroke, and are some varieties of attacks more dangerous than others?

PROSPECTIVE STUDIES: HOW GREAT IS THE DANGER?

Answers to these questions were few and far between. A major problem was the interventionist attitude of many physicians and surgeons. Despite the existing lack of knowledge, articles reported prophylactic interventions such as carotid surgery or drug treatment. Some authors flaunted the word 'prognosis' in the title but included only patients judged ineligible for surgical

---

[26] Marshall (1964), The natural history of transient ischaemic cerebro-vascular attacks.
[27] Shorvon and Compston (2019), *Queen Square*, 406–8.
[28] Williams and Wilson (1962), Major and minor syndromes of basilar insufficiency.
[29] Fisher (1967b), Vertigo in cerebrovascular disease; Williams (1967), Central vertigo.
[30] Stevens and Matthews (1973), Cryptogenic drop attacks: an affliction of women.

treatment after angiography,[31] or meanwhile prescribed anticoagulants.[32] Others more openly advocated uncontrolled or poorly controlled interventions, claiming early promise, or at least safety, of the therapeutic measures; the inevitable mishaps must have been buried in private archives.

Hospital-Based Studies

Nevertheless, two early and almost 'clean' studies of the natural history of transient ischaemic attacks appeared in 1964; the picture these painted was not uniform, but at least not alarming. John Marshall (1922–2014), Reader and later Professor at the Institute of Neurology in London,[33] followed 61 patients with transient ischaemic attacks of the brain (some also had attacks of unilateral blindness). The abbreviation 'TIAs' was commonly used, Marshall wrote; it therefore must have been buzzed around in hospital corridors before he introduced it into the scientific literature. After a period of almost four years on average, only a single major stroke episode had occurred.[34] It should be added that about half of the attacks were classified as vertebrobasilar, while the criteria for that category were rather liberal (vertigo, visual field defects, diplopia, and drop attacks). In another group of patients under Marshall's care, of at least the same size, in whom brain infarction had been the first event and who reported TIAs in retrospect, the average interval between the first TIA and stroke had been shorter than the average follow-up period in the first group of patients, those who had presented with TIAs. This sounded reassuring but may well be interpreted as another proof of the difference between tracking back from calamitous disease to remembered events and, conversely, follow-up after a possible warning symptom.

The second early prospective study came from the North Staffordshire Royal Infirmary in Stoke-on-Trent, where (Enid) Joan Acheson (1926–2019), a mother and future consultant in renal medicine in Manchester,[35] had joined the stroke project of Edward Charles Hutchinson (1921–2002). They followed up 82 patients who had been referred by their general practitioner because of repetitive attacks of cerebral ischaemia (duration of less than one hour; isolated vertigo excluded), for an average period of 40 months. In that interval, as many as half of them (42) experienced a stroke – somewhat more often in the carotid than in the posterior circulation – but almost half of these 42 patients were said to function normally, while 11 were moderately or severely disabled and 12 were

---

[31] Regli (1971), Die flüchtigen ischämischen zerebralen Attacken; Ziegler and Hassanein (1973), Prognosis in patients with transient ischemic attacks.

[32] Baker, et al. (1968), Prognosis in patients with transient cerebral ischemic attacks.

[33] Shorvon and Compston (2019), Queen Square, 447–8.

[34] Marshall (1964), The natural history of transient ischaemic cerebro-vascular attacks.

[35] https://history.rcplondon.ac.uk/inspiring-physicians/enid-joan-acheson (Munk's roll).

dead.[36] If their results are recalculated as an annual risk of disabling stroke or death, this rate would be around 12 per cent, but of course the confidence interval for such a small sample is wide.

Community-Based Studies

The two hospital-based studies begged the question of whether the outlook for patients with TIAs who, for some reason, are *not* referred to a neurologist is better, the same, or worse than for those who are. In the 1960s, one community-based study was carried out, though not without its own bias, in a retirement community in California, where residence was restricted to persons aged 52 years or older; the medical records of about 90 per cent of this population were registered at the local clinic. Over a period of some six years, 44 patients were identified with a first definite TIA (duration of less than 24 hours) and followed up for an average period of over two years (27.4 months). Unfortunately, a minority of the group had been treated with anticoagulants, at least for some time, and two underwent carotid endarterectomy. At the end of the study period, nine patients had a definite stroke, two a possible stroke, and six had died ('none due to cerebral thrombosis'). This roughly corresponded to a 17 per cent annual rate of stroke or death, again in a small sample.[37]

Two other community-based studies deserve mention. Records from the Mayo Clinic on the fate of 73 patients with TIAs in or near Rochester, Minnesota, over a period of 15 years, indicated 27 strokes and 26 deaths from causes other than stroke,[38] or an annual rate of stroke or death of 5–6 per cent, but six subjects were lost to follow-up. And in a rural and biracial community in Georgia, a sample of almost 2500 persons was followed up for an average period of more than seven years. Of 28 subjects with definite or probable TIAs, only two had a stroke in the study period, while three died of heart disease;[39] calculation of an annual rate would be even more meaningless than for those above.

In summary, the scarce studies on the natural history of TIAs are difficult to interpret because of the inconsistencies of several key factors: first of all the population – community or hospital, secondly the criteria for the diagnosis of TIA or stroke, and thirdly the tendency of patients and physicians to prefer some kind of intervention, despite attendant uncertainties, over watchful

[36] Acheson and Hutchinson (1964), Observations on the natural history of transient cerebral ischaemia.

[37] Friedman, *et al.* (1969), Transient ischemic attacks in a community.

[38] Goldner, *et al.* (1971), Long-term prognosis of transient cerebral ischemic attacks.

[39] Karp, *et al.* (1973), Transient cerebral ischemia.

waiting. It is no wonder that estimates of the toll of stroke after a TIA showed wide variations, but at any rate, such events occurred more often than in the general population.

Evidently, sentiments of whether or not transient focal deficits of the brain or the eye might eventually end up in permanent loss of function were highly dependent on ideas about the pathophysiology of the fleeting phenomena. Several explanations were offered in the course of time.

EARLY EXPLANATIONS OF TRANSIENT ISCHAEMIC ATTACKS

At the beginning of the twentieth century, the relationship between TIAs and atherosclerosis was not yet part of common medical knowledge. As recounted in Chapter 9, the notion of abnormal constriction of cerebral arteries by sympathetic hyperactivity once again enjoyed some popularity.

Arterial Spasm

An example is the explanation of William Russell (1852–1940), a physician and later Professor of Medicine in Edinburgh. In a clinical lecture published in 1909, he recited the case of a 50-year-old farmer with intermittent attacks of hemiplegia; then he proposed:

> In this condition the closing of the blood channels is initiated by the channels themselves, and is effected by means of their muscular coat. It is a local closing, and may be partial or total – that is to say, it may only lessen the amount of blood passing, or it may completely arrest the flow of blood to the part. As a result there is either impairment or complete suspension of function, until the vessel opens and permits the blood to resume its course.
>
> That such local closing of arterial channels is possible is seen in the local syncope of 'dead fingers,' in the 'local syncope' of Raynaud's disease, in some cases of migraine, in the vessels of the retina in quinine blindness, and in temporary partial blindness seen to be due to the closing of a branch of the retinal artery. A corresponding explanation is required for the phenomena which were exhibited in Mr M's case [a farmer]. His case it only one of many I could give you.[40]

After some hesitation, William Osler (1849–1919), one of the most influential physicians of his time,[41] also came round to the idea of spasm as causing attacks of transient aphasia or paralyses in hypertensive patients.[42]

---

[40] Russell (1909), Intermittent closing of the cerebral arteries.
[41] Bliss (1999), *William Osler: A Life in Medicine*.
[42] Osler (1911), Transient attacks of aphasia and paralyses.

Some ophthalmologists who examined patients during attacks of monocular blindness offered similar views. Early examples are the Philadelphian Professor of Ophthalmology William Campbell Posey (1866–1934)[43] and Robert Alexander Lundie (1855–1918),[44] a general practitioner in Edinburgh with a special interest in diseases of the eye. The 'anaemic portion' of a retinal branch Arthur Benson had seen, in 1894, moving to the periphery in the 32-year-old mariner (see above) reminded Lundie of the 'spasm' he observed in 1906 in an 88-year-old gentleman:

> When I saw him, within half-an-hour of the onset of the attack, he greeted me with: 'It is going off; I can see a little now'. I found that the upper part of the field had some perception; but the lower part remained quite blind.
>
> On ophthalmologic examination (it was unfortunately only possible to use the indirect method), I found that the media were clear, the appearances natural, and the vessels normal except the upper main branch of the retinal artery. In this there was an interruption of the column of blood just beyond the margin of the disc, in a section of the vessel somewhat less in length than one disc-diameter. The position of this part of the vessel could be traced as a whitish streak; but it seemed entirely empty. [. . .] I could almost fancy that a tiny transparent finger and thumb were nipping the artery, just as one nips an Indian-rubber tube.[45]

Additional first-hand reports of temporary narrowing of retinal arteries appeared,[46] some with the additional observation that the occluded artery slowly refilled, while the 'contracted area' moved to the periphery of the retina.[47] Arterial spasm was sometimes invoked as the cause, even in autopsied cases of brain softening, if the arteries in question failed to show thrombosis or occlusion.[48]

Vasospasm Contested

Sir George Pickering (1904–1980), a pioneer of the idea that hypertension is one end in the normal distribution of a continuous variable rather than a disease ('essential hypertension'), argued in 1948 that attacks of 'transient cerebral paralysis' in patients with chronic hypertension were strikingly similar

[43] Zentmayer and Rowan (1934), William Campbell Posey; Posey (1902), Transient monocular blindness.
[44] JT (1919), Robert Alexander Lundie.
[45] Lundie (1906), Transient blindness due to spasm of the retinal artery.
[46] Harbridge (1906), Spasm of the central artery of the retina; Foerster and Guttman (1933), Cerebrale Complicationen bei Thrombangiitis obliterans; Sanders (1939), Intermittent occlusion of the central retinal artery.
[47] Weiss (1912), Amaurosis fugax durch Krampf der Retinalgefässe.
[48] Yates (1954), Cerebral pathology following carotid spasm.

to those in patients with mitral stenosis and auricular fibrillation. He designated the former as 'hypertensive encephalopathy', but clearly distinguished them from patients with convulsions and coma – to whom the term applies in current practice. Having chosen the leading medical journal in the USA, where many adhered to the theory of vasospasm, he made a convincing case against the idea of spasm:

> In chronic hypertension attacks of localised sensory or motor attacks of brief duration are probably not due to cerebral arterial spasm but to sudden organic arterial occlusion, for example by a thrombus. The speed and completeness of recovery from paralysis will depend on the size of the final infarct and on its position. The arguments for this hypothesis are: 1. The cerebral arteries have comparatively poorly developed muscular walls. 2. They constrict feebly to known vasoconstrictor agents. 3. In 11 patients with chronic hypertensive encephalopathy no sharp dividing line was found between attacks in which paralysis lasted only a few minutes and attacks from which complete recovery did not occur. 4. In 11 patients embolic occlusion of cerebral arteries produced attacks that were precisely similar in kind and range to those occurring in hypertension.[49]

Three years later, Fisher identified the role of atherosclerotic narrowing of neck arteries in patients with ischaemic stroke, some of whom had had transient attacks before. Yet his finding did not in itself elucidate the manner in which intermittent ischaemia was produced. Different explanations were still possible. Fisher initially implicated failure of collateral pathways. Another view was that these episodes represented a disturbance in the balance between the propulsive forces generated by the heart and the resistance generated by stenotic arteries in the neck, 'misery perfusion'. This view appealed particularly to vascular surgeons, used as they were to treating elderly males with intermittent claudication in the legs.

The Haemodynamic Theory

But surgeons were not the only proponents of this view. In 1951, Derek Denny-Brown (1901–1981),[50] a New Zealand-born neurologist who worked in several English-speaking parts of the world before settling in Boston, was disappointed with the therapeutic effects of vasodilator drugs and stellate blocks. Presenting several cases of transient episodes associated with stenosis or occlusion in extracerebral arteries, he proposed:

---

[49] Pickering (1948), Transient cerebral paralysis in hypertension, 430.
[50] Shorvon and Compston (2019), *Queen Square*, 448–55.

The transient cerebral disorders which are cited as examples of 'vaso-spasm' have in common a defective collateral circulation. The primary event is occlusion of a cerebral vessel, not by spasm but by endarteritis. The repeated transient disorders reflect the sensitivity of the tissue, thus indirectly supplied by collateral vessels, to fluctuations in systemic blood pressure.[51]

Almost 10 years later, Denny-Brown reiterated the role of hypotension in the pathogenesis of temporary focal ischaemia, especially if collateral pathways were inadequate, referring to experimental work he had performed in the meantime with John Stirling Meyer (1924–2011).[52] In Los Angeles, the cardiologist Eliot Corday (1913–1999) and the neurosurgeon Sanford F. Rothenberg (1919–1991), collaborating in clinical and experimental studies, also concluded that 'cerebral vascular insufficiency' was largely the result of a combination of arterial narrowing and low blood pressure.[53]

Hypotension: Near-Fainting, Rarely TIAs

However, two sets of observations argued against 'misery perfusion' as the key factor. The first was an experiment with induced hypertension in patients with TIAs, performed in the 1960s at the National Hospital in London by Robert (Evan) Kendell (1935–2002),[54] future Professor of Psychiatry in Edinburgh, together with John Marshall. They studied 23 patients with 'TIAs', represent-ing nearly all their patients with this diagnosis in the course of one year. In 10 of them, the attacks were attributed to the carotid territory, and in the other 13 to the posterior circulation – always more complex than only vertigo or blurring of vision. In these experiments, the patient was strapped to a tilt table and brought into an upright position; then the blood pressure was artificially lowered by intravenous injection of hexamethonium. Only one of the 23 patients experienced the same symptom as the attack that had brought him under medical attention (pain, numbness, and weakness of the left arm). Other patients had focal symptoms, but these were different from their previous attacks (5 patients) or these appeared only after near-fainting (6 patients), or they had no symptoms at all (11 patients).[55] The conclusion of Kendell and Marshall 'that hypotension is not an important causal factor in the genesis of transient cerebral ischaemic attacks', though branded 'a sweeping

[51] Denny-Brown (1951), Recurrent cerebrovascular symptoms.
[52] Denny-Brown (1960), Recurrent cerebrovascular episodes.
[53] Corday, *et al.* (1953), Cerebral vascular insufficiency; Rothenberg and Corday (1957), Etiology of transient cerebral stroke.
[54] https://history.rcplondon.ac.uk/inspiring-physicians/robert-evan-kendell
[55] Kendell and Marshall (1963), Hypotension in the genesis of transient focal cerebral ischaemic attacks.

statement' by an upset Denny-Brown,[56] was supported by fresh evidence, as well as by a more attractive hypothesis.

The new testimony against hypotension came a decade later, from 'experiments of nature'. Several studies revealed a close relationship between severe bradycardia or tachycardia and symptoms of diffuse cerebral ischaemia, variously described by patients as near-fainting, giddiness, blurred vision, or blacking out. Physicians in Atlanta, Georgia, performed long-term (10 hours) electrocardiographic monitoring on a group of 28 patients with paroxysmal symptoms of this kind; they found serious cardiac arrhythmias in eight of them versus only two in a group of 11 patients with attacks of focal brain ischaemia.[57]

Also, Robert L. Reed (1940–) and Robert G. Siekert (1924–2014) from the Mayo Clinic published on a vast series of 290 patients who had received artificial pacemakers for cardiac dysrhythmias; in 235 of them, the rhythm disorder had provoked symptoms of generalized neurological dysfunction, against only two patients with focal cerebral symptoms.[58]

In that same year, the cardiologist P. Michael McAllen (1916–2009), collaborating with John Marshall, reported eight patients with near-fainting attacks who had made long peregrinations in the medical system before serious dysrhythmia was uncovered by long-term electrocardiographic recording or, as a chance finding, on a standard electrocardiogram; they formed half of all patients in whom a pacemaker was fitted in the same time span.[59] Somewhat unfortunately, the authors used the term 'TIAs' for these giddy spells – correctly as far as semantics go, were it not that, in the meantime, a large part of the medical community had adopted the abbreviation to designate attacks of presumed *focal* brain ischaemia, as Siekert was not slow to point out.[60]

All in all, drops in blood pressure seemed an uncommon cause of TIAs, despite the celebrated London patient of 1954, in whom attacks of tachycardia no longer caused ischaemia of the brain and the eye after resection of a nearly occluded carotid segment (see p. 288).[61]

ARTERY-TO-ARTERY EMBOLISM

Fisher's work on cerebral infarction in the 1950s had established that thrombotic clots, or parts of these, could become disengaged from atheromatous lesions of extracranial arteries and cause brain softening by blocking a major or

[56] Denny-Brown (1963), Transient focal cerebral ischaemia.
[57] Walter, *et al.* (1970), Transient cerebral ischemia due to arrhythmia.
[58] Reed, *et al.* (1973), Rarity of transient focal cerebral ischemia in cardiac dysrhythmia.
[59] McAllen and Marshall (1973), Cardiac dysrhythmia and transient cerebral ischaemic attacks.
[60] Siekert (1973), Cardiac dysrhythmia and transient cerebral ischaemic attacks; McAllen and Marshall (1973), Cardiac dysrhythmia and transient cerebral ischaemic attacks.
[61] Eastcott, *et al.* (1954), Reconstruction of internal carotid artery.

minor branch downstream. The question was, could a similar phenomenon be invoked to explain cerebral TIAs? At any rate, in 1868, the ophthalmologist Hermann Knapp had strongly suggested this for the eye.

White, Moving Segments in the Retina

Fisher, once more, expanded Knapp's observation by adding a dynamic element, in a report of serial events in the retina during an attack of monocular blindness, published in 1959.

> A 54-year-old pharmacist had had recurrent headaches ten to fifteen years before admission. He had developed right hemiparesis two years before which had gradually cleared. For one and a half years, the patient had had brief episodes of partial or total blindness in his left eye once or twice a day. These attacks increased in frequency and duration, and, ten days before admission, he had numbness on the right side of his face, accompanied by complete loss of speech. [...] On neurologic examination, he had slight right facial weakness, a trace of dysarthria, and a definite, although mild, reduction of position sense in the fingers and toes on the right.[62]

Angiography had shown marked narrowing of the left carotid sinus. Apparently, Fisher had arranged to meet as soon as a new episode of blindness occurred, for Fisher caught his first view of the patient's left retina 20 minutes after the onset of a new attack. He then patiently followed the course of events. What he saw (Figure 10.1) deserves to be read in full but has to be summarized here. A segment of whitish material initially blocking the bifurcation of the central retinal artery moved in the course of one hour from the bifurcation to the periphery, especially in the superior temporal branch. Somewhat later, Fisher observed a second episode, though less completely. All the while, he was very careful in the interpretation of what he had seen:

> As the white segment migrated distally, it appeared to be temporarily halted at bifurcations, and our immediate impression was that a pale, intravascular substance had become arrested like an embolus. However, since the whiteness was possibly produced in some other way, the white segment has purposely not been alluded to as representing intravascular material in the descriptions. [...] Spasm, a process often evoked to explain transient retinal ischemia, was an alternative interpretation. However, the idea that vasospasm might disappear from the proximal end of an affected segment of artery and at the same time appear and advance at the distal end

[62] Fisher (1959), The fundus oculi in transient monocular blindness, 333–4.

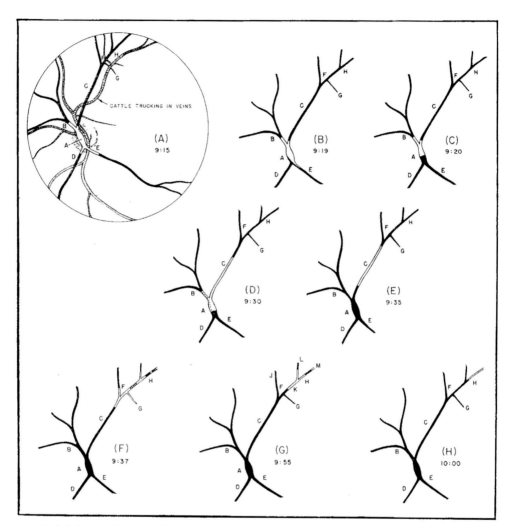

10.1 Ophthalmoscopic observations during an attack of blindness in the left eye (from Fisher, 1959). A summary of Fisher's highly detailed legend is: initially, at 9.15, a white, bloodless section at the bifurcation of the central retinal artery, in the stems of the superior and inferior retinal arteries, and in a short adjacent section of each of the four retinal arteries; also, a striped pattern in the column of blood of several veins in the upper retina. In the course of 45 minutes, the white appearance moved to the periphery, especially along the superior temporal branch. *Source:* By permission of *Neurology*.

of the segment – remaining unaltered between – would severely test our already too elastic conceptions of the capabilities of cerebral vasospasm.[63]

Only after having reviewed all other possibilities – fluctuation in the systemic blood pressure, progressive thrombosis, multiple emboli from the heart, or changes related to the upright posture, Fisher proposed:

[63] Fisher (1959), The fundus oculi in transient monocular blindness, 339.

We are tempted to generalize and suggest that intracranial transient ischemic episodes – at least some instances – will also find their explanation in the occurrence of local cerebral embolism or micro-embolism analogous to the process witnessed in the retinal circulation of our patient.[64]

Platelet Emboli

The next step in the understanding of TIAs, at least ocular TIAs, took place two years later and involved Dr Ralph Ross Russell (1928–) (Box 10.2).[65] At the time, his contribution to the understanding of intracerebral haemorrhage (Chapter 5) was still to come. He wrote the following case history in 1961, while based in Oxford at the Department of Medicine led by George Pickering:

A lorry-driver, aged 54, went to his doctor complaining of episodes of tingling and clumsiness in the right hand and arm, but nothing abnormal was found. [...] He continued to complain of intermittent symptoms in the right hand and also mentioned to his workmates that his vision was blurred from time to time. [...]

On the day of admission at 5 P.M. he was dressing to go out and complained to his wife that his collar seemed tighter than usual. After a struggle he managed to fasten it and bent down to put on his shoes. At that moment he gave a groan and toppled to the floor. For a few seconds he was motionless and appeared to be unconscious, but quickly came round and tried to get up. It was at once apparent that the right arm and leg were weak and clumsy, and although he spoke freely he made many mistakes with words. He managed to explain to his wife that he could not see out of the left eye and kept rubbing it with his left hand. [...] He was admitted to hospital at 8 P.M., three hours after the stroke.[66]

The patient's fundi were first examined at 8:30 P.M. The events witnessed in the retina of the left eye very much resembled those described by Fisher. Yet there were a few differences: this time the 'white material' moved to a lower retinal branch, and at the time of its completely disappearance (10:15 P.M.) the attack had lasted over five hours; a quarter of an hour later a new 'white body' appeared at the disc and moved downwards, now vanishing in little more than half an hour.[67]

[64] Fisher (1959), The fundus oculi in transient monocular blindness, 347.
[65] Ross Russell (2003), From the retired.
[66] Ross Russell (1961), Retinal blood-vessels in monocular blindness, 1422.
[67] Ross Russell (1961), Retinal blood-vessels in monocular blindness, 1423.

Box 10.2 Ralph Ross Russell (1928–).

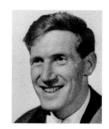

He was born in Edinburgh, the son of Robert Ross Russell and Elizabeth Ross Russell (née Hendry). His choice of medicine was not influenced by examples in his family. He graduated in Cambridge in 1958, having studied at that university for the MA degree and as a clinical student in Oxford; at that time, Cambridge did not have a clinical school. He then received a scholarship to work in the department of the Regius Professor of Medicine in Oxford. The incumbent at the time was Sir George Pickering, a world expert on hypertension. Since Pickering was busy debunking the vasospasm theory of TIAs of the brain, he encouraged Ross Russell to explore the subject further. It was from Oxford that Ross Russell documented two cases of arterio-arterial thrombo-embolism, from the internal carotid artery to branches of the ophthalmic artery. In 1961, he obtained his doctorate in medicine at the University of Oxford. Soon afterwards he received a grant from the National Institute of Neurological Diseases and Blindness (USA) to work at the Neurology Unit and the Mallory Institute of Boston City Hospital, with Derek Denny-Brown, and the Department of Neurology at Massachusetts General Hospital. There he studied micro-aneurysms of cerebral arterioles and their relationship with hypertension.

In 1963, he was appointed as a consultant at the National Hospital for Neurology and Neurosurgery, as it was then called, in combination with appointments at St Thomas Hospital and Moorfields Eye Hospital. In that position, he regularly encouraged younger neurologists to undertake further studies, especially in relation to cerebrovascular disease, the visual system, or both. He was senior author of a paper for *The Lancet* reporting on the disappearance of frequent attacks of monocular blindness during treatment with aspirin. Among his other papers is a report on loss of voluntary eyelid closure. In 1976, he published a book on vascular disease of the central nervous system and was the editor of the second edition, in 1983. With Marie-Germaine Bousser (Paris), he wrote a monograph on cerebral venous thrombosis. He retired from the National Hospital in 1993. Juniors recall his kind and modest personality.

Source: Portrait courtesy of Dr Ross Russell and family.

Endarterectomy of the left carotid artery began almost immediately afterwards (at 11:30 P.M., six-and-a-half hours after the stroke). The specimens removed from the carotid artery at operation were of three kinds:

(1) a portion of the intima of the artery with attached thrombus from the site of endarterectomy; (2) numerous small pieces of dark recent thrombus which were removed piecemeal from the cervical portion of the internal carotid; (3) a larger thrombus forming a cast of the cavernous part of the carotid artery with a smaller branch 3 cm. long joining the main trunk at its distal end [*i.e. the cerebral part of the internal carotid artery*]. This branch was probably an incomplete cast of the ophthalmic artery and its branches. [. . .] The cast of the upper carotid artery was composed

of dark laminated thrombus, but the branch was lighter in colour and the terminal filaments were white, friable, and threadlike. [...] The mass is probably largely composed of agglutinated platelets.[68]

Sadly enough, the eventual outcome was fatal five weeks later, owing to several complications. Autopsy confirmed the presence of a thrombus in the left middle cerebral artery, without any evidence of local atheroma.

Emboli: Platelets, Cholesterol Crystals, or Fibrinous Clots

So Ross Russell's observations in 1961 confirmed Fisher's careful 'attempt at generalization' two years before, on two counts. In the first place, the 'moving white segments' in the retina of patients with transient monocular blindness indeed represented intravascular material, that is, clumps of blood platelets. Secondly, the finding of retinal platelet emboli in a patient who had shortly before become hemiparetic by a fibrinous embolus in the territory of the same atheromatous carotid artery strongly supported the idea that TIAs of the brain might represent embolism from the same source as those of the eye.

In the same year, Robert W. Hollenhorst (1913–2008), an ophthalmologist at the Mayo Clinic in Rochester, Minnesota, having examined the eyes of more than 200 patients with occlusive disease within the carotid arterial system, found in 11 per cent of them bright plaques, ranging from an isolated finding to several dozens. The plaques were orange, yellow, or copper-coloured, situated at various bifurcations of retinal arterioles (Figure 10.2). About their nature, he wrote:

> It is probable that these bright plaques are embolic crystals of cholesterol arising from ulcerating atherosclerotic lesions situated on the cardiac valves or in the endothelium of the aorta or carotid arteries. Their nature has not been ascertained, as none of the eyes involved have been examined pathologically. [...] From the following observations, it appears that some of these plaques are definitely crystals: (1) they often reflect the light brightly in only one direction, and if the ophthalmoscopic light is turned at a different angle or if the eye is compressed, the bright yellow reflection may diminish or disappear; (2) when the segment of artery in which the plaque rests is made to pulsate by compressing the globe, the bright reflection may flash on and off with each pulsation; (3) occlusion of an arteriole by even large plaques is infrequent; (4) pieces may break off from proximal plaques and may lodge successively at smaller, more distal bifurcations and finally may disappear entirely from the retinal circulation.[69]

---

[68] Ross Russell (1961), Retinal blood-vessels in monocular blindness, 1425.
[69] Hollenhorst (1961), Bright plaques in the retinal arterioles, 255.

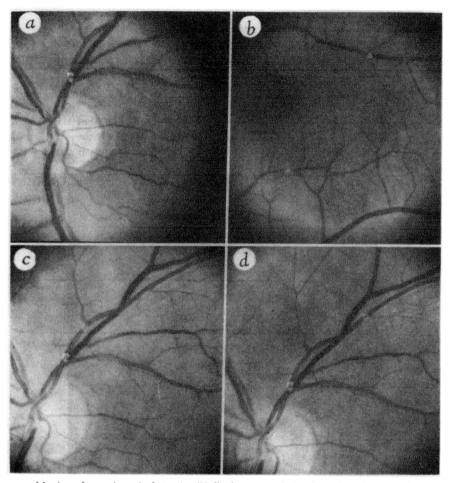

10.2 Moving plaques in retinal arteries (Hollenhorst, 1961). His legend reads: 'a and b. Left
retina on November 20, 1959. A fresh orange plaque is seen at the first fork above the optic disc;
two emboli are noted in the superior macular arteriole and one in the inferior macular arteriole.
c. Left retina on November 23. Note the additional plaque at the second fork of the superior
temporal arteriole. d. Left retina on November 25. The second plaque has moved to the third
fork of the superior temporal arteriole.'

Microscopic examination of embolic material in the retinal vessels was possible
in the case of another unfortunate patient, described by David J. McBrien and
colleagues at St Thomas' Hospital, London. After transient attacks of left-sided
weakness and blindness of the right eye, he underwent endarterectomy but
became suddenly comatose two days later, with profound left hemiplegia;
death followed within hours. Histological examination showed agglutinated
platelets in the retinal arteries.[70] The report did not contain information about
the intracerebral arteries, which prompted M. Rufus Crompton (n.d.), a

[70] McBrien, *et al.* (1963), The nature of retinal emboli.

pathologist at St George's, to comment that clumps of platelets might be responsible for transient attacks, but that in his experience, emboli causing strokes were fibrinous in nature.[71] At any rate, medical attention shifted more and more to embolism and its prevention.

PREVENTION OF STROKE: THE PROMISE AND THE PROBLEMS

Naturally, the identification of atheroma in the neck arteries as potential sources of emboli in the form of aggregated blood platelets, cholesterol crystals, or firm, fibrinous clots generated therapeutic hopes. Treatments preventing further TIAs should automatically prevent strokes, it was thought. Medical, as well as surgical, options were available; both showed some promise.

The Promise

The medical treatments on offer had in common that they were aimed at counteracting the process of clotting, although physicians at the Mayo Clinic found TIAs could be associated with an excess of red blood cells.[72] Fisher had already mentioned the potential of anticoagulant drugs in his 1951 article on carotid occlusion, referring to transient attacks preceding cerebral infarction.[73] Two years later, he published the case of a 70-year-old lady in whom anticoagulants had repeatedly arrested almost daily attacks of right-sided weakness without language disorder – and used the occasion to take another poke at the theory of vasospasm, which still had its adherents:

> If it is agreed that in the present instance the periodic transient episodes were typical of the vasospastic phenomena which herald the onset of some strokes, then it follows that the process of vasospasm has been altered and even prevented by anticoagulant therapy.[74]

In 1958, Fisher reported further encouraging results with this treatment, in a few scores of patients with TIAs: anticoagulant drugs, mostly coumarin derivatives, almost invariably led to their disappearance; patients who were alternately on and off anticoagulants fared better while receiving the drugs.[75] These preliminary conclusions were subsequently confirmed in London,[76] but not in

---

[71] Crompton (1963), Retinal emboli in stenosis of the internal carotid artery.
[72] Millikan, et al. (1960), Carotid and vertebral-basilar insufficiency associated with polycythemia.
[73] Fisher (1951), Occlusion of the internal carotid artery, 377.
[74] Fisher and Cameron (1953), Concerning cerebral vasospasm.
[75] Fisher (1958), The use of anticoagulants in cerebral thrombosis.
[76] Marshall and Reynolds (1965), Withdrawal of anticoagulants.

Newcastle.[77] Parenthetically, controlled studies of anticoagulants in patients with presumed cerebral infarction were downright disappointing.[78]

Whereas 'anticoagulants' in its literal sense imply every type of drug interfering with the clotting cascade, in clinical practice the term has become restricted to a subgroup of drugs interfering with fibrin formation, notably coumarins (vitamin K antagonists) and heparin derivatives. 'Antiplatelet agents' constitute another group; they antagonize the aggregation of blood platelets. Dipyridamole was the first compound of this type to be tested in a controlled clinical trial, set up by the research group of Hutchinson and Acheson in Stoke-on-Trent, of 169 patients with TIAs (about one-third of the total) or presumed ischaemic stroke (two-thirds). The number of events after an average period of two years showed no appreciable difference between the treatment group and the control group, not even for TIAs and strokes together.[79] In contrast, Michael Harrison (1936–2019),[80] with others at the National Hospital, found that attacks of transient monocular blindness were much diminished in frequency in two patients treated with aspirin, an old analgesic with a newly discovered antiplatelet action.[81] Similar effects transpired from an observational study by Mark Dyken (1928–2021) and his colleagues in Indianapolis,[82] in patients with TIAs of the brain.

Surgical treatment, mostly carotid endarterectomy, had its proponents too. At first, the operations sprang from the idea that removal of atheromatous material prevented ischaemic stroke by improving blood flow, as was the case in leg arteries. Walking indeed causes a large increase in local oxygen consumption and blood flow, but thinking does not. Also, it emerged in the mid-1960s that stenosis of an artery in the neck compromises blood flow to the brain only if it is very tight (less than 5 mm^2 of the remaining lumen), or if the collateral pathways are also diseased.[83] Gradually the opinion gained ground that ulcerated plaques might be a source of emboli, even if not associated with appreciable stenosis.[84]

Unclear Answers

The main aim of treatment, whether medical or surgical, is not merely to prevent further TIAs, but above all to prevent disabling ischaemic stroke. Yet

[77] Pearce, et al. (1965), Long-term anticoagulant therapy.
[78] Fisher (1958), The use of anticoagulants in cerebral thrombosis; Hill, et al. (1960), Long-term anticoagulant therapy; Hill, et al. (1962), Trial of long-term anticoagulant therapy.
[79] Acheson, et al. (1969), Controlled trial of dipyridamole in cerebral vascular disease.
[80] Limb (2019), Michael Harrison.   [81] Harrison, et al. (1971), Aspirin in amaurosis fugax.
[82] Dyken, et al. (1973), Carotid transient ischemic attacks and antiplatelet aggregation therapy.
[83] Brice, et al. (1964b), Effect of constriction on carotid blood-flow; Brice, et al. (1964a), Haemodynamic effects of carotid artery stenosis.
[84] Moore and Hall (1970), Importance of emboli from carotid bifurcation.

potential damage was also part of the equation. As indicated above, some patients died after endarterectomy, while published successes may well have been outnumbered by unpublished deaths. Physicians encountered the same dilemma, despite the optimistic tenor of an observational study from the Mayo Clinic claiming that brain infarction occurred less commonly in patients on continuous treatment with anticoagulants (for some reason) than patients not treated or treated only for limited time (for some other reason).[85] Only properly controlled studies could assess the balance between benefit and harm.

A first attempt at random allocation of anticoagulant treatment, performed at the Bellevue Hospital of Cornell University, New York, ran more or less aground due to a combination of two setbacks: patients dropping out for practical reasons, and haemorrhagic complications – often serious and occurring especially in older age groups.[86] Two other controlled studies were undertaken across multiple centres; one was coordinated from Massachusetts General Hospital in Boston and included groups with more serious cerebrovascular disease than TIA, and the other by the US Veterans Administration. Neither study found benefits of treatment in the occurrence of deaths; the number of new ischaemic or haemorrhagic events was too small to allow conclusions.[87]

At that point, in the mid-1970s, this narrative on the history of ischaemic stroke associated with diseased arteries comes to an end, at least in this book. There was growing awareness of the importance of preventing vascular damage in general, such as control of blood pressure across the population. But therapeutic advice was more difficult for patients with stroke warnings. This also applied to patients with atrial fibrillation, usually resulting from rheumatic heart disease. In this situation, cardiologists often recommended prophylactic treatment with anticoagulants;[88] neurologists tended to be more hesitant, even after a first stroke.[89]

Two Obstacles

Physicians seeking an answer to the question of whether stroke can be prevented in patients with TIAs by therapeutic measures, such as anticoagulants, antiplatelet agents, or endarterectomy, were faced with two difficulties.

The first was the novelty of designing therapeutic trials. In the course of the nineteenth century, physicians had grown accustomed to the idea that

[85] Siekert, et al. (1961), Anticoagulant therapy in intermittent cerebrovascular insufficiency.
[86] Groch, et al. (1959), Problems of anticoagulant therapy in cerebrovascular disease.
[87] Baker (1962), Anticoagulant therapy in cerebral infarction; Anonymous (1961), Anticoagulant therapy in cerebrovascular disease.
[88] Szekely (1964), Anticoagulant prophylaxis in rheumatic heart disease.
[89] Adams, et al. (1974), Mitral stenosis: survival with and without anticoagulants.

assessment of treatment efficacy was possible by comparing groups of patients,[90] and in 1948, an iconic trial of streptomycin in pulmonary tuberculosis had shown the way.[91] Yet the field of cerebrovascular disease was no exception to the rule that most methodological slip-ups have to be committed before they are recognized, as rules of trials are sometimes counterintuitive. The branch of science now called clinical epidemiology required not only mathematics, but also elements of philosophy, bordering on plain common sense.[92] For example, neurologists had to learn that strokes were not the only vascular events to be taken into account during follow-up.

The second, and seemingly insurmountable, problem was the similarity of symptoms in ischaemic and haemorrhagic stroke. After all, medical treatment often consisted of tampering with the balance between clotting and bleeding. Sure, in a patient with sudden hemiplegia who dies within hours, a haemorrhage is highly probable, and if such deficit takes place in the dominant hemisphere but is not accompanied by problems of language or sensation, many would think of lacunar ischaemia, but most strokes are somewhere in between these two extremes and the cause is anybody's guess.

It was up to the next generation to come up with solutions for these challenges.

[90] Matthews (1995), *Quantification and the Quest for Medical Certainty*.
[91] Medical Research Council (1948), Streptomycin treatment of pulmonary tuberculosis.
[92] Schwartz, *et al.* (1970), *L'essai thérapeutique chez l'homme*.

ELEVEN

SACCULAR ANEURYSMS

SUMMARY

Descriptions of superficial haemorrhages and of saccular aneurysms at the base of the brain appeared separately in the medical literature, before the first report of a ruptured basal aneurysm in 1813 (Blackall). This first patient was young, a recurrent characteristic in many later observations. Since the diagnosis was made only at autopsy, a fatal outcome seemed to be the rule, until preceding episodes of sudden, unusually severe headache were recognized (Stumpff, Wichern). A distinctive feature of ruptured aneurysms of the internal carotid artery was attendant oculomotor palsy (Stumpff); this allowed the first diagnosis during a patient's life, in 1920 (Symonds). Less specific were neck stiffness, retinal haemorrhages (Litten), caused by rupture of swollen veins (Terson, Manschot), and, after the introduction of lumbar puncture (Quincke, 1891), the demonstration of bloodstained cerebrospinal fluid.

The recognition of non-fatal episodes prompted attempts to try and prevent rebleeding through operative means. If the side of the aneurysm was known, carotid ligation could be undertaken, or sometimes even exploration and wrapping of the rupture site with muscle tissue (Dott, 1931). Later in the 1930s, when angiography made it possible to visualize an aneurysm, metal clips were applied to its neck (Dandy). The intra-arterial route was first explored in the early 1970s (Serbinenko). Direct surgical approach at an early stage was often followed by ischaemic complications ('vasospasm'); controlled trials of treatment remained largely inconclusive, partly by the difficulty of accounting for a patient's preoperative state.

Saccular aneurysms develop on large arteries at the base of the brain. Unlike micro-aneurysms, located on arterioles in deep regions, they are visible to the naked eye – hence the attribute 'saccular'. Their walls are often thin and may rupture. Given the location at the basal surface, haemorrhages after rupture first invade the subarachnoid space, hence the term 'subarachnoid haemorrhage'. Nonetheless, the impetus of arterial blood may also invade and destroy brain tissue, while the sudden increase in pressure may cause secondary ischaemia.

Before the connection between saccular aneurysms and superficial brain haemorrhages became known, these two abnormalities were described separately from each other.

SUPERFICIAL HAEMORRHAGES OR SACCULAR ANEURYSMS, APART

Haemorrhages at the Surface of the Brain

Some of the earliest brain haemorrhages on record were located at its base. In those cases, it is possible that an aneurysm was either overlooked or destroyed by the force of the bleeding. Examples are two of the four case histories in Wepfer's 1658 book on apoplexies,[1] and at least one of the several haemorrhages in Morgagni's famous work, a century later.[2] Morgagni also referred to a case he had read about,[3] in a scientific periodical from Basle.[4] Actually the report was a reprint of a thesis submitted in 1719, by Joh. Martinus Ott (n.d.) from Schaffhausen. Ott had described not only a superficial haemorrhage, but also a ruptured artery – perhaps an aneurysm:

> A blacksmith, seventy years old but still muscular, having been busy for several years with moulding cast iron, felt already two years before his death that a swelling appeared in his left flank; it came to distend his abdomen to a considerable degree. [...] He had learned to soften his food before ingestion. While the symptoms were worsening by the day, difficulty of breathing supervened, not responding to any treatment. At last, he had an apoplectic attack; his right eye was motionless, ingestion of food and swallowing extremely difficult, and his right side completely paralysed, as were the instruments of speech. This led to his death after six days, in the month of January, 1717.[5]

[1] Wepfer (1658), *Observationes Anatomicae*, 1–15 (patients 1 and 3).
[2] Morgagni (1761), *De Sedibus et Causis Morborum*, vol. I, 14 (epist. II, paragr. 19).
[3] Morgagni (1761), *De Sedibus et Causis Morborum*, vol. I, 22 (epist. III, paragr. 18).
[4] Ott (1751), Historia renis sinistri maxime tumidi.
[5] Ott (1719), Historia renis sinistri maxime tumidi, 5.

The dissection was carried out by Dr Burgauer:

> The brain, having been taken out, showed in the left hemisphere a lateral Willisian branch of the left carotid artery, tumescent with pitch-black blood, like dry gangrene; this vessel had ruptured and could be seen to have inundated the entire hemisphere with blood that was black like ink, down to the depth of the ventricles.[6]

So, apart from the superficial location, there was 'a ruptured carotid artery' and a 'paralysed eye', though on the 'wrong' side.[7] Presumably Ott thought he had made an error and that the eye should be affected on the same side as the arm and leg. Similarly, he was at a loss to explain, through body position and leakage of blood, why the hemiplegia was on the contralateral side; 'Valsalva's law', as Morgagni called it, was not yet known (see p. 100). The abdominal swelling was the actual subject of the thesis; it was a greatly enlarged left kidney, to the size of 'a bucket with one handle', compressing the stomach and the descending colon; the surface was irregular.

The first known illustration of a superficial haemorrhage appeared in 1812 (Figure 11.1), in the book on comatose diseases by John Cheyne (1777–1836) (see Box 3.4, p. 107); it also contained engravings of intracerebral haemorrhage (see Chapter 5).[8] The engraver used drawings made by the anatomist Charles Bell (1774–1842). Other reports of 'spontaneous' superficial haemorrhages at the base of the brain continued to appear,[9] even after the origin from ruptured aneurysms had become known.

Aneurysms

Morgagni did not describe aneurysms of brain arteries, but speculated about their existence, especially in the case of a certain Cardinal Ramazzini, an acquaintance. The prelate had shown him aneurysms on the back of both of his hands; soon afterwards he had become blind in one eye, and then in the other, followed by a fatal apoplexy; autopsy was not performed.[10]

Francisco Biumi (n.d.) from Milan performed, in the 1760s, the dissection of a 52-year-old woman who had suddenly died from an unknown cause; one carotid artery had widened in an aneurysmatic fashion within the cavernous

---

[6] Ott (1719), Historia renis sinistri maxime tumidi, 7–8.

[7] Ott (1719), Historia renis sinistri maxime tumidi, 15–16.

[8] Cheyne (1812), *Cases of Apoplexy and Lethargy*.

[9] Serres (1819), Nouvelle division des apoplexies, 302–11; Johnson (1824), Meningeal apoplexy; Wilks (1859), Sanguineous meningeal effusion; Froin (1904), Les hémorragies sous-arachnoidiennes; Forsheim (1913), Spontane Subarachnoidalblutung; Goldflam (1923), Spontane subarachnoidale Blutungen; Hyland (1933), Thrombosis of intracranial arteries.

[10] Morgagni (1761), *De Sedibus et Causis Morborum*, vol. I, 18 (epist. III, paragr. 8).

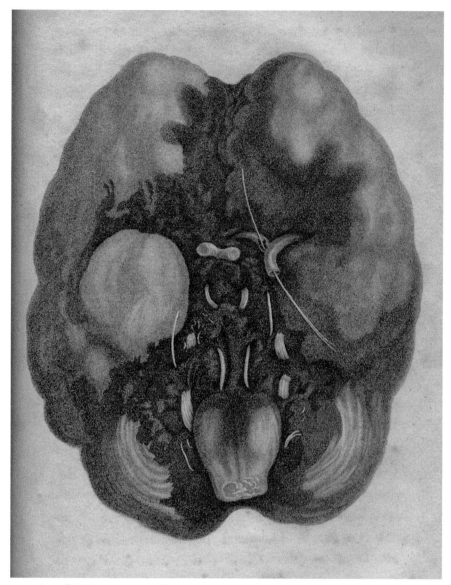

11.1 Superficial haemorrhage (Cheyne, 1812; engraving by J. Stewart). The original legend reads: 'This plate represents the base of the brain covered extensively with a coagulum of blood, owing to a rupture of the anterior artery of the cerebrum of the left side. The rupture of the vessel is sufficiently distinct without any letter of reference. The nerves have a peculiar appearance emerging from the dark coagulum.'

sinus, 'Vieussens's receptacle'.[11] Some authors have therefore gallantly, but inaccurately, credited Biumi with the first description of a brain aneurysm. However, there is a difference between common arterial widening and saccular aneurysms, which always occur at a site of arterial branching. Furthermore,

[11] Biumi (1765), Carotis aneurysmatica.

although the arterial wall in the cavernous sinus may indeed rupture, the effusion is limited to a duplicature of the dura mater, filled with venous blood; the result is an arteriovenous fistula, with peculiar symptoms of its own, as shown later.[12]

The true honour should probably go to Dr Gilbert Blane (1749–1834). In 1800, he contributed several cases of brain disease to the *Transactions of a Society for the Improvement of Medical and Chirurgical Knowledge*, a title typifying the Enlightenment. One of these stories was his post-mortem finding in a lady who had died at the age of 69 in a state of 'mania and fever':

> [...] there was no appearance in the brain itself that could in any way account for the symptoms. [...] But the morbid appearance in this case which was so singular, and to which the symptoms of complaint seem chiefly referrible, was two bulbs about five-eighths of an inch in diameter, filling up the hollow on each side of the *sella turcica*, which were evidently dilatations of the carotid arteries, and from their being filled with *laminae* of coagulated blood, there could be no doubt of their being aneurisms of these arteries. The dissection was made by Mr. Hunter, assisted by Mr. Home, in the presence of Dr. Jenner and myself, and all concurred in opinion, that these tumors were aneurisms. The one on the left side was the largest.[13]

The complaints Dr Blane associated with the parasellar aneurysms were visual symptoms, not the patient's terminal disease. Matthew Baillie (1761–1823) added Blane's observation to later editions of his own book on *Morbid Anatomy*, first published in 1793. He commented on the peculiarity of 'an aneurysm in both arteries in the same situation, and at the same time'.[14]

Soon after Cheyne's book illustrating a basal haemorrhage and Blane's account of aneurysmal dilatation of brain arteries, another British physician described the combination of these two abnormalities.

RUPTURED ANEURYSMS: A DIAGNOSIS MADE AT AUTOPSY

A Ruptured Aneurysm in a Patient with Dropsy

The first reported patient with a ruptured aneurysm was a young woman. She came under medical attention because of generalized skin oedema ('anasarca'). Her physician was John Blackall (1771–1860) (Box 11.1),[15] a distinguished practitioner in Exeter. In 1813, he published a treatise on 'dropsies', an umbrella term for 'accumulations of serous fluid which take place in the

---

[12] Coe (1855), Aneurism of carotid artery.   [13] Blane (1800), Case of aneurisms.
[14] Baillie (1812), *Morbid Anatomy*, 456–7.
[15] Anonymous (1860), The late John Blackall, M.D.

Box 11.1 John Blackall (1771–1860).

John was the sixth son of Theophilus Blackall, prebendary of Exeter cathedral, who died when John was 10 years of age. The mother Elizabeth Ley energetically managed the education of her four surviving sons. John studied medicine at Balliol College, Oxford, spent his clinical rotations on the wards of St Bartholomew's Hospital in London, and graduated in 1797. Back in Exeter, it proved difficult to compete with the established physicians; after a few years, Blackall moved to Totnes, a nearby market town, but he returned in 1807 to 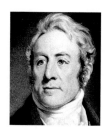 fill a vacancy at the local hospital. From then on, his reputation steadily increased. Caution was said to be one of his main characteristics; one could not be in his society, it was said, without feeling he was no ordinary person.

In his student days, Blackall had become interested in the phenomenon of albuminuria. Later on, he noticed its relation to dropsy, venous congestion, and kidney disease. In 1813, he published his well-known book on dropsy, which went through three subsequent editions. One year later, he obtained the degree of Medical Doctor in Oxford; in 1815, he was elected Fellow of the Royal College of Physicians. The Londoner Richard Bright, his junior by 18 years, definitively established the role of kidney disease in albuminuria and dropsy.

During the epidemic of Asiatic cholera of 1832, Blackall applied himself to his duties with untiring energy. He did not relinquish his practice until he had reached the age of 80 years.

Source: Portrait courtesy of Wellcome Foundation.

---

cellular membranes and circumscribed cavities of the body.'[16] Certain forms of it were associated with coagulable urine. One of Blackall's case histories ended with a fatal apoplexy:

> E. J. ætat. 20, [. . .], after unusual exposure to cold, became anasarcous, and complained of pain in her left side, with cough. [. . .]
>
> Soon after she had been put under my care, she was attacked suddenly, and without any apparent cause, by a most violent vomiting and diarrhoea, with head-ach of the most excruciating kind, a sensation as if the scalp were lifted by an internal force, some indistinctness of vision, intolerance of light, &c. She continued many days in the most excessive agony, the pupils neither fixed nor at all dilated, and the understanding suffering now and then only a momentary eclipse. [. . .] About twenty-four hours before death she fell into an apoplectic stupor.
>
> On examining the head, we found the veins of the pia mater turgid; in each of the lateral ventricles about half an ounce of blood loosely and recently coagulated, with some serum; the third and fourth ventricles

---

[16] Blackall (1813), *Observations on Dropsies*, i.

filled with a similar substance; and the brain itself in the immediate neighbourhood of these last considerably injured in its texture. The haemorrhage was traced to the basilary artery, which nearly at its bifurcation was dilated into an aneurismal sac of the size of a horse-bean, and appeared to have opened into the cavities of the brain at the communication between the third and fourth ventricles. A considerable quantity of pretty firmly coagulated blood was found under the membrane covering the tuberculum annulare[17] and medulla oblongata.[18]

One of the surgeons who performed or attended the autopsy in Exeter, a certain Mr Barnes, sent an eyewitness account to his colleague Joseph Hodgson (1788–1869) in London. Hodgson reproduced additional information in his book of 1815 on diseases of blood vessels:

> On the basis of the brain there was an extensive effusion of blood underneath the subarachnoid coat, and the cerebral substance was in some places lacerated by the effusion. In detaching the coagula to discover the point from which the blood had proceeded, an opening was made into an aneurysmal sac, [...] communicating with the trunk of the basilary, where it divides into the cerebellic and posterior cerebral arteries. [...] It was particularly thin, and had given way at the upper part, from which point the blood had forced its way into the ventricles and underneath the arachnoid membrane.[19]

In a footnote added during the production of his book, Hodgson alluded to a similar story of a young man who had died by a bleeding aneurysm, as large as a cherry, located at one of the anterior cerebral arteries.[20]

In the following two decades, more reports of ruptured saccular aneurysms saw the light; some of these were regarded as 'the first' by later reviewers, occasionally by the author himself, for example Étienne Serres (1786–1868), a physician at the Pitié. As recounted in Chapter 5, he published in 1819 'a new division of apoplexies': a cerebral and a meningeal type, with and without hemiplegia, respectively. Among his cases of meningeal apoplexy was a ruptured aneurysm of the basilar artery in a 59-year-old coppersmith.[21] In 1826, he republished the story, together with that of a second patient, a female merchant whose fatal haemorrhage originated from an aneurysm of the anterior cerebral artery.[22]

A year before Serres' second paper, Thomas Spurgin (1798–1864), a surgeon in Saffron Walden, Essex, contributed the story of a 57-year-old labourer with

[17] Nowadays called 'the pons' (of Varolio).
[18] Blackall (1813), *Observations on Dropsies*, 132–5.
[19] Hodgson (1815), *Diseases of Arteries and Veins*, 76–8.
[20] Hodgson (1815), *Diseases of Arteries and Veins*, 133.
[21] Serres (1819), Nouvelle division des apoplexies, 314–17.
[22] Serres (1926), Rupture des anévrysms, 421–31.

a ruptured aneurysm of the right anterior cerebral artery.[23] More case reports
appeared in the next decade, to start with in the atlas of Richard Bright
(1789–1858); it showed the first illustration of an aneurysm, pea-sized, arising
from a branch of the middle cerebral artery in a boy of 19 years who worked as
a collier (Figure 11.2).[24] Other communications in the early 1830s concerned a
54-year-old retired soldier with an aneurysm of the basilar artery,[25] a man of
45 years with 'a delicate constitution' who had bled from an aneurysm of the
middle cerebral artery, and – in the same publication – a 30-year-old bricklayer
whose aneurysm was at the anterior cerebral artery.[26] Even in these early
examples, the haemorrhage had not always been confined to the subarachnoid
space since blood had also invaded brain tissue or the ventricular system, a
finding to be confirmed time and again.[27]

Rebleeding

In most recognized cases of aneurysmal haemorrhage, the illness unfolded in a
single stage: sudden headache, mostly with a disturbance of consciousness,
followed by death a few days later. In 1836, a certain Armin Stumpff (n.d.)
described a biphasic disease course in the thesis he submitted at the University
of Berlin – written in Latin. The patient was a 20-year-old carpenter:

> On September 4, 1835, while at work, he was suddenly seized with
> headache and dizziness, so intense that he was knocked down and
> senseless for some time. When he had come round, the patient com-
> plained about extremely severe, throbbing headache everywhere in the
> head, which kept him from sleeping and eating. Because of the increasing
> pain he was admitted to the Charité Hospital on the 8th of the same
> month. [...] On September 18 the pain had almost entirely disappeared.
> [...] On September 24 the patient was discharged from hospital, not yet
> completely cured but much relieved.
>
> On November 22 he was readmitted to the Charité's Department for
> Diseases of the Eye because of increasing pain in the region of his right
> eye, while the light troubled him on that side and the right eyelid had
> recently started to droop.
>
> The patient went to sleep, without any sign that apoplexy was immi-
> nent. In the middle of the night the patients near to him suddenly awoke
> by the patient's stertorous and snorting respiration, with convulsions of
> his entire body. [...] After a brief pause, while he lay down in a state of

[23] Spurgin (1825), Aneurysm of the anterior cerebral artery.
[24] Bright (1827–31), *Reports of Medical Cases*, vol. II, part 1, 266–7; part 2, plate XIX.
[25] Jennings (1836), Aneurism of the basilar artery.
[26] King (1835), Aneurysms of the cerebral arteries.
[27] Richardson and Hyland (1941), Subarachnoid and intracerebral haemorrhage.

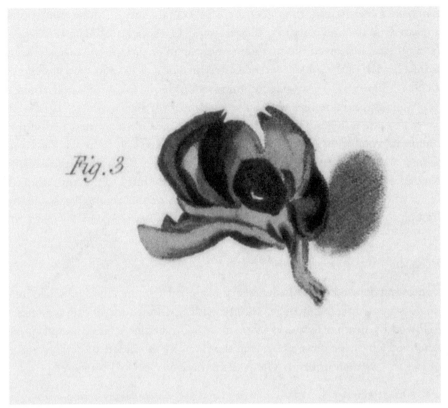

11.2 Ruptured aneurysm (from Bright, 1827–31). Drawing by C. J. Canton, engraving by W. T. Fry. The original legend is as follows: 'Small aneurysmal sac containing a clot of blood. This had taken place in one of the larger branches of the middle artery of the brain, and by its bursting had produced effusion of blood upon the surface of the brain, and consequent apoplexy.

A summary of the corresponding case history is: A boy of 19, collier, complained of being unwell; while sitting on the chamber utensil he suddenly exclaimed 'Oh my head' and passed into an insensible state. A few hours later the attending physician, Dr Streeter, found he spoke again, though languidly, with some, but not very severe headache. Eight days later the considerable pain in the head returned; the next morning the insensibility also returned and he died.'

unconsciousness, the convulsions returned with increased force and ended in death.[28]

Autopsy showed a ruptured aneurysm at the right internal carotid artery. Stumpff must have assumed two separate episodes of bleeding, though he did not explicitly state it. He was more intrigued by the involvement of cranial nerves (see below). At any rate, since the diagnosis of aneurysmal haemorrhage was made only at autopsy, the condition seemed almost invariably fatal and temporary recovery was therefore a very improbable event. At least this

---

[28] Stumpff (1836), De aneurysmatibus arteriarum cerebri, 9–11.

emerged from the writing of Byrom Bramwell (1847–1931), about a second
episode in a 50-year-old washerwoman from Edinburgh:

> The fact that the patient lived a fortnight after the first extravasation, and,
> indeed, practically recovered from the effects of the first rupture, is
> remarkable; for recovery after large meningeal haemorrhage, such as this
> was, is of the greatest rarity.[29]

Later publications again recounted episodes of sudden headache a few days or
weeks before a fatal haemorrhage. In 1912, Heinrich Wichern (1878–1940), a
perceptive physician in Bielefeld,[30] chronicled patients with ruptured aneurysms from his own practice and that of colleagues. In several patients, the
clinical features, pathological findings, or both were indicative of repeated
occurrences:

> This example leaves no room for any doubt that indeed a brain aneur-
> ysm, once perforated, can occlude and can later give rise to one or more
> further haemorrhages.[31]

As new observations confirmed Wichern's opinion,[32] there grew a general
awareness that aneurysms might burst on successive occasions. In the middle of
the twentieth century, when the diagnosis during life was still often delayed,
one-third of more than 400 patients had at least one episode of rebleeding; the
interval between the first and second haemorrhage was less than one week in
almost half of these.[33]

The scientific publications that followed in the rest of the nineteenth
century and the beginning of the next century were often compilations of
published cases, with fresh examples, but lacking new insights.[34] After 1907,
when the tally was already over 550 cases,[35] authors seemed to have lost count.
A few of these aneurysms were not saccular, but fusiform,[36] a rare variant not
discussed here any further. Gradually the attention shifted to the cause of
aneurysm formation and to the means of recognizing the clinical features of
their rupture.

---

[29] Bramwell (1886), Aneurism of the right internal carotid artery.
[30] Koppe (1950), Dr. med. Heinrich Wichern.
[31] Wichern (1912), Hirnaneurysmen, 236–9.
[32] Fearnsides (1916), Intracranial aneurysms, 262–6.
[33] McKissock and Paine (1959), Subarachnoid haemorrhage, 360.
[34] Brinton (1852), Report on cases of cerebral aneurisms; Gull (1859), Aneurisms of cerebral
     vessels; Lebert (1866), Ueber Aneurysmen der Hirnarterien; Gouguenheim (1866), Tumeurs
     anévrysmales du cerveau; Durand (1868), Des anévrysmes du cerveau, 3–56; Bartholow
     (1872), Aneurysms at the base of the brain; Peacock (1876), Intracranial aneurisms; von
     Hofmann (1894), Aneurysmen der Basilararterien; Beadles (1907), Aneurisms of the larger
     cerebral arteries; Fearnsides (1916), Intracranial aneurysms.
[35] Beadles (1907), Aneurisms of the larger cerebral arteries.
[36] Gull (1859), Aneurisms of cerebral vessels, 284; Griesinger (1862), Aneurisma der Basilararterie.

Why and When Aneurysms Develop

Hans Eppinger (1848–1916) implicated degenerative changes of the intimal layer, combined with a rent in the elastic lamina,[37] but other studies soon revealed that the wall of saccular aneurysms lacked a muscular layer. This explained their development at arterial branching sites, where the normal continuity of the *lamina muscularis* was necessarily interrupted.

Another striking characteristic was the young age of many patients; for example, a two-year-old child, having died of broncho-pneumonia, was found to harbour an aneurysm of the anterior communicating artery.[38] In adults, the common absence of atherosclerosis and high blood pressure also hinted at other causes. All this led to the idea of a congenital defect, or 'an inherent weakness due to a congenital abnormality in the structure of the arteries at their points of junction',[39] alone or combined with acquired factors.[40] The notion of a hereditary component was reinforced by occurrence in identical twins, siblings, or offspring.[41]

Finding vegetations of heart valves at post-mortem in some patients with ruptured aneurysms led physicians to implicate embolism with partial obstruction of a brain artery as the primary event,[42] especially in young patients (Figure 11.3).[43] An expert on the subject was G. Newton Pitt (1853–1929), a consultant at Guy's Hospital.[44] He went as far as suggesting, in 1890, that the great majority of cerebral aneurysms developed in this way:

> We are, therefore, justified in stating that the cause of four-fifths of all cerebral aneurysms is the retention of an embolus from a patch of fungating or granular endocarditis at the bifurcation of a vessel. Inflammatory changes take place in the clot, which in most cases softens and disappears, the wall of the vessel also inflames and dilates; the dilatation may take place at the set of the embolus occasionally on the distal, at other times on the proximal side of the obstruction, which may be complete. The more common condition is probably disappearance of the clot, with softening at the spot. In the great majority of the cases the middle cerebral was the vessel which was affected.[45]

[37] Eppinger (1887), *Pathogenesis der Aneurysmen*, 524–7.
[38] Turnbull (1915), Alterations in arterial structure, 248.
[39] Turnbull (1915), Alterations in arterial structure, 248.
[40] Wichern (1912), Hirnaneurysmen, 261.
[41] Brisman and Abbassioun (1971), Familial intracranial aneurysms; Fairburn (1973), 'Twin' intracranial aneurysms; Wilson and Cast (1973), 'Twin' intracranial aneurysms.
[42] Ponfick (1873), Ueber embolische Aneurysmen; Wichern (1912), Hirnaneurysmen, 231–6; Turnbull (1915), Alterations in arterial structure, 243–4.
[43] Church (1869), Contributions to cerebral pathology, 202–7; Church (1870), On the formation of aneurysms.
[44] Anonymous (1929), G. Newton Pitt.
[45] Pitt (1890), On cerebral embolism and aneurysm.

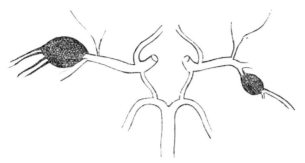

11.3 Embolic aneurysm in both middle cerebral arteries (from Pitt, 1890). The case history is, in summarized form: a man, aged 18, was admitted with severe heart disease; he developed headache, delirium, and numbness, with coldness on the left side, dying three weeks later. On the right side, there was a ruptured aneurysm of the middle cerebral artery, with a patch of softening in the temporo-sphenoidal lobe containing bloodstained fluid and clot. There was a small aneurysm of the opposite vessel.

It should be kept in mind, however, that the clinical course in patients with fatal haemorrhages from a septic aneurysm was very much different from that in 'idiopathic' cerebral aneurysms: many of these patients would already be ill from heart disease before an embolus lodged in a brain artery; also, brain ischaemia had often caused hemiplegia or other deficits before such rupture occurred. Aneurysms from septic emboli, curiously, but traditionally, named 'mycotic aneurysms', a term referring to fungi, developed not only at the circle of Willis, but also in smaller arterial branches of the brain or meninges. Their frequency decreased dramatically in the course of the twentieth century; in the autopsy series of Dorothy Russell (1895–1983), representing the years 1912–52 in London Hospital, one-quarter of all ruptured aneurysms was of bacterial origin,[46] whereas in the Newcastle series of John Walton (1922–2016), reported a decade into the era of antibiotics, this ratio was 1:30.[47]

Syphilis causing rupture of a saccular brain aneurysm secondary to granulomatous arteritis had been diagnosed several times,[48] but was much less common than septic emboli from the heart or emboli from syphilitic aneurysms of the aorta.[49]

Symptoms and Signs

The dominant symptom of subarachnoid haemorrhage from saccular aneurysms was, and still is, a sudden and often violent headache – 'a bolt from a blue

[46] Russell (1954), Intracranial haemorrhage, 689.
[47] Walton (1956a), *Subarachnoid Haemorrhage*, 17.
[48] Chvostek and Weichselbaum (1877), Syphilitische Endarteriitis; Wichern (1912), Hirnaneurysmen, 253–5; Turnbull (1915), Alterations in arterial structure, 250.
[49] Fearnsides (1916), Intracranial aneurysms, 237.

sky'. Many stories echo the intensity of the pain. Loss of consciousness could occur, for a shorter or longer period.

Neck stiffness was already a commonly recognized sign by the early twentieth century; some patients spontaneously complained of neck pain or kept their head in retroflexion.[50]

Oculomotor palsy associated with rupture of an aneurysm of the internal carotid artery in its terminal part was a prominent feature in the young carpenter whose fatal illness Stumpff related in 1836;[51] it did not take long before other reports associated a third nerve palsy with an aneurysm of the internal carotid artery, at its junction with the posterior communicating artery; yet, all these observations were made in retrospect.[52]

Retinal haemorrhages are a story by itself. On inspection of the eye in one of the earliest post-mortem observations of a ruptured aneurysm, in 1825, the sheath of the optic nerve was found 'thickened and distended with blood'.[53] A few decades later, Moritz Litten (1845–1907),[54] at the Charité in Berlin, found preretinal haemorrhages on ophthalmoscopy in both eyes of a patient who eventually died of subarachnoid haemorrhage.[55] He supposed that simultaneous bleeding had occurred from arterial micro-aneurysms in the brain and in the retina. However, Alfred Terson (1838–1925), an ophthalmologist in Toulouse, maintained that blood surrounding the optic nerve could not enter the eye. In 1900, he documented an instance of extensive bleeding into the vitreous body in a patient who had probably sustained an intracerebral haemorrhage; vision did not improve until 10 months later. Terson suggested that retinal veins were the source of retinal and vitreous haemorrhages, congested as they were by the pressure around the optic nerve.[56] Pathological proof of this came from Willem Arnold Manschot (1915–2010), later Professor of Ophthalmic Pathology in Rotterdam; he made a systematic study of the eye in subarachnoid haemorrhage.[57]

[50] Wichern (1912), Hirnaneurysmen, 239–44.
[51] Stumpff (1836), De aneurysmatibus arteriarum cerebri, 10–11, 25, 28–32.
[52] France (1846), Examples of ptosis, 46–7; Hare (1850), Paralysis of the motor oculi; Lebert (1866), Ueber Aneurysmen der Hirnarterien, 231, 404; Gouguenheim (1866), Tumeurs anévrysmales du cerveau, 40–2, 88–9; Hale-White (1894), Intracranial aneurysm in young subjects; Fearnsides (1916), Intracranial aneurysms, 249–52; Bramwell (1931), Aneurism of the circle of Willis and oculo-motor paralysis.
[53] Spurgin (1825), Aneurysm of the anterior cerebral artery, 444.
[54] Pagel (1901), *Ärzte des neunzehnten Jahrhunderts*, 1024.
[55] Litten (1881), Apoplexie des Gehirns und der Retina.
[56] Terson (1900), Hémorrhagie dans le corps vitré.
[57] Manschot (1944), The fundus oculi in subarachnoid haemorrhage; Manschot (1954), Subarachnoid hemorrhage, intraocular symptoms.

Hemiplegia, with or without dysphasia, sometimes occurred through invasion of brain tissue, mainly with ruptured aneurysms of the middle cerebral artery.[58]

Large aneurysms, at any location at the base of the brain, could sometimes reach sufficient magnitude to mimic the symptoms of a brain tumour, without rupturing.[59]

A murmur associated with a cerebral aneurysm, audible to the patient and heard by others through applying an ear or a stethoscope to the patient's head, was a symptom the surgeon–pathologist Cecil F. Beadles (1867–1933) found frequently mentioned in textbooks; he suspected it was one of those statements 'originally resting on very slender evidence, but acquiring a spurious importance by constant repetition'. His scepticism included 'hissing sounds' heard by patients.[60]

FROM SYMPTOMS TO DIAGNOSIS

The future laryngologist Achille Gouguenheim (1839–1901) wrote in his doctoral thesis on brain aneurysms (1866) that he had never witnessed a cure after rupture of a brain aneurysm.[61] He might have written, instead, that the diagnosis had so far been made only at autopsy. Heinrich Wichern from Bielefeld wrote in 1912, in the same article where he had drawn attention to the occurrence of rebleeding after initial survival, how difficult the diagnosis was during life:

> Though we are able, on looking back from the autopsy findings before us, to recognise certain features of the clinical course as the result of aneurysmal haemorrhage, this does not at all imply that, conversely, the presence of these symptoms allows the clinician to make a diagnosis of a ruptured aneurysm.[62]

Indeed, the combination of headache and meningeal irritation could – and still can – suggest inflammation instead of haemorrhage. More clues were needed to dispel the notion of an inexorably lethal disease and to raise the doctor's suspicion of such a disease.

The Cerebrospinal Fluid

In 1891, Heinrich Quincke (1842–1922) introduced the lumbar puncture – initially not as a diagnostic, but as a therapeutic procedure, with the purpose of

---

[58] Durand (1868), Des anévrysmes du cerveau, 14–19.
[59] Nebel (1834), Aneurysmata duo rariora, 28–37; Beadles (1907), Aneurisms of the larger cerebral arteries, 293–308.
[60] Beadles (1907), Aneurisms of the larger cerebral arteries, 318–21, 327–32.
[61] Gouguenheim (1866), Tumeurs anévrysmales du cerveau, 49.
[62] Wichern (1912), Hirnaneurysmen, 239.

withdrawing excess cerebrospinal fluid in children with hydrocephalus.[63] Initially there were concerns about the risks of the method; a presentation in 1902 by Léon Laruelle (1876–1960) from Gand prompted the comment 'Young man, you are a murderer' from Arthur van Gehuchten (1861–1914), the highly esteemed Professor of Neurology in Louvain.[64] Nevertheless, the technique was soon adopted as an aid to the diagnosis of diseases of the nervous system, especially in the diagnosis of meningeal infections, but also in order to detect meningeal haemorrhage.

What the lumbar puncture could show, however, was merely the presence of blood in the cerebrospinal fluid – not its origin. Subsequent autopsy could show a ruptured aneurysm, as in the earliest communication of Fernand Widal (1862–1929),[65] but this was a far-from-specific finding. The 30-odd patients with haemorrhagic spinal fluid Widal's pupil Georges Froin (1874–1932) described in his thesis had nearly all bled from a ruptured arteriole in the deep regions of the brain or from contusions by trauma.[66] In an early report from Lund of five autopsied patients with superficial haemorrhages, a ruptured aneurysm was the origin in two of them.[67] If a patient recovered, as happened in a case reported from Constantinople, the episode of subarachnoid haemorrhage might be classified as 'spontaneous', whereas an aneurysm was not considered.[68]

A useful discovery was the importance of the colour of the cerebrospinal fluid after it had been left standing for some time or if it was centrifuged. Professor Louis Bard (1857–1913) from Geneva found, in 1901, that the supernatant fluid was yellow, owing to a pigment derived from haemoglobin. On repeated puncture, the normal, clear aspect of the spinal fluid returned in the course of a fortnight.[69] Jean-André Sicard (1872–1929) investigated this phenomenon more systematically – he called the method *chromodiagnostic* – and noted its usefulness in distinguishing between a preceding haemorrhage and blood cells introduced by the needle.[70]

Oculomotor Palsy Attributed to Unruptured Carotid Aneurysm

The observations of oculomotor palsy resulting from a ruptured carotid aneurysm, by Stumpff in 1836 and by later authors, were all made after death. As Wichern had mused, it was another matter to suspect a ruptured aneurysm in a

---

[63] Quincke (1891), Die Lumbalpunktion des Hydrocephalus.
[64] '*Jeune homme, vous êtes un assassin*' (Minkenhof (1953), Bacteriële meningitides).
[65] Widal (1903), Le diagnostic de l'hémorragie meningée.
[66] Froin (1904), Les hémorragies sous-arachnoïdiennes.
[67] Ingvar (1916), Hémorragies méningées.
[68] Conos and Xanthopoulos (1912), Hémorrhagie méningée curable.
[69] Bard (1901), Liquide céphalorachidien hémorragique.
[70] Sicard (1901), Chromodiagnostic du liquide céphalorachidien.

hospital bed. In 1875, Jonathan Hutchinson (1828–1913),[71] a physician in London, came a little closer.[72] Mrs S, 40 years old, presented with a drooping eyelid on the left side, restricted movement of all rectus muscles, curiously most of abduction, and a wide, fixed pupil. These symptoms had developed in about one year, accompanied by worsening of the patient's usual headaches. Within a few months, the paralysis of the rectus muscles became complete. Hutchinson thought an aneurysm was a more likely diagnosis than a tumour, and proposed ligation of the carotid artery; the patient declined this treatment. Eleven years later, she died of an abdominal abscess related to an arterial aneurysm; the post-mortem confirmed the presence of a carotid aneurysm, with the size and shape of 'a bantam's egg'.[73]

The Diagnosis in a Live Patient

Some reviewers have awarded the laurels for this feat to Edvard Bull (1845–1925) in Christiania, now Oslo. In 1877, he chronicled the case history of a 17-year-old girl; in that same year, she was struck by severe headache while straining at stools. Bull found an oculomotor palsy, at first partial, then complete; her condition gradually improved, until five weeks later, when she became suddenly unconscious and died the same day. In the discussion section of the article, he explained how the combination of symptoms and signs might lead to the diagnosis of a ruptured aneurysm of the carotid artery that was eventually found at autopsy. Though writing that he had been less confident about the eventual outcome of the girl's illness than her parents,[74] it remains uncertain whether he actually suspected an aneurysm as the source of harm before dissection demonstrated it.

It was the year 1920 that witnessed at any rate the most celebrated instance of aneurysm rupture diagnosed *intra vitam*. The physician in question was the young British neurologist Charles Symonds (1890–1978) (Box 11.2).[75] He published the story three years later; in an addendum, he graciously conceded the priority to James Collier (1870–1935),[76] who, in 1922, had in a textbook chapter briefly alluded to the diagnosis in a young patient who had recovered.[77] Symonds saw his landmark patient during a fellowship he spent

---

[71] Parish (2007), Hutchinson, Jonathan.
[72] Hutchinson (1875), Aneurysm of the internal carotid.
[73] Bantam chicken: *poule naine, Zwerghuhn, pollo nano, krielkip.*
[74] Bull (1877), Akut Hjernaneurisma – Okulomotoriusparalyse – Meningealapoplexi.
[75] Symonds (1970), Autobiographical introduction; Shorvon and Compston (2019), *Queen Square*, 239–49.
[76] Symonds and Cushing (1923), Contributions to the clinical study of cerebral aneurysms, 16.
[77] Collier and Adie (1922), Diseases of the nervous system, 1352.

Box 11.2 Charles Symonds (1890–1978).

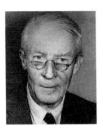

Charles (Putnam) Symonds was the son of Canadian-born Sir Charters Symonds, a surgeon at Guy's Hospital, and Fanny Marie Shaw. As a medical student at Oxford, Charles was attracted to neurology by reading Sherrington's *The Integrative Action of the Nervous System*. In Guy's Hospital, he came under the spell of Arthur Hurst (1879–1944) and his clinical demonstrations of nervous diseases. In the First World War, he served as a dispatch motorcyclist, was wounded, and returned home. He graduated in 1915, then served with the Medical Corps, collaborating with the future neurophysiologist Edgar D. Adrian (1889–1977). He went through the ranks at the National Hospital, then the almost exclusive gateway to neurology in the UK. In 1920, his young wife died and Symonds went to the USA, as an intern in psychiatry with Adolf Meyer (1866–1950) in Baltimore, and in neurosurgery with Harvey Cushing (1869–1939) in Boston.

Having returned to England with his American second wife Edythe Eva Dorton – they were to have two sons – Symonds became a physician at Guy's Hospital, and from 1926 also at the National Hospital. He contributed to several neurological conditions, including encephalitis lethargica, functional nervous disorders, cerebral venous thrombosis, and cough headache. At the outbreak of World War II, Symonds once more joined the army, as a captain in the Royal Air Force. Initially he established a military hospital for head injuries in Oxford, together with the neurosurgeon Hugh Cairns (1896–1952). Later he collaborated with Denis Williams (1908–1990) in studying psychological disorders precipitated by flying duties. He left the Royal Air Force as an air vice marshal and was knighted in 1946. Symonds retired from Guy's Hospital in 1955, and from consulting practice in 1963. In the late 1970s, a neurology registrar in London was surprised to find that the quiet gentleman on his ward was an erstwhile famous neurologist.

Source: Portrait courtesy of 'Journal of Neurology'.

in Boston, with the neurosurgeon Harvey Cushing (1869–1939).[78] He made the following notes:

> B.J.H., a married woman, aged 52, was admitted to the medical wards of the Peter Bent Brigham Hospital on August 30, 1920, complaining of headache and vomiting. She was thought to have a cerebral tumour and was transferred to the service of Dr Cushing. [...]
>
> In April 1919 the patient had an illness, causing her to take to her bed for four weeks, which was diagnosed as influenza. With this was associated severe headache, pain in the back of the neck radiating into her back, and vomiting. [...] In December 1919 she first noticed diplopia, which has since become permanent.

---

[78] Fulton (1946), *Harvey Cushing: A Biography*.

About August 14, 1920, she was seized with a sudden severe pain in the right supra-orbital region, which has persisted; for the first three days this was accompanied by frequent vomiting. A few days after the onset of this attack it was noted that her right eyelid was drooping. [...] There is complete right-sided ptosis at rest. [...] The right pupil is larger than the left [...]; it does not react to light or in accommodation. [...] There is complete paralysis of all muscles innervated by the right third and fourth cranial nerves.

On the morning of September 2, the patient experienced a sudden exacerbation of the orbital pain, with loss of consciousness for twenty minutes. New episodes of unresponsiveness occurred during the night and in the next morning; at noon she was comatose.

A right sub-temporal decompression was performed by Dr Cushing the same afternoon. A tense dura was disclosed, which on being opened revealed recently clotted blood extending over the whole hemisphere and apparently coming from the base of the skull. [...] She died early on the morning of September 4.

The autopsy was performed the same afternoon. On removing the brain the whole sub-dural and sub-arachnoid spaces were found full of recently coagulated blood. This washed away easily under the tap, disclosing a small saccular aneurysm about 8 mm in circumference at the junction of the right internal carotid and posterior communicating arteries.[79]

Symonds had made a drawing of the anatomical situation (Figure 11.4). Later, in an informal note, he described the details of his interaction with Cushing at the time:

When I had suggested the diagnosis of intracranial aneurysm in a case on which he was about to operate, he was, to say the least, sceptical. But when he explored the parasellar region there was uncontrollable haemorrhage, and the patient died [the] next day. Now it happened that the only time that Cushing could attend the post-mortem was on the following afternoon, on which most of us, and, as it transpired, Cushing himself had tickets for a great baseball match. His edict was that the post-mortem should be held at that time and that we should be present; and we were. When the aneurysm was disclosed he handed me the brain in a basin saying: 'Symonds, you made the correct diagnosis: either this was a fluke or there was reason in it. If so, you will prove it. You will cease your ward duties as from now, and spend all your time in the library.'[80]

---

[79] Symonds and Cushing (1923), Contributions to the clinical study of cerebral aneurysms, 139–44.
[80] Symonds (1970), Autobiographical introduction, 8.

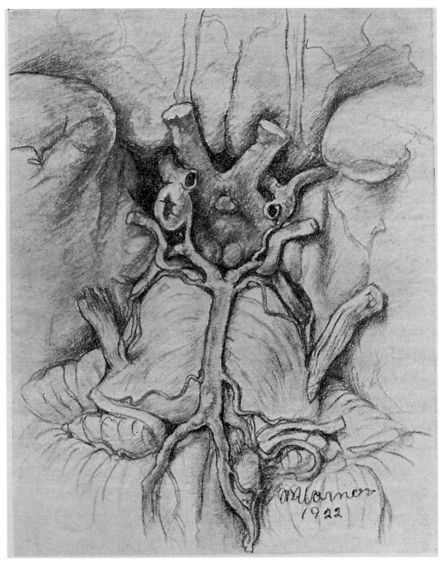

11.4 A saccular aneurysm suspected during life, in 1922 (from Symonds, 1923). The original legend reads: 'Drawing of the base of the brain, showing the aneurysm at the junction of right internal carotid and posterior communicating arteries.'

Cushing's mandate resulted in a paper in which Symonds recounted, apart from the above case history, four later patients in whom the diagnosis had been made during life; in two, the aneurysm had been confirmed post-mortem, and the other two survived.[81] Cushing added a postscript with four other fatal episodes of aneurysm rupture he had retrieved from the records and in whom the diagnosis had been made only in retrospect. A year later, Symonds wrote a

[81] Symonds and Cushing (1923), Contributions to the clinical study of cerebral aneurysms.

Box 11.3 Norman M. Dott (1897–1973).

Norman (McOmish) Dott was a descendant of the Huguenots named D'Ott who fled from Flanders to Scotland at the end of the seventeenth century. He was born in Colinton, five miles outside of Edinburgh, as the third child and first son of Peter Dott, a self-educated art dealer, and Rebecca Morton, well read and religious. As a boy, Norman had the most improbable pets, but he was also fascinated by machinery. Apprenticed to an engineering firm when barely 16 and driving his newly acquired motorbike in the busy streets 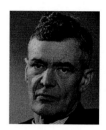 of Edinburgh, he crashed into a motored taxi. In hospital, the attending surgeon managed to save his left leg despite multiple fractures. During his stay in hospital, Norman became converted to surgery; after his discharge, he went right back to school in order to learn Latin. He entered the University of Edinburgh in October 1914, soon after the outbreak of the First World War – his bad leg kept him from the battlefields where several schoolmates lost their lives. As a second-year student, he once sneaked into the Western Infirmary of Glasgow to see William Macewen operate.

   Having qualified in 1919, Dott was a resident house surgeon in Edinburgh and assisted Edward Albert Sharpey-Schafer (1850–1935) in experimental work on the pituitary gland. In 1923, he sailed to Boston on a Rockefeller Fellowship to spend a year with Harvey Cushing (1869–1939). After his return, Dott regularly sought Cushing's advice in his attempts to establish a neurosurgical service in Edinburgh. In 1931, he married his secretary Margaret Robertson. Operations took place in cramped facilities, until in 1938, a neurosurgical ward could be opened, thanks to the St Andrew Biscuit Works. Dott developed new techniques and surgical instruments, gradually turning the department into a centre of excellence. In the Second World War, he organized a 'Brain Injuries Unit' at Bangour Hospital. In 1947, the University of Edinburgh appointed him to a professorship. The City of Edinburgh conferred the Freedom of the City on him in 1962.

Source: © National Galleries of Scotland.

---

review article on subarachnoid haemorrhage, including a discussion of causes other than aneurysm, the aspect of the cerebrospinal fluid, and clinical features.[82]

   Soon the diagnosis of ruptured aneurysm was made more often during life. This is how Norman M. Dott (1897–1973) (Box 11.3),[83] still a young neurosurgeon in 1933, expressed his feelings about the poor outcomes he had met with:

> From observation of a number of cases with single attacks and spontaneous recovery and return to health, and of a number with recurrent bleedings with intervals of days or weeks which ended fatally, we began to appreciate the sinister significance of a recurrence and the possibility of satisfactory and indefinite survival in its absence.[84]

[82] Symonds (1924), Spontaneous subarachnoid haemorrhage.
[83] Rush and Shaw (1990), *With Sharp Compassion.*
[84] Dott (1933), Intracranial aneurysms, 223.

This sentiment, that recurrent bleeding might be averted, led to the beginning of a therapeutic era – not just for the management of aneurysmal haemorrhage, but for the entire field of cerebrovascular disease. For the first time in history, physicians' actions truly could, and in some cases did, change the course of cerebrovascular disease for the better.

SURGICAL OCCLUSION OF ANEURYSMS

Initially, the operative procedure was limited to attempts at relieving the pressure on the small, fragile clot that formed the only barrier against renewed bleeding. In the words of Dott, looking back in 1969: 'We answered by carrying out some "blind" carotid ligations in cases that we could diagnose clinically.'[85]

Finding and Wrapping the Aneurysm

Yet the results of carotid ligation were often disappointing, especially in patients with multiple bleeding episodes. In 1931, another strategy presented itself to Dott, writing two years later:

> We were accustomed to deal successfully with quite formidable intracranial haemorrhages during operations by applying to the bleeding point a fragment of fresh muscle which formed a secure scaffolding for the clot, and became organised into fibrous tissue with it. Why not expose a bleeding aneurysm and deal with it after this fashion?

Indeed, an occasion had presented itself 'to put these speculations to the test of practice':

> The patient was a healthy active man of 53. For several years he had suffered from recurrent left frontal headaches with simultaneous drooping of the left eyelid. [...] Then he had a typical attack of spontaneous subarachnoid haemorrhage with the characteristic sequelae of meningeal irritation and cerebral compression. Lumbar puncture showed blood in the cerebrospinal fluid. [...] He was recovering well, when, eight days after this attack, there was a further haemorrhage. Again he made a good recovery. On the fourteenth day, while at stool, he had a third and more serious haemorrhage with collapse for some hours, and then recovery with a residual left oculomotor paresis and some degree of aphasia. [...] From former experiences we felt certain that the illness would end fatally from further bleeding, and decided to operate in the hope of averting this.

[85] Dott (1969), Intracranial aneurysm formation, 1.

Dott approached the aneurysm via a left frontal flap. It was a difficult matter, he wrote, to elevate the tense and oedematous brain, and to identify the basal structures, wholly covered with clots:

> The left optic nerve was found, and the internal carotid artery was defined at its outer side. This vessel was closely followed upwards, outwards and backwards to its bifurcation into the middle and anterior cerebral arteries. As this point was being cleared of tenacious clot, a formidable arterial haemorrhage filled the wound. With the aid of suction apparatus held close to the bleeding point, we were able to see the aneurysm. It sprang from the upper aspect of the bifurcation junction: it was about 3 mm. in diameter; blood spurted freely from its semi-detached fundus. Meanwhile a colleague was obtaining fresh muscle from the patient's leg. A small fragment of muscle was accurately applied to the bleeding point and held firmly in place so that it checked the bleeding and compressed the thin-walled aneurysmal sac. Thus it was steadily maintained for twelve minutes. As the retaining instrument was then cautiously withdrawn, no further bleeding occurred. [. . .]
>
> It is now over two years since the operation. The patient has so fully recovered that he is able for the responsible legal and social duties on which he was formerly engaged.[86]

Dott had made a sketch of the aneurysm, published only much later (Figure 11.5).[87] Looking back in 1969, he disclosed his special relationship with the patient:

> I was then still a surgical paediatrician as well as a surgical neurologist. The Chairman of the Board of the Children's Hospital was an able middle-aged legal gentleman who ruled the medical staff as with a rod of iron - sometimes with whips of scorpions. [. . .]
>
> He made a good recovery and was thus protected from further haemorrhage. Additionally, either his haemorrhages or my endeavours provided a beneficent leucotomy effect, and, consequently, a most harmonious Board-Staff relationship pertained thereafter. In addition to his onerous legal and hospital administrative duties he thereafter took an active part in founding Edinburgh's Orthopaedic Hospital. He died some 12 years later, full of years, from a heart infarct, while deer stalking in the Scottish Highlands.[88]

Different Approaches

A little later in the 1930s, cerebral angiography allowed preoperative visualization of the aneurysm (Figure 11.6).[89] This enabled Dott and other

---

[86] Dott (1933), Intracranial aneurysms, 223–5.
[87] Todd, *et al.* (1990), Norman Dott's contribution to aneurysm surgery.
[88] Dott (1969), Intracranial aneurysm formation, 2–4.
[89] Dott (1933), Intracranial aneurysms, 228–9.

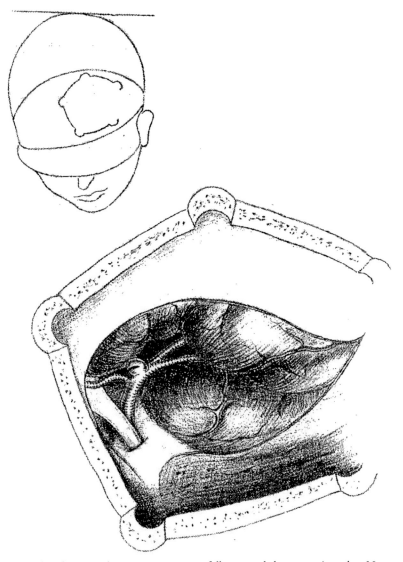

11.5 The first saccular aneurysm successfully treated by operation, by Norman Dott; presumably he made the drawing himself. A left frontal flap exposed a proximal aneurysm of the middle cerebral artery (from Todd *et al.*, 1990).

neurosurgeons to adapt their interventions to the shape and location of the aneurysm: ligation of the common or internal carotid artery, wrapping the aneurysm with muscle or ligating its neck, or, especially with aneurysms of the anterior cerebral artery, clipping of the parent vessel.[90]

---

[90] Falconer (1951), Surgical treatment of intracranial aneurysms; Dott (1969), Intracranial aneurysm formation.

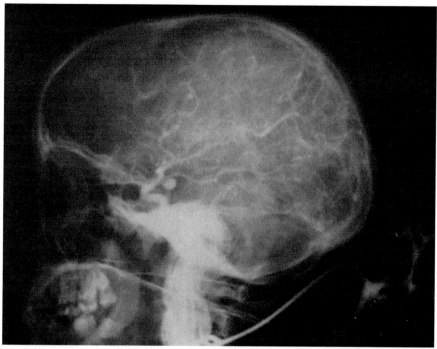

11.6 Angiogram made with Thorotrast® (thorium dioxide) in 1933, showing an aneurysm of the carotid artery at the junction with the posterior communicating artery, in a 23-year-old woman. She was treated by means of carotid ligation; 24 years later, she died from carcinoma of the hepatic duct (from Dott, 1969). *Source:* By permission of *Clinical Neurosurgery.*

In 1937, the Boston neurosurgeon Walter Dandy (1886–1946),[91] another pioneer, introduced the use of a metal clip to occlude the neck of ruptured aneurysms located at the terminal part of the internal carotid artery (Figure 11.7).[92] Aneurysms of the middle cerebral artery or the basilar artery, however, long defied attempts to occlude them;[93] as operative and anaesthesiologic techniques developed, even rupture sites at these difficult locations became within the reach of the neurosurgeon.[94] An important advance was the introduction of intraoperative microscopy, with Hugo Krayenbühl (1902–1985) and Gazi Yasargil (1925–) in Zurich as central figures.[95]

[91] McCarthy (2007), Dandy, Walter Edward.
[92] Dandy (1938), Aneurysm cured by operation.
[93] Dandy (1944), *Intracranial Arterial Aneurysms*, 129–31.
[94] Norlén and Olivecrona (1953), Aneurysms of the circle of Willis; Gass, *et al.* (1958), Eradication of middle cerebral aneurysms; Drake (1961), Aneurysms of the basilar artery; Drake (1968), Further experience with aneurysm of the basilar artery; Robinson (1971), Ruptured aneurysms of the middle cerebral artery; Drake (1971), Ruptured intracranial aneurysms.
[95] Yasargil and Fox (1975), The microsurgical approach to intracranial aneurysms.

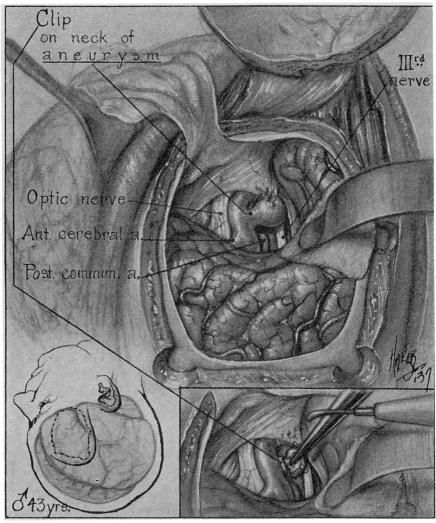

11.7 Clipping of an aneurysm (Dandy, 1938). The legend (Dandy, 1944, p. 113) reads: 'Typical aneurysm of the intracranial internal carotid artery, showing the narrow neck of the sack and the bulging aneurysm; also the point of rupture. The inset shows the clip placed upon the neck of the aneurysm, and the aneurysm itself shrivelled with the electric cautery.'

Brain Swelling and the Timing of Operation

Rebleeding was not the only problem. During the operation, the brain frequently appeared 'tense and oedematous', in Dott's words, or even 'red, swollen and angry',[96] as Charles Drake (1920–1998) in London, Ontario, put it; often the swelling continued after the operation and could prove fatal. This oedema, probably ischaemic in origin, was generally attributed to reactive

---

[96] Sundt (1975), Ischemic complications after subarachnoid hemorrhage, 424.

arterial spasm, especially in the region of the ruptured aneurysm.[97] However, the purported role of arterial narrowing, though widely accepted and the subject of quite a few experimental studies,[98] was not accepted by all. Other determinants of secondary brain ischaemia emerged,[99] while some even flatly denied there was a correlation with arterial narrowing.[100]

Whether or not the term 'vasospasm' as shorthand for 'delayed cerebral ischaemia' was correct or not, there was no doubt that this complication was a major cause of death and disability in the early phase after aneurysm rupture, the more so after craniotomy.[101] Some neurosurgeons therefore recommended to delay operation beyond the first or the first two weeks.[102] Of course, such a policy entailed the risk of rebleeding in the waiting period, so there were dangers in either strategy. In 1971, a courageous trial in Helsinki, involving 178 patients in good condition, showed that after a median period of more than 40 days, craniotomy had probably nothing more to offer.[103] Others advocated hypothermia during the surgical procedure,[104] but conclusive evidence for the benefits of cooling was lacking.

The Intra-arterial Route

An endovascular route to aneurysms, via intra-arterial catheterization, was a far less invasive method than intracranial surgery but, of course, posed many technical problems. F. A. Serbinenko (1928–2002), from the Burdenko Institute of Neurosurgery in Moscow,[105] was an early proponent of this approach.[106] He used an inflatable balloon attached to the catheter, introduced by direct puncture of an extracerebral artery or via the transfemoral route. Initially the purpose was temporary occlusion of blood vessels, mainly for diagnostic purposes prior to embolization; sometimes the aim was to induce clotting of fistulas or other vascular anomalies. The next step was partial occlusion of aneurysms, by means of detachable balloons.

---

[97] Ecker and Riemenschneider (1951), Spasm of the intracranial arteries.
[98] Echlin (1968), Current concepts of vasospasm; Gurdjian and Thomas (1969), Cerebral vasospasm; Odom (1975), Cerebral vasospasm.
[99] Crompton (1964a), Pathogenesis of infarction following rupture of cerebral aneurysms.
[100] Millikan (1975), Cerebral vasospasm and ruptured intracranial aneurysm.
[101] Crompton (1964b), Infarction following rupture of cerebral aneurysms.
[102] Norlén and Olivecrona (1953), Aneurysms of the circle of Willis; Drake (1971), Ruptured intracranial aneurysms.
[103] Troupp and af Björkesten (1971), Controlled trial of late surgical versus conservative treatment.
[104] Botterell, et al. (1956), Hypothermia in the surgical management of intracranial aneurysms; McKissock, et al. (1960a), Hypothermia in the surgical treatment of aneurysms.
[105] Teitelbaum, et al. (2000), Fedor A. Serbinenko.
[106] Serbinenko (1974), Balloon catheterization and occlusion.

Controlled Trials

Whether operative intervention was at all beneficial remained a matter for debate.[107] Wylie McKissock (1906–1994),[108] the founder of a neurosurgical team at Atkinson Morley's Hospital in London, mounted controlled clinical trials in the years around 1960. This showed an advantage for operative treatment of aneurysms at the internal carotid–posterior communicating artery,[109] and also for aneurysms of the middle cerebral artery, at least in men.[110] However, for aneurysms of the anterior artery or the anterior communicating artery, they found no difference between surgical and conservative treatment.[111] Meanwhile, neurosurgical journals began to abound with series from single centres, uncontrolled and without information on referral patterns or other selection criteria.

In the 1960s, several centres in North America and some in Europe decided to collate their results according to the same protocol. Initially this cooperative undertaking was an observational study.[112] Its sequel was designed as a randomized controlled trial comparing operative aneurysm occlusion with carotid ligation and bed rest;[113] stratification was planned for the site of the aneurysm (of the anterior circulation only) and for the interval between rupture and intervention.[114] However, the eventual report was mainly concerned with surgical subgroups.[115] The overall survival rates in the four treatment groups, published as a book chapter,[116] were difficult to interpret by differences in the period of follow-up (one, three, or five years). Also, the initial condition of patients, which proved an important determinant of outcome, was probably not balanced between the four groups.

Grading of Patients

Indeed, quite apart from the method of treatment, the eventual outcome depended not only on the location and size of the aneurysm, the patient's

[107] Logue (1956a), Aneurysms on the anterior cerebral and anterior communicating artery; Falconer (1959), Surgery of intracranial aneurysms (correspondence); Logue (1956b), Surgery of intracranial aneurysms; Walton (1956b), Surgery of intracranial aneurysms.
[108] Bell (1996), Wylie McKissock.
[109] McKissock, et al. (1960c), 'Posterior-communicating' aneurysms.
[110] McKissock, et al. (1962), Middle-cerebral aneurysms.
[111] McKissock, et al. (1965), Anterior communicating aneurysms.
[112] Locksley, et al. (1966), Cooperative study of intracranial aneurysms. II. General survey; Sahs, et al., ed. (1969), Intracranial Aneurysms and Subarachnoid Hemorrhage.
[113] Sahs (1974), Report on a randomized treatment study. I. Introduction.
[114] Nibbelink and Knowler (1974), Cooperative study of intracranial aneurysms. II. Design.
[115] Nibbelink, et al. (1977), Intracranial aneurysms and subarachnoid hemorrhage. IV-A. Regulated bed rest; Henderson, et al. (1977), Intracranial aneurysms. IV-B. Regulated bed rest – statistical evaluation.
[116] Graf, et al. (1981), Long-term follow-up evaluation of randomised study.

age, and the interval between haemorrhage and operation, but also – and perhaps above all – on the patient's overall 'brain status', in terms of level of consciousness and presence of focal neurological deficits.[117] In properly designed comparative studies, grouping of patients according to such prognostic variables might allow a realistic assessment of treatment results.

A first criterion was the presence or absence of coma;[118] attempts at finer distinctions followed. Botterell and colleagues divided their patients into five categories: 'moribund or near moribund, with failing vital centres and extensor rigidity' (grade 5); 'major neurological deficit and deteriorating or older patients with less severe neurological deficit but pre-existing degenerative cerebrovascular disease' (grade 4); 'a drowsy patient with a neurological deficit' (grade 3); 'a drowsy patient without significant neurological deficit' (grade 2); and 'a conscious patient with or without signs of blood in the subarachnoid space' (grade 1).[119] In the 1970s, the so-called Hunt and Hess classification came into use, which also attempted to quantify the inflammatory response of the meninges, as follows: 'asymptomatic, or minimal headache and nuchal rigidity' (grade 1); 'moderate to severe headache, nuchal rigidity, no neurological deficit other than cranial nerve palsy' (grade 2); 'drowsiness, confusion, or mild focal deficit' (grade 3); ' stupor, moderate to severe hemiparesis, possibly early decerebrate rigidity and vegetative disturbances' (grade 4); and 'deep coma, decerebrate rigidity, moribund appearance' (grade 5).[120]

Clearly, all these terms leave much room for variation among different observers. Some words were semi-quantitative ('mild, moderate, severe'); other denominations served to capture degrees of unconsciousness ('drowsiness, stupor, coma'), a predicament with which physicians had been grappling for ages, or they suggested impending death (moribund, decerebrate rigidity). It was in 1974 that the neurosurgeons Graham Teasdale (1940–) and Bryan Jennett (1926–2008) in Glasgow devised a new method for assessing the level of consciousness in all forms of brain disease, from trauma to tumour. Their method no longer referred to abstractions in the doctor's mind, but merely recorded three aspects of the patient's responses to stimuli: eye opening, arm movement, and speech.[121] After all, it was on such responses that the old terms were implicitly based. Importantly, the total score (3–14) only indicates a certain rank order, not a true mathematical value that can be averaged, added up, etc.

[117] McKissock, *et al.* (1960b), Results of treatment of intracranial aneurysms; Graf (1971), Patients with nonsurgically-treated aneurysms.
[118] McKissock, *et al.* (1960b), Results of treatment of intracranial aneurysms.
[119] Botterell, *et al.* (1956), Hypothermia in the surgical management of intracranial aneurysms, 34.
[120] Hunt and Hess (1968), Surgical risk in the repair of intracranial aneurysms.
[121] Teasdale and Jennett (1974), Assessment of coma.

Despite the great advance in recording the level of consciousness, the 'Glasgow Coma Score' could not solve all problems. Other important prognostic factors remained: time after rupture, age, neurological deficits, blood pressure, and concomitant disease.[122]

All in all, in the mid-1970s, the management of patients with ruptured aneurysms remained a tough subject for therapeutic studies. It depended on some evidence and on much optimism. Prompt diagnosis was a first condition. Some reports suggested that survivors of aneurysmal haemorrhage often mentioned previous headache episodes;[123] this led to the notion of 'warning leaks', but it remained uncertain whether such preliminary symptoms could be distinguished from common, non-specific forms of headache.

[122] McKissock, *et al.* (1960b), Results of treatment of intracranial aneurysms.
[123] Waga, *et al.* (1975), Warning signs in intracranial aneurysms.

TWELVE

CEREBRAL VENOUS THROMBOSIS

SUMMARY

Brain disease caused by purulent clots obstructing venous sinuses in children was the first and, for a long time, the only recorded variant of cerebral venous thrombosis. These early cases were secondary to septic inflammation, either elsewhere in the body (de Haen, 1759) or in the mastoid region (Abercrombie, 1818). In 1829, Tonnellé recorded more clinical and morphological details in a large series of children with cerebral phlebitis. Soon afterwards, Bright and Cruveilhier confirmed and illustrated the attendant changes in brain tissue.

Thrombosis of cerebral veins could also occur without local inflammation; in children by obstruction of venous outflow in the neck or chest (Tonnellé), and in adults mostly through states of dehydration or emaciation (Gowers). The diagnosis during life was difficult because the symptoms were non-specific, except with isolated thrombosis of veins in the Rolandic area. Angiography facilitated the diagnosis, but treatment remained controversial. With time, causal associations with other factors became apparent: puerperium, haematological disorders, head trauma, and contraceptive agents. A transient syndrome of headache and papilloedema, often accompanied by neurological deficits ('pseudotumor cerebri'; Nonne, 1904), was later attributed to partial thrombosis of venous sinuses, at least in some patients (Symonds: 'otitic hydrocephalus'). Eventually, a group of patients remained in whom elevated pressure of the cerebrospinal fluid was, by definition, unrelated to thrombosis ('idiopathic intracranial hypertension').

Some may wonder why, among the many categories of cerebrovascular disease distinguished in recent decades, only cerebral venous thrombosis has been singled out for a discussion of its history. The answer is simple: thrombotic obstruction of cerebral veins, of sinuses in particular, has been known for a long time – but inflammatory in origin. For example, this is what Gregor Nymmann (1592–1638) saw in 1629 in the region of the *torcular Herophili*: 'thick, sanguineous fluid, often also mixed with viscous phlegm, solidified and quite compact, very suitable for obstructing it'.[1] Nymmann, not yet familiar with the circulation of blood, regarded the *torcular* as the hub of the brain vessels, where obstruction caused apoplexy. Indeed, inflammatory obstruction of venous sinuses may well have accounted for a proportion of strokes in the seventeenth century. A more precise description appeared in the next century.

INFLAMMATORY OBSTRUCTION OF VENOUS SINUSES

A Young Girl with Apoplexy and Convulsions

In the middle of the eighteenth century, the Bürgerspital in Vienna was on its way to becoming an important teaching centre. The empress Maria Theresia (1717–1780) had invoked the help of Gerard van Swieten (1700–1772) for the modernization of health care in her realm. Van Swieten, in turn, appointed Anton de Haen (1704–1776) (Box 12.1) as the chief physician at the hospital. Both had been taught by Boerhaave in Leiden; both were also Roman Catholics, always an impediment to careers in the northern part of the Low Countries. In 1759, de Haen included the following story in the chapter on apoplexy in his *Ratio Medendi*, published annually:

> On July 6, 1759, I performed dissection on a little girl who had suffered from continuous headache. *Continuous*, I say, for from the time she could speak she perpetually complained about it. The principal site of it, she indicated, was mostly behind the right eye. Otherwise, she was cheerful, lively, always busy running, jumping and playing; she never suffered from cough, breathlessness or fatigue, according to the observations of her worthy parent, a Viennese physician. She died when she was six-and-a-half years of age. Eight days before her death she was sometimes found a bit dull and forgetful, yet otherwise quite healthy. Four days before her death she was seized by apoplexy and convulsions of the right arm. The convulsions ceased during the last two days of her life, but finally apoplexy put a peaceful end to her life, without notable fever.
> The dura mater was intact, the pia showed extreme varicosity over the entire surface of both hemispheres. In the longitudinal sinus, from its very

[1] Nymmanus (1629), *Tractatus de Apoplexia*, 103.

> ### Box 12.1 Anton de Haen (1704–1776).
>
> de Haen was born in The Hague, as the seventh child of the family; his father was said to be in the fishing trade. The family belonged to the Jansenist section of the Roman Catholic Church, with an ascetic lifestyle and pessimist ethics. The movement separated from the Catholic Church in 1723 and eventually evolved into the Old-Catholic Church; Anton stayed true to this faith all his life. After secondary education at the Jansenist seminary in Amersfoort, he studied humaniora and medicine in Louvain and graduated in 1735 in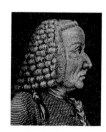
> Leiden, where he greatly enjoyed Boerhaave's clinical teaching. For the next 19 years, he was a private practitioner in The Hague. Around 1740, he married Magtildis Lauerenburg; they remained childless. De Haen published three medical treatises; one of these was about *colica Pictonum* ('colic of Poitou'), known in Britain as 'Devonshire colic', later attributed to chronic lead poisoning, mostly through additives of wine.
>
> In 1754, de Haen and his family left The Hague for Vienna, probably instigated by van Swieten. As Director of the Bürgerspital, he transformed it to a teaching hospital, very much like Boerhaave's 'St Caecilia Gasthuis' in Leiden. In addition, he was appointed Professor of Practical Medicine at the University of Vienna; van Swieten, supported by Empress Maria Theresia, had reorganized its medical faculty and reduced the influence of the Jesuit order. From 1756 onwards, de Haen published an annual volume, entitled *Method of Treatment (Ratio Medendi)*. Included subjects were specific disease conditions, results of dissections, animal experiments, and technical innovations such as electrotherapy and thermometry. Gradually he fell out with van Swieten, probably because de Haen felt constrained with respect to teaching and publishing. He did not easily change his mind and always remained a staunch opponent of 'variolation'. In 1776, he became incapacitated by 'dropsy' and died in that same year.

beginning to where it connects with the lateral sinuses, a white structure was present, like a white worm. [...] It continued into the lateral sinuses.[2]

De Haen also found abnormalities in the girl's chest. There were adhesions (*concretiones*) between the lungs and the pleura, diaphragm, and pericardium, as well as between the lobes themselves. These were not easy to disconnect, such as with 'serous' or 'cellular' adhesions, but tough and sticky; they had to be carefully released with a knife.

De Haen regarded the white, worm-like longitudinal structure as a 'pure polyp' (*merus polypus*). He apparently used this term in the sense of *coagulum*, since its nature manifested itself most clearly, he wrote, where it branched into the lateral sinuses; there, the white colour was tinged with the redness of

---

[2] de Haen (1759), *Ratio Medendi*, 172–4.

blood, with protruding 'sanguineous fibres'. His opinion was confirmed when he had ordered to preserve the white structure in water instead of in alcohol: after four days, it had almost completely dissolved. Referring to 'polyps' found elsewhere in the body of other patients, de Haen implicated either pressure or stagnation as its cause. He seemed to regard the polyp and the pulmonary disease as unrelated conditions; his comment on the absence of fever suggests he was not thinking of an inflammatory disorder.[3]

Similar case reports did not appear until half a century later, when the practice of post-mortem investigation had become more widespread – not only in Paris, but also in Edinburgh.

Purulent, Cheesy Matter

John Abercrombie (1780–1844), an important figure in the history of brain softening (see Box 6.3, p. 201), was interested in diverse diseases of the brain. In 1818–19, he wrote a series of articles on the subject; the first of these was on 'Chronic inflammation of the brain and its membranes'. His 'case 17' is relevant here:

> August 3, 1816. Miss S. aged 16, complained of severe headach, which extended over the whole head; had an oppressed look, and great heaviness of the eyes; pulse 120; tongue clean and moist; face rather pale. She had been liable to suppuration of the ears; and the left ear had been discharging matter for three weeks; had complained of headach for a fortnight; confined to bed for two days. [*treatments, daily notes on changes*]
> 5th – some vomiting, severe attacks of shivering; [...] 7th – a dull, vacant look; [...] 10th, 11th – strength failing, a tendency to stupor, and occasional delirium; 12th – more comatose, but sensible when roused; knew those about her a few minutes before her death.
> *Dissection.* The pia mater was highly vascular, as if minutely injected. [...] The veins were very turgid, and at one place, on the posterior part, there was a slight appearance of extravasated blood under the pia mater. [...] The left lateral sinus was remarkably diseased through its whole extent. When compressed it discharged purulent matter, and some thick cheesy matter; it contained no blood; its coats were much thickened, and its inner surface was dark coloured, irregular and fungous. At one place the cavity was nearly obliterated. The disease extended into the Torcular Herophili, and affected a little the termination of the longitudinal sinus. [...] The auditory portion of the bone was extremely carious; the cells of it were everywhere full of purulent matter, and communicated freely with the cavity of the ear.[4]

[3] de Haen (1759), *Ratio Medendi*, 175–8.
[4] Abercrombie (1818b), Chronic inflammation of the brain, 288–9.

In this first quarter of the nineteenth century, knowledge about microbes was still decades away. Inflammation was often regarded as a more or less unitary condition, characterized by redness, fever, pain, and swelling (*rubor, calor, dolor, tumor*). Pus occurred as a regular accompaniment, but opinions diverged on the question of whether purulent matter was a cause or an effect of inflammation.

Phlebitis

'One has hardly paid attention to diseases of veins'[5] was one of the opening sentences of François Ribes (1765–1845), an esteemed military surgeon during Napoleon's reign,[6] in an article on 'phlebitis' dating from 1825. His publication has been cited as the first report of cerebral venous thrombosis, but, as the preceding paragraphs attest, with little justification. Of the seven brief case histories Ribes presented, all adults, six patients had inflammatory disease of a vein in the arm or leg. The last patient, a 45-year-old man 'of great distinction', had a history of headache, melancholia, epilepsy, 'mental derangement', and delirium, extending over several years before he died after a recurrence of melancholia and epilepsy. The longitudinal sinus was filled by a firmly organized clot in its frontal third, while the rest of the sinus contained a mixture of clots, fluid blood, and membranous fragments; the walls of the sinus were thickened, red, and covered by an inflammatory membrane.[7]

Children with Pus in the Sinus or Elsewhere

The young nineteenth century saw many more examples of what de Haen had witnessed: sick children with inflammatory changes in the cerebral sinuses, as well as in other organs. A physician with extensive experience in this field was the young Louis Tonnellé (1803–1860) (Box 12.2),[8] who acquired it during his internship in the Parisian *Hôpital des Enfants*.

Tonnellé's essay, submitted in 1829 as part of his application for membership of the *Société royale de médecine*, dealt specifically with affections of the venous sinuses in the brain. It is remarkable for several other reasons. To begin with, apart from inflammatory forms of venous sinus thrombosis, the most common kind, he distinguished a non-purulent category, in which coagulation within venous sinuses was unrelated to inflammation – more about this below.

Furthermore, Tonnellé divided inflammatory lesions of the sinuses into two categories. In the first, the inflammatory process started in or near the wall of the sinus, such as in Abercrombie's 'Miss S', who had purulent ear disease.

---

[5] Ribes (1825), Recherches sur la phlébite, 5.
[6] Vesselle and Vesselle (2014), François Ribes.
[7] Ribes (1825), Recherches sur la phlébite, 35–7.   [8] Herpin (1860), Louis Tonnellé.

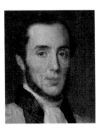

Box 12.2 Louis Tonnellé (1803–1860).

Tonnellé's life is intimately connected with the city of Tours. After his medical studies and internships in Paris, he returned to the town where he was born in 1803, on 6 Fructidor (24 August). His father Louis-Henry-Jérôme was a local physician and surgeon. After qualifying as a surgeon in 1826, Louis was appointed assistant physician at the general hospital in Tours. Five years later, having become chief surgeon, he and his colleague Pierre-Fidèle Bretonneau (1778–1862) spent much energy on establishing a School of Medicine and Pharmacy in Tours, which Tonnellé directed from 1841 to 1855.

In the course of his career, Tonnellé took an active part in caring for the indigent population of Tours, via his membership of the municipal council; in the hospital, he established a service for free medical consultation. He was highly regarded for his bedside teaching and published on surgical procedures and puerperal fever. In the cholera epidemic of 1849, he overexerted himself, to the detriment of his own health. After an attack of 'paralysis' in 1855, he retreated to the fresh air of nearby Saint-Cyr-sur-Loire. In 1858, his son Alfred, a brilliant medical student, fell victim to typhus at the age of 21. After Louis himself had died two years later, his wife Pauline, who died in 1862, bequeathed the family's possessions to the city of Tours, in honour of her husband and son. This led to the foundation of an artisanal school, two homes for convalescent patients from the general hospital, and a primary school for girls, all situated in Saint-Cyr-sur-Loire.

Source: Portrait courtesy of *Université de Tours.*

Examples were a two-year-old girl with a purulent lesion on the scalp as the first sign of disease (Tonnellé's case 8), a girl of the same age with a purulent ulcer in the occipital region (case 9),[9] and a boy of 10 years with an impression fracture inflicted by the leg of a horse (addendum).[10] In most other children with fatal inflammatory sinus thrombosis in Tonnellé's series, autopsy showed inflammatory foci in other organs. Sometimes these were in the lungs (cases 6, 7, and 14), as in de Haen's 'little girl', with other children in the bowels (cases 10, 13, and 15) or in the leg (case 11); sometimes the source of inflammation remained unclear.

Tonnellé trod carefully in explaining the relationship between purulent lesions in internal organs and lethal inflammatory sinus thrombosis. He first considered the possibility that purulent inflammation might arise locally in blood, despite the recent trend towards 'solidism' in medicine. Nevertheless, he came down on the side of passive transport of pus, which eventually became stuck in the sinus.[11] He regarded pseudo-membranes, with or without pus, as a product of

[9] Tonnellé (1829), *Maladies des sinus veineux*, 39–48.
[10] Tonnellé (1829), *Maladies des sinus veineux*, 79.
[11] Tonnellé (1829), *Maladies des sinus veineux*, 63–6.

the vessel wall, and not of the clot;[12] Jean Cruveilhier (1791–1874), who was chairman of the committee examining the essay, contested this interpretation,[13] yet Tonnellé was admitted as a member of the *Société*.

Illustrations

Richard Bright (1789–1858), cited before because of his coloured illustrations of haemorrhage and softening in the brain, deserves to be mentioned again. He contributed a single case history, but with great detail and again an illustration. In 1828, he found inflammatory occlusion of the longitudinal sinus on dissection of a boy aged 20 months.

> On the 23rd of April 1828, having for some days had slight cough, but having been during the whole day in apparently higher spirits than usual, he fell asleep in his mother's arms, and awoke suddenly, screaming dreadfully, appearing to suffer great pain in his head. [...] I was called to the child by Mr. Mountford, who was in attendance, in the afternoon of May the 9th; [...] The child was very pallid and fretful; pulse 120; he was constantly throwing his head about, but never attempted to raise it from the pillow. There was no strabismus, and the pupils reacted to light; no convulsions; the head felt hot. [*new treatments, daily notes*]
>
> 11th. Suffered very severe convulsions in the night. [...] 12th. Much torpor, with occasional convulsions. [...] 13th. Greatly convulsed in the night. Constant convulsions during the time of our visit. [...] 14th. Night less disturbed by convulsions; does not seem conscious; and the right arm almost motionless and powerless, except that the fingers are convulsively clasped to and fro. [...] The feet are stiffly extended and turned inwards. [...] 15th. Passed a tranquil night, inclined to sleep, yet undoubtedly conscious of things around him. [...] 16th. The left arm and hand almost constantly convulsed; face not convulsed; he is perfectly conscious. [...] 17th. Is apparently approaching to a state of coma; [*evening*] Has lain nearly senseless nearly all the day, but swallowed his medicine very well two hours ago. [...] The child died about 11 o'clock; that is, two hours after the visit.[14]

Figure 12.1 shows the abnormalities in the brain, especially the 'yellow coagulum' filling the cortical veins and the haemorrhagic changes in the underlying cortex. Since Bright found the lateral ventricles distended, he included this case in a chapter on 'hydrocephalus'; the ventricular walls had a normal aspect. The findings in the rest of the body are more relevant:

---

[12] Tonnellé (1829), *Maladies des sinus veineux*, 69.
[13] Tonnellé (1829), *Maladies des sinus veineux*, 3–11.
[14] Bright (1827–31), *Reports of Medical Cases*, vol. II, part 1, 57–9.

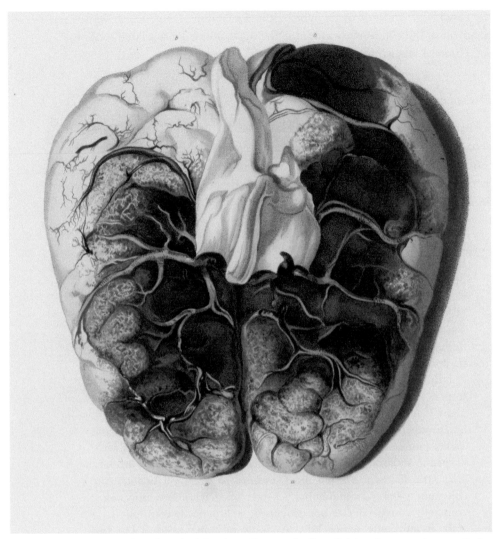

12.1 Venous sinus thrombosis in a boy of 20 months (from Bright, 1829–31, vol. 2, part I, plate v; coloured aquatint, drawn by Frederick Richard Say, engraved by William Say). The frontal lobes are at the bottom of the picture. The longitudinal sinus has been folded back and is uncoloured. The following text is from Bright. 'All the larger veins on the surface of both hemispheres running into the longitudinal sinus were seen round and hard, quite filled with yellow-coloured coagulum as if injected with wax, while the whole vertex was covered under the membranes with dark extravasated blood. [. . .] On carefully opening the longitudinal sinus the whole was full of a coagulum taking the exact form of the sinus [. . .].'

The lung on the right side was rather too firm, though still crepitant, and the lower edges were somewhat emphysematous. The left lung presented throughout every part a most complete specimen of pneumonic hepatization, of a pinkish or gray red colour: it was harder than liver, altogether impervious to air, and cut firm with a slightly granulated texture. The large bifurcation of the trachea, when the lung was squeezed, filled with puriform fluid. The pleura adhered firmly in the lower part to the ribs, and was, when torn away, found to be covered with a rough and completely scabrous false membrane.[15]

Bright, pondering on the relationship between the lesion in the brain and that in the chest, supposed that the lung disease had caused cerebral congestion:

> The evidence, as derived from dissection, of true inflammatory action in the arachnoid and pia mater is very small; indeed I doubt whether inflammation existed in that part, but am rather induced to ascribe the cerebral mischief to congestion, probably favoured by the entire obliteration of the lung on one side, in connection with an habitual peculiarity of the organization of the venous system of the brain.[16]

Bright did not comment on the 'yellow-coloured coagulum as if injected with wax' he found in the cortical veins running towards the superior longitudinal sinus (Figure 12.1), whereas Tonnellé had regarded these segments as purulent. Bright ended the story as follows: 'This case seems to throw some light on the congestive nature of some cases of softening of the brain.' Elsewhere he had intimated in cases of 'pale softening' that it 'produced in my mind an impression that the proper supply of blood had been cut off by some change in the vessels of the pia mater, or some obstruction in their passage through the cineritious substance'.[17] In other words, Bright distinguished two causes of brain softening: congestion and failure of the blood supply. In both cases, softened tissue could be infiltrated by blood.

Jean Cruveilhier, however, gave a different twist to the leaking capillaries: he did not regard them as the result of brain softening, but as its cause.

'Capillary Apoplexy'

Cruveilhier's important contributions to pathological anatomy have been mentioned before: he presented his case histories and interpretations with coloured lithographic illustrations, produced by artists such as Antoine Chazal (1793–1854). Subscribers received instalments in folio format (*livraisons*), with subjects more or less in the order they had occurred. Over the course of some 12 years (1829–42), 40 parts appeared. In the eighth *livraison*, so presumably around 1831, Cruveilhier included, under the title *Inflammation of the dural Sinus*, the case of a four-year-old girl, admitted because of drowsiness and groaning, diagnosed as pneumonia and ascariasis; she died five days after admission. Dissection of the brain showed purulent thrombosis of the superior

[15] Bright (1827–31), *Reports of Medical Cases*, vol. II, part 1, 61.
[16] Bright (1827–31), *Reports of Medical Cases*, vol. II, part 1, 62.
[17] Bright (1827–31), *Reports of Medical Cases*, vol. II, part 1, 192.

longitudinal vein and also of the superficial veins running towards it.[18] The accompanying illustration closely resembled Bright's figure (Figure 12.1).

In two later instalments, numbers 20 and 36, Cruveilhier presented four more patients with thrombosis of the superior longitudinal sinus and its tributary veins, in one case without clinical details; all four had inflammatory disease of internal organs.[19] Curiously enough, he now arranged them under the heading 'Capillary Apoplexy', a notion he had developed in the meantime, as explained in Chapter 6. He regarded it as a distinct form of apoplexy, more related to 'common apoplexy' (primary intracerebral haemorrhage) than to 'white softening'. For him, the haemorrhagic changes in brain tissue were the key phenomenon (Figure 12.2). Inflammatory obstruction of cerebral sinuses was always accompanied, he wrote, by intracerebral haemorrhage, as punctate ('capillary') haemorrhages or in solid form (*en foyer*).

1830s to 1930s: Increased Recognition, Few Cures

A century after Bright and Cruveilhier, when 'red softening' was generally explained as secondary infiltration of blood leaking from damaged capillaries into necrotic brain tissue, and when also, and more importantly, bacterial infection was recognized and even classified, the dramatic course of the disease was still unchanged. Expansion of health care institutions and the creation of medical specialties led to publication of large series of children with cerebral venous thrombosis. In 1937, a physician in Birmingham listed 32 fatal cases from his own experience and from hospital records, all but three associated with infectious disease of the skull or internal organs.[20] A series reported from Boston, in the same year, contained 80 such instances in children, almost invariably under three years of age. More than half of them had septic conditions: otitis media, mastoiditis, cellulitis of the scalp, or bacteraemia without meningeal localization.[21] Most other children in this group were in a state of 'severe nutritional disturbance'.

In isolated thrombosis of a lateral sinus, mostly as a complication of mastoiditis, the outcome could be favourable, sometimes after operation,[22] sometimes without. Recovery was regarded impossible if the superior longitudinal

---

[18] Cruveilhier (1829–42), *Anatomie pathologique*, vol. I, livraison VIII–2, 4.
[19] Cruveilhier (1829–42), vol. I, livraison XX–3, 4–5; Cruveilhier (1829–42), vol. II, livraison XXXVI–I, 1–6.
[20] Ebbs (1937), Cerebral sinus thrombosis in children.
[21] Bailey and Hass (1937), Dural sinus thrombosis in early life: recovery from the acute thrombosis of the superior longitudinal sinus and its relation to certain acquired cerebral lesions in childhood.
[22] Macewen (1904), Sinus thrombosis and recovery; Turner (1908), Operation for sigmoid sinus thrombosis.

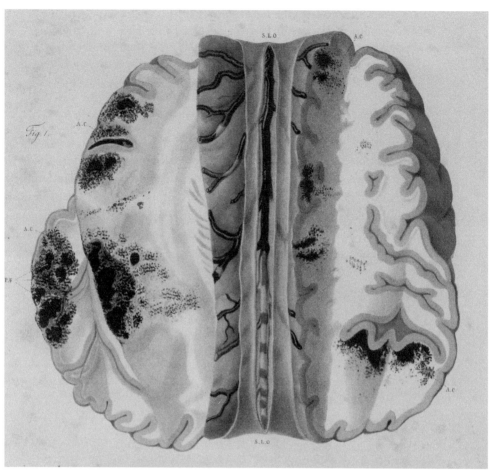

12.2 'Capillary apoplexy', associated with inflammatory thrombosis of the superior longitudinal sinus (from Cruveilhier 1829–42, livraison XXXVI–1, plate I). The corresponding part of the text is: 'The brain represented here belongs to a young girl of 22. [. . .] The corresponding clinical details have not been communicated. The numerous veins ending in the superior longitudinal sinus and this sinus itself are filled with very dense coagulated blood, partly black, partly without colour, everywhere tightly connected to the walls of the vessels. In the longitudinal sinus, the inflammation seems to have progressed from the back to the front, for the posterior half of the clot is pale, yellowish, and contains pus throughout its width. The convexity of the two hemispheres shows at its surface haemorrhagic stains, formed by blood that has infiltrated the grey matter, which has almost completely disappeared at these sites [. . .].'

sinus was involved. The same fatal outcome seemed attached to thrombosis of the internal cerebral veins in children with infection, emaciation, or both.[23] However, in 1933, the paediatrician Randolph K. Byers (1896–1988) and the pathologist George M. Hass (1907–2000), from Boston, dared to challenge this sombre outlook:

[23] Ehlers and Courville (1936), Thrombosis of internal cerebral veins in infancy.

There was every reason to believe that many patients with primary sinus thrombosis must survive. [...] These predictions have been advanced possibly without adequate proof. Nevertheless, if sinus thrombosis as a puzzling and often unsuspected complication of disease is constantly kept in mind, the etiology of certain instances of 'encephalitis', spontaneous subarachnoid hemorrhage, cerebral palsy, cortical atrophy, mental defectiveness, epilepsy and hydrocephalus may then become apparent.[24]

Subsequently, Hass, now writing with Orville T. Bailey (1909–1998) as first author, supported these views in a separate publication on three children. Though all three had eventually died, this occurred in a second phase of their illness. In each of the patients, the brain lesions caused by the sinus thrombosis had contributed to the fatal outcome, but a phase of stability, or even improvement, had preceded it, while at autopsy, the sinus had shown definite evidence of reorganization. Therefore, Bailey and Hass suggested that such a disorder might explain residual brain lesions in children:

We believe that the patients here reported give support to our contention that certain acquired cerebral defects are due to thrombosis of the superior longitudinal sinus and its sequelae. The possible relation of cerebral lesions secondary to sinus thrombosis and non-traumatic scars of the cerebrum associated with Jacksonian epilepsy is emphasized.

Thus far about 'septic' forms of cerebral sinus thrombosis, as they came to be called.

'PRIMARY' CEREBRAL VENOUS THROMBOSIS

Among the many purulent forms of dural sinus thrombosis Louis Tonnellé had observed during his internship at the Parisian children's hospital before returning to Tours, he recognized a few cases where the coagulation process was not induced by inflammation, at least not locally, but by changes within the vascular system elsewhere. In most of these patients, the blood flow was slowed down or even obstructed.[25]

Obstruction or Slow Flow

Tonnellé's first case of this kind was a girl of nine years, known to suffer from 'softening' of the first few cervical vertebrae, presumably by a tuberculous process. She started to stumble and faint, then became comatose, with convulsions on the left side, and soon died. The superior longitudinal sinus showed

[24] Byers and Hass (1933), Thrombosis of the venous sinuses.
[25] Tonnellé (1829), *Maladies des sinus veineux*, 15–30.

brown, clotted blood, as did most superficial veins, the right lateral sinus, and also the right jugular vein, which was completely enveloped by a tuberculous abscess. The left lateral sinus and the left jugular vein were still patent, but of much smaller calibre. Thus, the inflammatory lesion had caused thrombosis by obstructing the venous outflow in the neck, not by infecting the sinus. In the second patient, a two-year-old boy, the venous outflow of the brain was again obstructed by a massive tuberculous lesion in the vertebral column, but at the level of the superior vena cava. All sinuses, superficial veins, and jugular veins contained clotted blood; the surface of the brain was softened, with extensive extravasation.

A third patient, a child of two-and-a-half years of age, suffered from severe rickets, with disfigured limbs and a chest volume reduced by more than half. The boy had been admitted with severe dyspnoea; the heart action seemed weak. He died six weeks later, in a state of coma. The finding, on dissection, of solid clots in a tense superior longitudinal sinus and its tributary veins was a surprise; Tonnellé suggested weak action of the heart, especially a markedly dilated right ventricle, as the most probable explanation.

A last patient with non-septic sinus thrombosis in his series was a 14-year-old boy suspected of some disorder of the blood. He was hospitalized three weeks before his death because of jaundice and 'intermittent fever no longer responding to quinine sulphate'; dissection showed not only a coagulum in the longitudinal sinus, but also extreme splenomegaly and hepatomegaly.

Elusive Symptoms

In the case histories cited so far, the diagnosis was invariably a surprise. It could hardly be otherwise. As Tonnellé remarked, the symptoms largely reflected general features of brain disease: headache, disturbances of consciousness, convulsions, sometimes paralysis.[26] Even these symptoms could be obscured by those of an underlying illness, for example fever, abscesses, or general emaciation. At the other extreme, some early symptoms could be misinterpreted. Samuel Wilks (1824–1911), a physician at Guy's Hospital in the middle of the nineteenth century, recounted a striking example in a collection of his lectures published in 1878.

> A lady, below middle age, had been for some time a little out of health, when she was seized with headache, a complaint to which she was not used. When it had existed a week I saw her. The pain was all over the head, and especially at the back; it was constant, but with paroxysms of

[26] Tonnellé (1829), *Maladies des sinus veineux*, 76–8.

greater severity. She was anemic, had a weak pulse, temperature normal, no fever, no rigors, and, in fact, no feverish or other symptoms beside the headache. On the following day she was exactly the same but in addition had occasional sickness. On the next day she thought she had a little weakness in right arm and leg, but this passed off. During the next two days the headache continued, but there was no fever, and the pupils were rather contracted. Her intelligence remained intact. During this time she was seen by several of the most distinguished physicians in London, who, individually and separately, expressed their opinion that she was not suffering from any organic affection of the brain, as there was not a single symptom to indicate it, nor any acute inflammatory affection; in fact, that she was the subject of a functional disturbance only. On the day after this she became very sick, and towards evening sank into a half-conscious state. On the following day her limbs became rigid and limbs flexed, then convulsive twitchings came on, and she died. She had thus been ailing for about twelve days.

Post-mortem examination. The surface of the brain was turgid with blood; the vessels of the pia mater were everywhere tightly filled with coagulum, and felt like so many worms under the fingers. On opening the longitudinal sinus this was found to be completely closed by fibrin, which was adherent to the walls, and in some places softening in the centre; the lateral sinuses in the same manner were filled with fibrin; this was traced as far as the jugular veins, and there ceased.[27]

'A case like this is in the highest degree obscure, both as to its pathology and diagnosis,' Wilks commented. Given the poor specificity of the clinical features, early twentieth-century textbooks of the nervous system rarely mentioned the disease. One also looks in vain in the collections of clinical lectures published by Charcot, Brissaud, and Raymond; moreover, these demonstrations were largely based on outpatients.

It was otherwise in the textbook by William Gowers (1845–1915) (Box 12.3),[28] one of the outstanding neurologists at the 'National Hospital for the Relief and Cure of the Paralysed and Epileptic', opened at Queen Square, London, in 1860; his textbook was arranged according to anatomical structures, instead of according to symptoms. Gowers devoted several pages to sinus thrombosis, at least in the second edition of 1893. The superior longitudinal sinus was most commonly affected:

> External oedema and distension of veins may be present on the sides of the head and forehead. There may be epistaxis from the veins of the nose, which communicate with the anterior extremity of the sinus. In young

---

[27] Wilks (1878), *Diseases of the Nervous System*, 146–8.
[28] Shorvon and Compston (2019), *Queen Square*, 145–55; Scott, *et al.* (2012), *William Richard Gowers*.

Box 12.3 William Gowers (1845–1915).

William (Richard) Gowers was the only surviving child of William
Gowers, a shoemaker in Hackney, East London, and Ann Venables.
After his father's early death in 1852, his mother took him to live with
her brother, a gunmaker in Headington, Oxford; soon she left herself,
having to care for her ailing mother. Young William obtained a
scholarship to attend Christ Church College School in Oxford. On
a visit to Essex, he met the family physician Thomas Simpson in
Coggeshall, who offered him the position of apprentice. Since this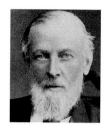
system of medical education was being phased out, Gowers also had to prepare for a
matriculation test in London. The local surgeon Harold Giles helped him to gain some
practical experience. Gowers then became a medical student at University College
Hospital, mentored by William Jenner (1815–1898), Professor of Medicine.

After graduation in 1870, he successfully applied for the position of registrar at the
National Hospital, Queen Square, established 10 years before. His industry and efficiency –
he was an astute record keeper and he zealously practised writing in shorthand – soon made
him assistant physician. Gowers' teaching in the room for outpatients attracted students
from University College. His methods of examination were detailed, but not obsessional;
also, he was an expert ophthalmoscopist. In 1875, he married Mary Baines, the daughter of a
Yorkshire businessman; they were to have two daughters and two sons. The couple lived at
50, Queen Anne Street, where William also had his consulting rooms.

Having become a consultant to the hospital in 1883, with the right to admit his own
patients, Gowers continued to collect and organize his personal observations. He published
extensively; he is most famous for his two-volume *Manual of Diseases of the Nervous System*,
first published in 1886. A skilled draughtsman, he provided his own illustrations. Gowers
was knighted in 1897, on the occasion of Queen Victoria's diamond jubilee. After
retirement in 1910, he was soon troubled by ill health. In 1914, both he and his wife
developed pneumonia and died within a few months.

Source: Portrait courtesy of Wellcome collection.

children, the fontanelle may be prominent, in striking contrast to its
previous depression if there had been collapse from diarrhoea.

Cerebral symptoms are chiefly general – apathy, somnolence, and
coma; vomiting and convulsions, usually general, but sometimes local;
rigidity of the neck, and sometimes of the muscles of the back. In adults,
convulsions are less common than delirium, quiet or active. There is
usually headache. [...] Unilateral symptoms are usually due to the
extension of the thrombus into veins over one hemisphere, and then
there may be unilateral convulsions, often beginning locally, and loss of
power on one side.[29]

---

[29] Gowers (1893), *A Manual of Diseases of the Nervous System*, vol. II, 453.

Gowers did not mention 'disc congestion' in this context. Yet, being an expert ophthalmoscopist, he wrote elsewhere that such swelling could be seen in softening as a result of arterial disease.[30]

NEW CAUSES OF 'PRIMARY' VENOUS SINUS THROMBOSIS

The complete stagnation of venous outflow of the brain that had caused thrombosis in Tonnellé's first two children without suppurative disease was quite rare. Much more common were situations of general weakness and wasting, such as in the child with rickets. Gowers wrote about the role of these 'poor states of the blood and circulation':

> *Primary thrombosis* usually occurs in association with general malnutrition and prostration, and hence is often termed 'marantic thrombosis'. It occurs at all ages, but most frequently in children, and next in frequency in the very old. In children, it is met with up to fourteen years of age, but the chief liability is during the first six months of life, and the chief cause is severe and exhausting diarrhoea. It may, however, follow any prostrating malady, lung disease, long-continued suppuration, or acute specific diseases. In adults, it occurs occasionally during the last stage of phthisis, sometimes from acute diseases, in the puerperal state, as a result of gout, or in the course of cancer.[31]

The Puerperium, Cortical Veins, and Possible Survival

Gowers's perceptive though casual mention of childbirth had not escaped the authors of a paper on cerebral venous thrombosis in the puerperal phase that appeared in the early 1940s. J. Purdon Martin (1893–1984), consultant neurologist at the National Hospital, Queen Square, and Harold L. Sheehan (1900–1988), pathologist in Glasgow and specialist in disorders of pregnancy, presented five case histories.[32] In the preceding century, when purulent infections in general were rampant in the puerperal period,[33] a few single case reports had drawn attention to non-septic cerebral venous thrombosis after childbirth.[34] Three of Martin and Sheehan's cases came to necropsy; two had died a few weeks after confinement, and the third three years later, from an

---

[30] Gowers (1882), *Manual and Atlas of Medical Ophthalmoscopy*, 131–3.
[31] Gowers (1893), *A Manual of Diseases of the Nervous System*, vol. II, 450.
[32] Martin and Sheehan (1941), Primary thrombosis of cerebral veins (following childbirth).
[33] Ribes (1825), Recherches sur la phlébite; Kluyskens (1876), Maladies inflammatoires pendant les couches.
[34] Témoin (1860), *La Maternité de Paris, 1859*; Béhier (1874), Coagulations veineuses, suite de couches; Scougal (1888), Hemiplegia nine days after parturition; Collier (1891), Thrombosis of cerebral veins.

unrelated disease. Of the two surviving patients, the diagnosis was confirmed on exploratory operation in one; in the other example, the diagnosis was presumed because of similarity of symptoms and circumstances with those in the 'verified cases'. The authors hoped to alert the medical readership to consider this diagnosis in cases one might otherwise perhaps regard as 'late eclampsia' or 'cerebral embolism'.

A further important aspect in this publication was that thrombosis could be limited to superficial veins running towards the longitudinal sinus, without involvement of the sinus itself; this was how the diagnosis was made in the patient who underwent an exploratory operation. Before that time, isolated thrombosis of cerebral veins had been reported in three isolated case reports; all three had involved men and the diagnosis had been established by means of an exploratory operation showing an affected vein in the Rolandic area.[35]

The repeated association of cerebral venous thrombosis with the puerperal period, Martin and Sheehan pondered, could not be explained by infection or by complications of the delivery, which had been uneventful in all cases. Another essential element of Martin and Sheehan's paper is that they made the diagnosis in two young women who survived. Apart from one surviving young mother, they included a history not associated with parturition, of an 18-year-old girl recovering from typhoid fever; one morning she had seven epileptic fits, with residual stupor. For about a week, she could see and feel touch, but was unable to read and recognize objects with her left hand; eventually she was restored to full health. The authors also tried to understand why recovery after occlusion of veins is often better than in arterial thrombosis or haemorrhage, an observation that was to be confirmed again and again:

> The first is that the lesion is on the surface of the brain, where a larger lesion is required to produce the same degree of paralysis than if the lesion is, say, in the internal capsule. Secondly, in cases in which haemorrhage occurs the blood is effused under a lower pressure than in cases of arterial bleeding and so causes less disruption of fibres.[36]

Twenty-five years later, in 1966, three authors from King's College Hospital in London reviewed 177 previously published cases of puerperal sinus thrombosis, of whom the large majority had died; four histories of their own, of whom three survived, showed a more hopeful trend.[37]

---

[35] Dowman (1926), Thrombosis of the Rolandic vein; Waggoner (1928), Thrombosis of a superior cerebral vein; Davis (1933), Thrombosis of a superior cerebral vein; Irish (1938), Thrombosis of the superior cerebral vein.

[36] Martin and Sheehan (1941), Primary thrombosis of cerebral veins (following childbirth), 353.

[37] Carroll, et al. (1966), Cerebral thrombophlebitis in pregnancy and the puerperium.

Trauma

It was not unexpected that thrombosis of the superior longitudinal sinus could result from penetrating skull wounds. Lesions of this kind occurred in the trenches of the First World War, as documented by Gordon Holmes (1876–1965) and Percy Sargent (1873–1933).[38] Despite the risk of infection, some patients survived.

The diagnosis of cerebral sinus thrombosis is less obvious when a closed head injury without initial sequelae is followed by progressive headache. Papilloedema or lumbar puncture could indicate an increased pressure of the cerebrospinal fluid, and X-rays might reveal the presence of a linear skull fracture crossing a longitudinal or lateral sinus. In 1946, Arthur D. Ecker (1913–2006), a neurosurgeon in New York, described 2 of the 11 examples of this kind he had encountered.[39] A later author even suspected thrombosis of a cerebral sinus after head trauma without a demonstrable skull fracture, on the basis of temporarily raised cerebrospinal fluid pressure.[40] The advent of angiography made it possible to confirm the thrombotic origin in similar cases.[41]

Imaging: Venography and Serial Angiography

In 1937, an otorhinolaryngologist from Stockholm, Paul Frenckner (1896–1967), addressed his colleagues in London about his new radiographic technique for visualizing the lumen of the dural sinuses. After experiments in Rhesus monkeys, he had drilled a hole and injected contrast in the lateral sinus of two patients with otogenic infections in whom he suspected thrombosis. Having thus made the diagnosis, an operation followed; the outcome was favourable in one patient, but fatal in the second. His presentation met with some scepticism;[42] a few took up the procedure.

A more promising diagnostic procedure was the venous phase of cerebral angiography, technically demanding, but less invasive. Hugo Krayenbühl (1902–1985) from Zurich pioneered this approach in 1954.[43] Since the diagnosis of venous thrombosis depended on the *absence* of a contrast agent in venous structures, one had to be quite certain that the defective filling was not related to the method of injection or to the timing of the radiographs (Figure 12.3). Once the feasibility of this method was confirmed,[44] it became the standard in

---

[38] Holmes and Sargent (1915), Injuries of the superior longitudinal sinus.
[39] Ecker (1946), Linear fracture across the venous sinuses.
[40] Beller (1964), Benign post-traumatic intracranial hypertension.
[41] Kinal (1967), Traumatic thrombosis of dural venous sinuses.
[42] Frenckner (1937), Sinography.   [43] Krayenbühl (1954), Cerebral venous thrombosis.
[44] Askenasy, *et al.* (1962), Thrombosis of the longitudinal sinus.

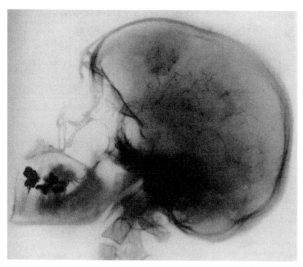

12.3 Cerebral venous thrombosis demonstrated by angiography (capillary phase; from Krayenbühl, 1954). The capillaries did not reach the cortical surface and a phlebogram was not obtained. A summary of the case history is as follows. A 50-year-old man, in good health, had a motor car accident and sustained a fracture of the left humerus and a bump on the left side of the forehead. A fortnight later, he developed severe thrombosis of the left leg and was treated with oral anticoagulants. About eight weeks after the accident, he was discharged from hospital and the anticoagulant treatment was tapered. The next day, he complained of increasing headache, with vomiting. In the course of the following two days, he felt pins and needles on the right side, then jerking on that same side. Finally, a left-sided hemiplegia occurred, with coma. Angiography (venous phase above) failed to show filling of venous structures. The patient died one day later. Autopsy showed thrombosis of all dural sinuses, the sinus rectus, and most cerebral veins.

the 1960s; in that same period, direct puncture of the carotid artery was gradually replaced by catheter techniques.

Hormonal, Haematological, and Other Uncommon Factors

After the Second World War, the 'face' of cerebral sinus thrombosis changed in a dramatic fashion, at least in the industrialized part of the world. The most important factor was the advent of antibiotics; infections as the cause became the exception rather than the rule. In 1956, two authors from London, an otorhinolaryngologist and a neurosurgeon, mused:

> This paper may figure almost as a memorial to a disease which is now nearly extinct in its original form but still appears occasionally so disguised that it is not so easily recognisable.[45]

---

[45] Reading and Schurr (1956), Thrombosis of the sigmoid sinus; past and present.

Several reviews marked this same transition – not only a well-known article by Henry Barnett (1922–2016) and Herbert Hyland (1900–1977),[46] but also monographs.[47] The later post-war years also saw the virtual disappearance of what had of old been the second main cause of cerebral venous thrombosis, the 'marantic' variant, essentially tantamount to dehydration. Apart from aged patients dying from congestive heart failure or a terminal phase of cancer,[48] most later cases were associated, if not with the puerperal phase, with hormonal contraceptives,[49] or with rare coagulopathies such as paroxysmal nocturnal haemoglobinuria.[50]

A brief word on treatment. Oral anticoagulants were occasionally given,[51] whereas others strongly discouraged their use, given the common finding of haemorrhagic infarction.[52] This controversy was to continue into the next millennium.

Although this story of cerebral venous thrombosis stops around 1975, as in other chapters of this book, it is unavoidable to pay attention to a related form of the disease. This variant was not mentioned in Gowers' summary of symptoms, because it is rarely, if ever, fatal and therefore difficult to recognize.

A RELATED SYNDROME: HEADACHE AND PAPILLOEDEMA

'Pseudotumor Cerebri'

In 1904, Max Nonne (1861–1959), Chief of Neurology at the Eppendorf Hospital in Hamburg, later Professor of Neurology at Hamburg's newly founded university, described a series of eight remarkable patients. They presented with a syndrome of gradually developing headache, papilloedema, often also unilateral weakness or convulsions, and raised pressure of the cerebrospinal fluid on lumbar puncture; combinations of these symptoms strongly suggested a brain tumour. Yet, in the course of several months or years, they miraculously recovered. In a few other patients with similar symptoms, who subsequently died of intercurrent disease or complications of an exploratory operation, inspection of the brain surface failed to reveal relevant abnormalities.[53]

---

[46] Barnett and Hyland (1953), Noninfective intracranial venous thrombosis.
[47] Garcin and Pestel (1949), *Thrombo-phlébites cérébrales*; Kalbag and Woolf (1967), *Cerebral Venous Thrombosis*.
[48] Towbin (1973), Latent cerebral venous thrombosis.
[49] Atkinson, *et al.* (1970), Intracranial venous thrombosis and oral contraception.
[50] Johnson, *et al.* (1970), Cerebral venous thrombosis in nocturnal hemoglobinuria.
[51] Brookfield (1974), Primary cerebral venous thrombosis.
[52] Barnett and Hyland (1953), Noninfective intracranial venous thrombosis.
[53] Nonne (1904), Pseudotumor cerebri.

Nonne was at a loss to interpret these serious, yet transient clinical features. He distinguished two sets, though combinations were common. The first consisted of headache and papilloedema through raised pressure of the cerebrospinal fluid; he termed this 'hydrocephalus'.[54] The role of the fluid was largely known at the time; careful anatomical and experimental studies of Axel Key (1832–1901) and Gustaf Retzius (1842–1919) from Stockholm had shown, in 1875, that intrusions of arachnoid villi into the dural sinus served as an outlet for the cerebrospinal fluid produced by the choroid plexus.[55] In 1893, Heinrich Quincke (1842–1922) in Kiel had suggested that the subarachnoid space might have been overfilled in some of his patients – a condition he called 'serous meningitis', though there was no fever.[56]

The second category of symptoms Nonne's patients showed was unilateral brain dysfunction: mostly hemiparesis, sometimes hemiconvulsions. Of course, Nonne had no reason to suspect thrombosis of cerebral sinuses, then known as an invariably fatal condition. He ended up by naming the condition 'pseudotumor cerebri'.

'Otitic Hydrocephalus'

And yet, almost as an afterthought, Nonne added the history of a young woman whose disease course he could interpret only by assuming that 'a benign sinus thrombosis from ear disease had been followed by hydrocephalus, with subsequent resorption'.[57] Charles Symonds (1890–1978), starring in Chapter 11 on cerebral aneurysms, also used the term 'hydrocephalus' to indicate increased pressure of the cerebrospinal fluid in three patients with suppurative ear infections: 'otitic hydrocephalus'.[58] His patients had no neurological deficits other than a sixth nerve palsy. At that time, Symonds regarded thrombosis of the lateral sinus as only one of the possible causal factors; later he became more restrictive.[59] Repeated lumbar puncture was his preferred treatment.

Other reports followed. In 1937, the neurosurgeon Walter Dandy presented 22 cases of what he called 'intracranial pressure without brain tumour'.[60] Remarkably enough, none of them showed signs of transient brain dysfunction, unlike all eight patients in Nonne's series. Dandy probably regarded such signs as an exclusion criterion. Ventriculography was among his extensive investigations and showed the internal brain spaces were narrowed rather than

[54] Nonne (1904), Pseudotumor cerebri, 189–91.
[55] Key and Retzius (1875–6), *Anatomie des Nervensystems*, vol. I, 179–87.
[56] Quincke (1893), Über Meningitis serosa.
[57] Nonne (1904), Pseudotumor cerebri, 213–14.   [58] Symonds (1931), Otitic hydrocephalus.
[59] Symonds (1956), Otitic hydrocephalus.
[60] Dandy (1937), Intracranial pressure without brain tumor.

widened; therefore, Dandy criticized the term 'hydrocephalus'. He remained undecided on whether the increased pressure resulted from an extra volume of the cerebrospinal fluid, blood, or both. He treated most patients by operative decompression in the temporal region.

For a long time, the role of the sinuses in the pseudotumor syndrome remained unclear, despite the association between pseudotumor and suppurative ear disease suggested by Nonne and confirmed by Symonds. This changed by the finding, in 1951, of the pseudotumor syndrome not only in thrombosis of the lateral sinus, but also in three patients with partial thrombosis of what was now called the superior sagittal sinus. The authors were the New York neurosurgeons Bronson S. Ray (1904–1993) and Howard S. Dunbar (n.d.).[61] In two of their three patients, the diagnosis was confirmed by direct venography. Treatment was operative: clearing the sinus in one, subtemporal decompression in the other. The third patient presented with fever and unilateral convulsions; he was medically treated and recovered. The authors suggested that venography might explain 'the symptom complex variously called pseudotumor cerebri, serous meningitis, and otitic hydrocephalus'.[62] This suggestion proved only partially correct, when in a new series of patients with pseudotumor, the same authors found evidence of thrombosis in only 10 of 24 patients.[63]

Serial angiography was applied somewhat less sparingly than the more invasive method of direct venography in patients with pseudotumor; again, thrombosis of the lateral sinus could be found in some patients with headache after an episode of mastoiditis.[64]

'Idiopathic Intracranial Hypertension'

Thus, thrombosis of one or more cerebral sinuses proved to be the underlying cause in at least a proportion of pseudotumor syndromes, but its demonstration depended on invasive radiographic procedures. However, in the third quarter of the twentieth century, notions about the pseudotumor syndrome began to move away from thrombosis and cerebral sinuses.

It started with the name. John Foley (1917–2011), at the time first assistant of neurology at St George's Hospital in London, again criticized the term 'hydrocephalus' to indicate raised cerebrospinal fluid pressure in patients with the pseudotumor syndrome, and instead proposed the term 'benign

---

[61] Ray and Dunbar (1951), Thrombosis as a cause of pseudotumor cerebri.
[62] Ray, *et al.* (1951), Dural sinus venography, 485.
[63] Davidoff (1956), Pseudotumor cerebri, 608.
[64] Greer (1962), Benign intracranial hypertension. I. Mastoiditis and lateral sinus obstruction; Gills, *et al.* (1967), Benign intracranial hypertension.

intracranial hypertension'.[65] This denomination firmly puts emphasis on the raised pressure. Focal signs were rare in Foley's own series of 60 patients, whereas in Nonne's eight patients, the very occurrence of transient hemiparesis or hemiconvulsions had prompted him to name the condition 'pseudotumor'. Seven subsequent series of 'benign intracranial hypertension', altogether with more than 500 cases in the period up to 1975, did not even mention hemispheric deficits,[66] reported these as absent,[67] or explicitly excluded such patients.[68]

Another change was the decreasing proportion of patients with antecedent ear infection or head trauma. In Foley's series of 1955, either condition had occurred in about a quarter of all patients, slightly less often in a series from Glasgow (1974),[69] and – otitis alone – from New York City (1956).[70] All other reports mentioned above either reported the absence of previous infection and trauma, or excluded patients with such a history.

Nowadays, the condition is often called 'idiopathic intracranial hypertension',[71] which explicitly rules out cerebral sinus thrombosis or any other specific cause. It predominates in women, especially obese women, and has also been attributed to a variety of drugs and systemic conditions.[72] Nevertheless, its gradual metamorphosis from Nonne's 'pseudotumor', later regularly explained by partial sinus thrombosis, to 'idiopathic intracranial hypertension', for which absence of any underlying disease condition is a requirement, is a useful example of the changeable nature of medical diagnoses.

The story of 'pseudotumor cerebri' is not the first example in the history of cerebrovascular disease, or of medicine, where the significance of a term is seen shifting, sometimes ending up by representing almost the opposite of its initial meaning. Nor will it be the last. After all, names of diseases do not refer to entities that exist by themselves. They only stand for ideas.

---

[65] Foley (1955), Benign forms of intracranial hypertension.

[66] Davidoff (1956), Pseudotumor cerebri; Guidetti, *et al.* (1968), 100 cases of pseudotumor cerebri.

[67] Paterson, *et al.* (1961), Pseudotumor cerebri; Johnston and Paterson (1974), Benign intracranial hypertension; Weisberg (1975), Benign intracranial hypertension.

[68] Lysak and Svien (1966), Pseudotumor cerebri; Wilson and Gardner (1966), Benign intracranial hypertension.

[69] Johnston and Paterson (1974), Benign intracranial hypertension.

[70] Davidoff (1956), Pseudotumor cerebri.

[71] Buchheit, *et al.* (1969), Papilledema and idiopathic intracranial hypertension.

[72] Weisberg (1975), Benign intracranial hypertension.

EPILOGUE

An X-ray is directed at the skull. Its energy is largely absorbed when it meets the dense layers of calcium. Whatever is left traverses brain tissue almost without resistance and is then once again decimated by the other side of the skull. If a morsel of energy is left at all, it makes virtually no imprint on the photographic plate: a blank spot. All X-rays together produce a negative outline of the skull. Though the brain has been traversed, it does not contribute to the image.

But, some people reasoned in the 1970s, suppose a tightly collimated bundle of X-rays circles around the skull, in a plane perpendicular to the body axis. Then, a given small part of the brain in this plane, say a square of 1.5×1.5 millimetres, with a depth of a few millimetres, will absorb a tiny portion of the X-ray energy not just once, but many, many times. And on the opposite side of the circumnavigated skull, one might measure what remained of all the linear routes the X-rays traversed while it was moving around. Finally, computer technology might make sense of those almost countless measurements and assign an absorption value not only to that single square, but also to all similar squares in the slice. That could perhaps allow the reconstruction of a slice of the living brain – or at least an image representing absorption values.

And so it happened. In the mid-1970s, computed tomography was developed. Extravasated blood is immediately recognizable because haemoglobin contains iron, with a high absorption value; it is white in the image, like

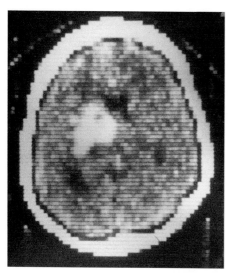

<small>EPILOGUE</small> Computed tomogram of a slice of the brain (from New and Scott, 1975). The white blob on the left side of the picture corresponds to haemorrhage in the region of the basal ganglia. The dark area on its upper right side, in the midline, represents the frontal horns of the lateral ventricles. The posterior horns of the lateral ventricles are also visible, lower down in the image, but that on the left side of the image is dilated and displaced, by obstruction of the cerebrospinal fluid produced there. *Source:* By permission of Lippincott, Williams & Wilkins.

the skull (Figure).[1] Infarcted brain tissue reacts at first normally, but after a few days, its absorption value decreases: it becomes darker than healthy brain tissue. Stroke was, of course, not the only disease in which the new diagnostic technique contributed to the treatment of patients. In 1979, the Nobel Prize for Physiology or Medicine was awarded for this work, to the engineer Godfrey Hounsfield (1919–2004; EMI industries, Middlesex) and the physicist Alan M. Cormack (1924–1998; Tufts University, Medford, Massachusetts).

Other new imaging techniques were to follow. But for stroke, the changes were immediate and dramatic. Haemorrhage could be distinguished from infarction with confidence. This opened the way for treatment.

A final word about the term 'stroke'.[2] For ages, people have used similar expressions in other languages, for example in French ('*attaque*'), Spanish ('*golpe*'), German ('*der Schlag*'), Italian ('*ictus*'), or Dutch ('*beroerte*'). The medical profession preferred the term 'apoplexy', but confusion set in after the occlusive variant became known in the middle of the nineteenth century: some doctors still called both kinds 'apoplexy', while others used it only for brain haemorrhage. In the course of the twentieth century, the term 'cerebrovascular accident' gained ground; it had a professional ring, while it veiled the remaining ignorance about what had actually happened. After the advent of computed tomography, that veil could be dropped.

---

[1] New and Scott (1975), *Computed Tomography of the Brain and Orbit.*
[2] Gunewardene (1932), 'The stroke in high arterial pressure'.

ACKNOWLEDGEMENTS

The contents of this book reflect, I hope, how excellent my teachers have been – in neurology, language, and history. Hans van Crevel (1931–2002) and Arthur Staal (1926–2016) in Rotterdam have been my role models in all aspects of academic medicine. More recently, the passion and erudition of Piet Gerbrandy, Charles Hupperts, Rodie Risselada, and David Rijser of the Department of Classical Languages at the University of Amsterdam made me forget that studying Latin had been undertaken as the means to an end. Back at the University of Utrecht, studying 'History and Philosophy of Science', I found the methods of historians of science more difficult to penetrate than those of physicians or linguists, despite the efforts of especially Frank Huisman and Dirk van Miert. I hope my 'history of ideas' has been contextualized at least to some extent, though surely many deeper layers have been left unexplored.

The preceding text would not have been written, had I not known that some fellow neurologists and friends shared my interest and were also willing to spend part of their time in commenting on preliminary versions of one or more chapters. They are, in alphabetical order: Marie-Germaine Bousser, Alastair Compston (first prize), Jaap Kappelle, Peter Koudstaal, Bart van der Worp, Rien Vermeulen, Olivier Walusinski, and Charles Warlow. Eva Graafstal assisted my struggles with a Norwegian text; Ad Stijnman guided a paragraph on reproduction techniques, and Max Viergever assisted me in radiological matters.

Living in a digital age was another sine qua non. Many organizations and institutions allowed my computer screen to conjure up a variety of texts that otherwise should have been leafed through in libraries all over Europe or even beyond: Bayerische Staatsbibliothek, *Bibliothèque interuniversitaire* (*BIU*) *de Santé*, Biodiversity Heritage Library, Gallica, Google books, HATHI Trust, Internet Archive, National Library of Medicine (USA), Springer Link, and Wellcome Library. They cannot be thanked enough.

I am greatly indebted to Utrecht University Library. Its rich collection of books and particularly journals allowed me easy access to the many primary sources I needed; the library staff were invaluable, whether manning its two nearby locations or transporting bound journals or other books from distant storage sites.

The contribution of the staff at Cambridge University Press cannot be praised highly enough; I owe special thanks to Anna Whiting, helpful Commissioning Editor, and to the production team headed by Katy Nardoni. The patient and diligent copy-editing of Joyce Cheung has spared me ever so many blushes, while Nigel d'Auvergne's indexing skills provide access from many angles.

Not least important, my wife Carien has supported me in our more than 50 years together; she has lovingly borne that even after retirement, I have still remained a bookworm.

REFERENCES

Aber, GA and CE Hutchinson. Edward Charles Hutchinson. *British Medical Journal* 2002;**325**:498.

Abercrombie, J. Researches on the pathology of the brain; part II, on apoplexy. *Edinburgh Medical and Surgical Journal* 1818a;**14**:553–92.

Abercrombie, J. Observations on chronic inflammation of the brain and its membranes. *Edinburgh Medical and Surgical Journal* 1818b;**14**:265–327.

Abercrombie, J. Researches on the pathology of the brain: part III, on paralysis. *Edinburgh Medical and Surgical Journal* 1819;**15**:1–33.

Abercrombie, J. *Pathological and Practical Researches on Diseases of the Brain and the Spinal Cord.* Edinburgh, Waugh and Innes, 1828.

Acheson, J, G Danta, and EC Hutchinson. Controlled trial of dipyridamole in cerebral vascular disease. *British Medical Journal* 1969;**1**:614–15.

Acheson, J and EC Hutchinson. Observations on the natural history of transient cerebral ischaemia. *The Lancet* 1964;**284**:871–4.

Ackerknecht, EH. *Rudolf Virchow: Arzt, Politiker, Anthropologe.* Stuttgart, Ferdinand Enke, 1957.

Ackerknecht, EH. *Medicine at the Paris Hospital 1794–1848.* Baltimore, MD, Johns Hopkins University Press, 1967.

Adam, JHC. De Apoplexia. Thesis Halae Magdeburgicae, 1728.

Adams, GF, JD Merrett, WM Hutchinson, *et al.* Cerebral embolism and mitral stenosis: survival with and without anticoagulants. *Journal of Neurology, Neurosurgery, and Psychiatry* 1974;**37**:378–83.

Albury, WR. Broussais, François-Joseph-Victor. In Bynum, WF and Bynum, H, eds. *Dictionary of Medical Biography.* Westport, CT, Greenwood Press, 2007, 266–8.

Alder, K. *The Measure of All Things.* London, Little, Brown, 2002.

Ameli, NO and DW Ashby. Non-traumatic thrombosis of the carotid artery. *The Lancet* 1949;**254**:1078–82.

Anders, HE and WJ Eicke. Über Veränderungen an Gehirngefässen bei Hypertonie. *Archiv für den gesamten Neurologie und Psychiatrie* 1939;**167**:562–75.

Anders, HE and WJ Eicke. Die Gehirngefässe beim Hochdruck. *Archiv für Psychiatrie und Nervenkrankheiten* 1940;**112**:1–44.

Anderson, RM and MM Schechter. A case of spontaneous dissecting aneurysm of the internal carotid artery. *Journal of Neurology, Neurosurgery, and Psychiatry* 1959;**22**:195–201.

Andral, G. *Clinique médicale – Maladies de l'Encéphale.* Paris, Deville Cavellin, 1833.

Andrell, O. Thrombosis of the internal carotid artery: a clinical study of 9 cases. *Acta Medica Scandinavica* 1943;**114**:336–72.

Anonymous. Observation d'hémiplégie, avec ramollissement du cerveau. *Nouvelle Bibliothèque Médicale* 1824;**6**:363–6.

Anonymous. Discussion du mémoire de M. Rochoux sur l'hypertrophie du coeur considérée comme cause de l'apoplexie et le système de Gall. *Archives Générales de Médecine* 1836;**II–II**:107–12.

Anonymous. Observation d'inflammation de la carotide interne, avec ramollissement du cerveau, suivie de réflections sur cette observation. *Gazette Médicale de Paris* 1838;**VI**:54.

Anonymous. Ramollissement du cerveau. *Archives Générales de Médecine* 1840;**III–8**:219–21.

Anonymous. The late John Blackall, M.D. *British Medical Journal* 1860;**1**:75–6.

Anonymous. Eliza Walker Dunbar, M.D. *British Medical Journal* 1925a;**2**:496–7.

Anonymous. Eliza Walker Dunbar M.D. Zürich, L.R.C.P.I., L.M. *Bristol Medico-Chirurgical Journal* 1925b;**42**:197–8.

Anonymous. G. Newton Pitt. *British Medical Journal* 1929;**1**:425–6.

Anonymous. An evaluation of anticoagulant therapy in the treatment of cerebrovascular disease. Report of the Veterans Administration cooperative study of atherosclerosis, Neurology Section. *Neurology* 1961;**11**:132–8.

Anonymous. Philippe Ricord (1800–1889), syphilographer. *JAMA* 1970;**211**:115–16.

Anonymous. Kein Gauß drin. *Hannoversche Allgemeine Zeitung*, 28 October 2013.

Arab, A. Hyalinose artériolaire cérébrale; essai de synthèse anatomo-clinique. *Schweizer Archiv für Neurologie, Neurochirurgie, und Psychiatrie* 1959;**84**:1–33.

Aretaeus. *De Causis et Signis acutorum, et diuturnorum Morborum, Libri quatuor; de Curatio acutorum, et diuturnorum Morborum, Libri quatuor.* Lugduni Batavorum, Apud Janssonios van der Aa 1735 [*c*.150].

Argyll Robertson, D. Four cases of spinal miosis: with remarks on the action of light on the pupil. *Edinburgh Medical Journal* 1869;**15**:487–93.

Aselli, G. *De Lactibus sive lacteis Venis, quarto Vasorum mesaraicorum Genere novo invento.* Mediolanum, Giovanni Battista Bidelli, 1627.

Askenasy, HM, IZ Kosary, and J Braham. Thrombosis of the longitudinal sinus. Diagnosis by carotid angiography. *Neurology* 1962;**12**:288–92.

Askey, JM. Hemiplegia following carotid sinus stimulation. *American Heart Journal* 1946;**31**:131–7.

Astruc, P. À propos du centenaire de la thermométrie clinique. *Progrès Médical* 1952;**80**:543–4.

Atkinson, EA, B Fairburn, and KW Heathfield. Intracranial venous thrombosis as complication of oral contraception. *The Lancet* 1970;**295**:914–18.

Auenbrugger, L. *Inventum novum ex Percussione Thoracis humani ut Signo abstrusos interni Pectoris Morbos detegendi.* Vindobonae, Joannis Thomas Trattner, 1761.

Bailey, OT and GM Hass. Dural sinus thrombosis in early life: recovery from the acute thrombosis of the superior longitudinal sinus and its relation to certain acquired cerebral lesions in childhood. *Brain* 1937;**60**:293–314.

Baillie, M. *A Series of Engravings, Accompanied with Explanations, which Are Intended to Illustrate the Morbid Anatomy of Some of the Most Important Parts of the Human Body.* London, J. Johnson and G. Nicol, 1803.

Baillie, M. *The Morbid Anatomy of Some of the Most Important Parts of the Human Body*, 4th edn, London, J. Johnson and G. Nicol, 1812.

Baker, RN. Anticoagulant therapy in cerebral infarction; report on cooperative study. *Neurology* 1962;**12**:823–35.

Baker, RN, JC Ramseyer, and WS Schwartz. Prognosis in patients with transient cerebral ischemic attacks. *Neurology* 1968;**18**:1157–65.

Ball, P. *The Devil's Doctor: Paracelsus and the World of Renaissance Magic and Science.* London, William Heinemann, 2006.

Barbé, A and J Lévy-Valensi. Lacunes de désintégration cellulaire dans un système nerveux d'hérédosyphilitique. *Revue Neurologique* 1908;**16**:339–40.

Barberis, I, NL Bragazzi, L Galluzzo, *et al.* The history of tuberculosis: from the first historical records to the isolation of Koch's bacillus. *Journal of Preventive Medicine and Hygiene* 2017;**58**:E9–12.

Bard, L. Du liquide céphalo-rachidien hémorragique. *Comptes Rendus des Séances et Mémoires de la Société de Biologie* 1901;**53**:747–8.

Barnett, HJ and HH Hyland. Noninfective intracranial venous thrombosis. *Brain* 1953;**76**:36–49.

Barré, J-A, D Philippidès, and F Isch. Thrombose de la carotide interne. Étude clinique, artério et encéphalographique. *Revue Neurologique* 1947;79:442–4, 662–4.

Bartholow, R. Aneurysms at the arteries at the base of the brain: their symptomatology, diagnosis and treatment. *American Journal of the Medical Sciences* 1872;**44**:373–86.

Battacharji, SK, EC Hutchinson, and AJ McCall. The circle of Willis: the incidence of developmental abnormalities in normal and infarcted brains. *Brain* 1967;**90**:747–58.

Bauhinus, C. *Theatrum anatomicum, novis Figuris aeneis illustratum et in Lucem emissum.* Francofurti, M. Becker, 1605.

Bauhinus, C. *Theatrum anatomicum.* Francoforti, Ioann. Theodorus de Bry, 1621.

Baumgarten, P. Über gummöse Syphilis des Gehirns und Rückenmarks, namentlich der Gehirngefässe, und uber das Verhältniss dieser Erkrankungen zu den entsprechenden tuberculösen Affectionen. *Archiv für pathologische Anatomie und Physiologie und für klinische Medicin* 1881;**86**:179–221.

Bayle, ALJ. *Traité des Maladies du Cerveau et de ses Membranes.* Paris, Gabon et Cie, 1826.

Bayle, F. *Tractatus de Apoplexia.* Tolosae, B. Guillemette, 1677.

Beadles, CF. Aneurisms of the larger cerebral arteries. *Brain* 1907;**30**:285–336.

Becquerel, A. Rapport sur le mémoire présenté par M. E. Bouchut à la Société Médicale des Hôpitaux. *Actes de la Société Médicale des Hôpitaux de Paris* 1850;**1**:44–50.

Béhier, J. Coagulations veineuses multiples, suite de couches. Ramollissement et hémorrhagie cérébrale. *Gazette des Hôpitaux Civils et Militaires* 1874;**47**:489–90.

Béhier, J and D Bourgeois. Sur la gangrène des membres dans la fièvre typhoide. *Bulletin de la Société Médicale des Hôpitaux de Paris* 1857;**III-1**:412–32, 488–92, 501–14.

Beitzke, H. Die Rolle der kleinen Aneurysmen bei den Massenblutungen des Gehirns. *Verhandlungen der Deutschen pathologischen Gesellschaft* 1936;**29**:74–80.

Bell, BA. Wylie McKissock: reminiscences of a commanding figure in British neurosurgery. *British Journal of Neurosurgery* 1996;**10**:9–18.

Beller, AJ. Benign post-traumatic intracranial hypertension. *Journal of Neurology, Neurosurgery, and Psychiatry* 1964;**27**:149–52.

Benda, CE. Désiré Magloire Bourneville. In Haymaker, W and Schiller, F, eds. *The Founders of Neurology.* Springfield, IL, Charles C. Thomas, 1970, 410–13.

Bennett, HJ. Pathological and histological researches on inflammation of the nervous centres. *Edinburgh Medical and Surgical Journal* 1843;**60**:376–99.

Benson, A. Recurrent temporary visual obscurations. *Transactions of the Eighth International Ophthalmological Congress.* Edinburgh, T. and A. Constable, 1894, 81–90.

Benton, AL and RJ Joynt. Early descriptions of aphasia. *Archives of Neurology* 1960;**3**:205–22.

Bertoloni Meli, D. *Visualizing Disease: The Art and History of Pathological Illustrations.* Chicago, IL, University of Chicago Press, 2017.

Beyer, J. Lycosthenes. www.bbkl.de/public/index.php/frontend/lexicon/L/Ly/lycosthenes-conrad-61950. [Accessed 27 April 2022]

Biemond, A. Thrombosis of the basilar artery and the vascularization of the brain stem. *Brain* 1951;**74**:300–17.

Biemond, A. *Hersenziekten,* 3rd edn, Haarlem, De Erven F. Bohn, 1961.

Binswanger, O. Die Abgrenzung der allgemeinen progressiven Paralyse. *Berliner medizinische Wochenschrift* 1894;**31**:1103–5, 1137–9, 1180–6.

Biumi, F. Carotis ad receptaculum Vieussenii aneurysmatica, etc. In Sandifort, E, ed. *Thesaurus Dissertationum programmatum, alioriumque opusculorum selectissimorum, ad omnem Medicinae Ambitum pertinentem.* Lugdunum Batavorum, S. and J. Luchtmans, P. v.d. Eijk, and D. Vijgh, 1778 [1765], 373–9.

Blackall, J. *Observations on the Nature and Cure of Dropsies.* London, Longman, Hurst, Rees, Orme, and Brown, 1813.

Blackwood, W, JF Hallpike, RS Kocen, *et al.* Atheromatous disease of the carotid arterial system and embolism from the heart in cerebral infarction: a morbid anatomical study. *Brain* 1969;**92**:897–910.

Blane, G. Case of aneurisms of the carotid arteries. *Transactions of a Society for the Improvement of Medical and Chirurgical Knowledge* 1800;193–8.

Bliss, M. *William Osler: A Life in Medicine.* Oxford, Oxford University Press, 1999.

Blom, P. *The Vertigo Years.* New York, NY, Basic Books, 2008.

Boerhaave, H. *Aphorismi de cognoscendis et curandis Morbis in Usum domesticae Doctrinae digesti*. Lugdunum Batavorum, Apud Johannem van der Linden, 1709.

Boerhaave, H. *Atrocis, nec descripti prius, Morbi Historia. Secundum medicae Artis Leges conscripta*. Lugdunum Batavorum, Boutestein, 1724.

Boerhaave, H and J van Eems. *Praelectiones academicae de Morbis Nervorum*. Lugduni Batavorum, Apud Petrum van der Eyk et Cornelium de Pecker, 1761.

Böhne, C. Über die Bedeutung der Hirnerweichung in der Pathogenese der kompakten apoplektischen Hirnblutung. *Zeitschrift für den gesamten Neurologie und Psychiatrie* 1931;**137**:611–20.

Bonetus, T. *Sepulchretum, sive Anatomia practica ex Cadaveribus Morbo denatis*. Genevae, Sumptibus Leonardo Chouët, 1679.

Bonner, TN. Rendezvous in Zurich; seven who made a revolution in women's medical education, 1864–1874. *Journal of the History of Medicine and Allied Sciences* 1989;**44**:7–27.

Borte, G. Leben und Wirkungsstätten von Julius Cohnheim. *Zentralblatt für Allgemeine Pathologie und Pathologische Anatomie* 1985;**130**:291–7.

Botterell, EH, WM Lougheed, JW Scott, *et al*. Hypothermia, and interruption of carotid, or carotid and vertebral circulation, in the surgical management of intracranial aneurysms. *Journal of Neurosurgery* 1956;**13**:1–42.

Bouchard, C-J. Étude sur quelques points de la pathogénie des hémorrhagies cérébrales. Thesis Paris, 1866.

Bouchut, E. Mémoire sur la nature du ramollissement cérébrale sénile. *Actes de la Société Médicale des Hôpitaux de Paris* 1850;**1**:37–43.

Bouley, BA. *Pious Postmortems: Anatomy, Sanctity, and the Catholic Church in Early Modern Europe*. Philadelphia, PA, University of Philadelphia Press, 2017.

Bouquin, C. Lithographie. In Fouché, P, *et al*., eds. *Dictionnaire encyclopédique du Livre*. Paris, Éditions du Cercle de la Librairie, 2005, 780–3.

Bourée, JBH. Essai sur l'apoplexie. Thesis Montpellier, 1804.

Bourneville. Études cliniques et thermométriques sur les maladies du système nerveux. Thesis Paris, 1872.

Bourneville. De l'hémianesthésie liée à une lésion d'un hémisphère du cerveau. *Presse Médicale* 1873;**1**:244–6.

Brain, WR. *Diseases of the Nervous System*, 6th edn, Oxford, Oxford University Press, 1962.

Bramwell, B. Case of aneurism of the right internal carotid artery. *Edinburgh Medical Journal* 1886;**32**:97–101.

Bramwell, E. A case of leaking aneurism of the circle of Willis and two cases of recurrent oculo-motor paralysis: a clinical comparison. *Edinburgh Medical Journal* 1931;**38**:689–95.

Breugelmans, R and K Gnirrep. Bibliografie. In Bosman-Jelgersma, HA, ed. *Petrus Forestus Medicus*. Duivendrecht, Drukkerij Stolwijk, 1997, 17–116.

Brewer, DB. Max Schultze (1865), G. Bizzozero (1882) and the discovery of the platelet. *British Journal of Haematology* 2006;**133**:251–8.

Brice, JG, DJ Dowsett, and RD Lowe. Haemodynamic effects of carotid artery stenosis. *British Medical Journal* 1964a;**1**:1363–6.

Brice, JG, DJ Dowsett, and RD Lowe. The effect of constriction on carotid blood-flow and pressure gradient. *The Lancet* 1964b;**283**:84–5.

Bricheteau, I. Considérations et observations sur l'apoplexie. *Journal Complémentaire du Dictionnaire des Sciences Médicales* 1818;**1**:129–52, 289–317.

Bricheteau, I. De l'influence de la circulation sur les fonctions cérébrales, et de la connection de l'hypertrophie du coeur avec quelques lésions du cerveau. *Journal Complémentaire du Dictionnaire des Sciences Médicales* 1819;**4**:17–37.

Bright, P. *Dr. Richard Bright*. London, The Bodley Head, 1983.

Bright, R. *Reports of Medical Cases, Selected with a View of Illustrating the Symptoms and Cure of Diseases by a Reference to Morbid Anatomy*. London, Longman, Rees, Orme, Brown, and Green, 1827–31.

Bright, R. Cases illustrative of the effects produced when the arteries and the brain are diseased, selected chiefly with a view to the diagnosis in such affections. *Guy's Hospital Reports* 1836;**1**:1–40.

Brigo, F, S Lattanzi, E Trinka, *et al.* First descriptions of tuberous sclerosis by Désiré-Magloire Bourneville (1840–1909). *Neuropathology* 2018;**38**:577–82.

Brinton, W. Report on cases of cerebral aneurisms. *Transactions of the Pathological Society of London* 1852;**3**:47–9, 49–51.

Brisman, R and K Abbassioun. Familial intracranial aneurysms. *Journal of Neurosurgery* 1971;**34**:678–82.

Brissaud, E and A Souques. Maladies de l'encéphale. In Bouchard, CJ and Brissaud, E, eds. *Traité de médecine*, vol. IX. Paris, Masson et Cie, 1904, 1–346.

Bristowe, JS. Analysis of seven cases of obstruction of the cerebral arteries. *Transactions of the Pathological Society of London* 1859a;**10**:44–58.

Bristowe, JS. Syphilitic (?) disease of the brain and liver; with obstruction by clots of cerebral arteries. *Transactions of the Pathological Society of London* 1859b;**10**:21–4.

Broadbent, WH. Absence of pulsation in both radial arteries, the vessels being full of blood. *Transactions of the Clinical Society* 1875;**8**:165–8.

Broadbridge, AT and EV Leslie. Cerebral angiographic contrast media; a comparison of hypaque 45% and urografin 60% and an assessment of the relative clinical toxicity of urografin 60%, hypaque 45%, diaginol 25% and diodone 35% in carotid arteriography. *British Journal of Radiology* 1958;**31**:556–60.

Broca, P. Remarques sur le siège de la faculté du langage articulé, suivies d'une observation d'aphémie (perte de la parole). *Bulletin de la Société Anatomique* 1861;**II–6**:330–57.

Brock, WH. *The Norton History of Chemistry.* New York, NY, W. W. Norton & Company, 1992.

Brookfield, DS. A case of primary cerebral venous thrombosis. *Postgraduate Medical Journal* 1974;**50**:765–6.

Brunner, JC. De apoplexia, post quinquennium recurrens fortissima à sanguine extravasato, cum capitis anatome. *Miscellanea Curiosa, sive Ephemeridum Medico-Physicarum Germanicarum*

Academiae Caesareo-Leopoldinae Naturae Curiosorum – Decuriae III 1694;**1**:271–8.

Buchheit, WA, C Burton, B Haag, *et al.* Papilledema and idiopathic intracranial hypertension. *New England Journal of Medicine* 1969;**280**:938–42.

Büchner, F. Zur Pathogenese der Hochdruckapoplexie. *Deutsche Medizinische Wochenschrift* 1936;**62**:369–71.

Bucquoy, J. *Des concrétions sanguines.* Paris, L. Leclerc, 1863.

Budínová-Smelá, J, J Lhotka, and F Marx. Thrombosis arteriae carotis internae. *Časopis lékařů českých* 1949;**88**:93–8.

Buess, H. Zur Geschichte des Embolie-Begriffs. In Leuch, O, *et al.*, eds. *Schweizerisches Medizinisches Jahrbuch 1946.* Basel, Benno Schwabe & Co, 1946, LVII–XX.

Bull, E. Akut Hjernaneurisma – Okulomotoriusparalyse – Meningealapoplexi. *Norsk Magazin for Laegevidenskaben* 1877;**7**:890–5.

Bull, JW, J Marshall, and DA Shaw. Cerebral angiography in the diagnosis of the acute stroke. *The Lancet* 1960;**275**:562–5.

Burckhardt, J. *Die Kultur der Renaissance in Italien.* Basel, Schweighauser, 1860.

Burdet, W. A wonder of wonders. *Pamphlet,* 1651.

Burrows, G. *On Disorders of the Cerebral Circulation and on the Connection between Affections of the Brain and Diseases of the Heart.* London, Longman, Brown, Green, and Longmans, 1846.

Burserius, JB. *Institutiones Medicinae practicae.* Mediolani, Typis imperialis Monasterii s. Ambrosii Majoris, 1781.

Butterfield, H. *The Whig Interpretation of History.* London, G. Bell and Sons, 1950 [1931].

Byers, RK and GM Hass. Thrombosis of the dural venous sinuses in infancy and childhood. *American Journal of Diseases of Children* 1933;**45**:1161–83.

Bylebyl, JJ. The School of Padua. In Webster, C, ed. *Health, Medicine and Mortality in the Sixteenth Century.* Cambridge, Cambridge University Press, 1979, 335–70.

Calmeil, LF. *De la Paralysie considérée chez les Aliénés*. Paris, J. B. Baillière, 1826.

Calverley, JR and CH Millikan. Complications of carotid manipulation. *Neurology* 1961;**11**:185–9.

Campbell, AW. The morbid changes in the cerebro-spinal nervous system of the aged insane. *Journal of Mental Science* 1894;**40**:638–48.

Caplan, LR. Charles Foix: the first modern stroke neurologist. *Stroke* 1990;**21**:348–56.

Caplan, LR. *C. Miller Fisher; Stroke in the 20th Century*. Oxford, Oxford University Press, 2020.

Capparoni, P. Domenico Mistichelli e la sua scoperta dalla decussatio pyramidum. *Atti e memorie della Accademia di storia dell'arte sanitaria* 1939;**5**:261–75.

Cardanus, H. *In septem Aphorismorum Hippocratis Particulas Commentaria*. Basileae, Henricus Petri, 1564.

Carlino, A. *Books of the Body: Anatomical Ritual and Renaissance Learning*. Chicago, IL, University of Chicago Press, 1994.

Carroll, JD, D Leak, and HA Lee. Cerebral thrombophlebitis in pregnancy and the puerperium. *Quarterly Journal of Medicine* 1966;**35**:347–68.

Carswell, R. *Pathological Anatomy: Illustrations of the Elementary Forms of Disease*. London, Longman, Orme, Brown, Green, and Longmans, 1838.

Carter, KC. *The Rise of Causal Concepts of Disease: Case Histories*. Farnham, Ashgate Publishing, 2003.

Casper, ST. *The Neurologists: A History of a Medical Specialty in Modern Britain, c.1789–2000*. Manchester, Manchester University Press, 2014.

Casserius, J and D Bucretius. *Tabulae anatomicae LXXIIX, omnes novae nec ante hac visae, Daniel Bucretius, Wratislawensis, Philos. et Med. D., XX quae deerant supplevit et omnium explicationes addidit*. Venetiis, Apud Evangelistam Deuchinum, 1627.

Castaigne, P, F Lhermitte, JC Gautier, et al. Internal carotid artery occlusion. A study of 61 instances in 50 patients with post-mortem data. *Brain* 1970;**93**:231–58.

Castaigne, P, F Lhermitte, JC Gautier, et al. Arterial occlusions in the vertebro-basilar

system. A study of 44 patients with post-mortem data. *Brain* 1973;**96**:133–54.

Catola, G. Lacunes de désintégration cérébrale. *Revue de Médecine* 1904;**24**:778–809.

Cerulli, G. *Riflessioni intorno ai Mali apopletici*. Napoli, Vincenzo Orsini, 1806.

Chao, WH, ST Kwan, RS Lyman, et al. Thrombosis of the left carotid artery. *Archives of Surgery* 1938;**37**:100–11.

Charcot, J-M. Rhumatisme articulaire aigu; phénomènes comateux; hémiplégie; infiltration d'une substance plastique concrète, contenant des globules pyoïdes dans plusieurs viscères, et en particulier dans le cerveau et la rate; lésions dyssentériques de la muqueuse de l'intestin grêle et du colon. *Comptes Rendus des Séances et Mémoires de la Société de Biologie* 1851;**3**:91–4.

Charcot, J-M. Gangrène du pied et de la jambe gauches; dépôts fibrineux multiples dans les reins, la rate, le foie; engorgements hémoptoiques dans les deux poumons. *Comptes Rendus des Séances et Mémoires de la Société de Biologie* 1855;**II–2**:213–20.

Charcot, J-M. Gangrène du pied et de la jambe gauches; dépots fibrineux multiples dans les reins, la rate, le foie; engorgements hémoptoiques dans les deux poumons; observation lue à la Société de Biologie. *Gazette Médicale de France* 1856;**III–11**:130–2.

Charcot, J-M. Note sur la température des parties centrales dans l'apoplexie liée à l'hémorrhagie cérébrale et au ramollissement du cerveau. *Comptes Rendus des Séances et Mémoires de la Société de Biologie* 1867;**IV–4**:92–3.

Charcot, J-M. Discussion, séance du 19 Juillet 1873. *Comptes Rendus des Séances et Mémoires de la Société de Biologie* 1873;**25**:283.

Charcot, J-M and B Ball. *Leçons sur les maladies des vieillards et les maladies chroniques*. Paris, Adrien Delahaye, 1868.

Charcot, J-M and C Bouchard. Nouvelles recherches sur la pathogénie de l'hémorrhagie cérébrale. *Archives de Physiologie Normale et Pathologique* 1868;**I**:110–27, 643–65, 725–34.

Charcot, J-M and C-É Brown-Séquard. Discussion (sur les localisations cérébrales).

Comptes Rendus des Séances et Mémoires de la Société de Biologie 1875–6;399–403 (1875), 1–3, 8–11, 13–17, 254–7.

Charcot, J-M and A Vulpian. Sur deux cas de sclérose des cordons postérieurs et de la moelle avec atrophie des racines postérieures (tabes dorsalis, Romberg; ataxie locomotrice progressive, Duchenne de Boulogne). *Comptes Rendus des Séances et Mémoires de la Société de Biologie* 1862;**III–4**:155–73.

Chevers, N. Remarks on the effects of obliteration of the carotid arteries on the cerebral circulation. *London Medical Gazette* 1845;new series-**1**:1140–51.

Cheyne, J. *Cases of Apoplexy and Lethargy, with Observations on the Comatose Diseases.* London, Thomas Underwood; Edinburgh, Adam Black; Glasgow, Walter Duncan; Dublin, Gilbert and Hodges, 1812.

Cheyne, J. Autobiographical sketch. In Cheyne, J, ed. *Essays on Partial Derangement of the Mind, in Relation to Religion.* Dublin, London, and Edinburgh, William Curry Jr and Co, Longman, Brown and Co, and Fraser and Co, 1843, 1–38.

Chiari, H. Ueber das Verhalten des Teilungswinkels der Carotis communis bei der Endarteriitis chronica deformans. *Verhandlungen der Deutschen pathologischen Gesellschaft* 1905;**9**:326–30.

Christian, HA. *Osler's 'The Principles and Practice of Medicine'.* New York, NY, D. Appleton-Century Company, 1944.

Church, WS. Contributions to cerebral pathology. *Saint Bartholomew's Hospital Reports* 1869;**5**:164–215.

Church, WS. On the formation of aneurysms, especially intracranial aneurysms in early life. *Saint Bartholomew's Hospital Reports* 1870;**6**:99–112.

Chvostek, F and A Weichselbaum. Herdweise syphilitische Endarteriitis mit multipler Aneurysmenbildung. *Allgemeine Wiener medizinische Zeitung* 1877;**22**:257–8.

Clarke, E and CD O'Malley. *The Human Brain and Spinal Cord: A Historical Study Illustrated by Writings from Antiquity to the Twentieth Century.* San Francisco, CA, Norman Publishing, 1996.

Clarke, JM. On the value of suspension in the treatment of tabes dorsalis. *The Lancet* 1891;**138**:114–17.

Coe, RW. Case of aneurism of the left internal carotid artery within the cranium. *Association Medical Journal* 1855;1067–9.

Cohn, B. *Klinik der Embolischen Gefässkrankheiten, mit besonderer Rücksicht auf die ärztliche Praxis.* Berlin, August Hirschwald, 1860.

Cohnheim, J. *Untersuchungen ueber die embolischen Processe.* Berlin, August Hirschwald, 1872.

Cole, FM and PO Yates. The occurrence and significance of intracerebral micro-aneurysms. *Journal of Pathology and Bacteriology* 1967;**93**:393–411.

Cole, W. Phaenomena in cadavere praenobilis cujusdam faeminae, apoplexia peremptae, inter dissecandum, Maii 12, 1679, observata. *Philosophical Transactions of the Royal Society of London* 1685;**15**:168–72.

Cole, W. *A Physico-medical Essay Concerning the Late Frequency of Apoplexies, Together with a General Method of Their Prevention and Cure.* Oxford, printed at the theater, 1689.

Collier, J and WJ Adie. Diseases of the nervous system. In Price, FW, ed. *A Textbook of the Practice of Medicine.* London, Henry Frowde and Hodder & Stoughton, 1922, 1279–579.

Collier, W. Thrombosis of cerebral veins. *British Medical Journal* 1891;**1**:521–2.

Compston, A. From the archives: 'Observations on intracranial aneurysms', by R. W. Ross Russell. *Brain* 2005;**128**:2219–21.

Compston, A. '*All Manner of Ingenuity and Industry*': *A Bio-bibliography of Dr Thomas Willis 1621–1675.* Oxford, Oxford University Press, 2021.

Comte, A. Des paralysies pseudo-bulbaires. Thesis Paris, G. Steinheil, 1900.

Conos, B and C Xanthopoulos. Hémorrhagie méningée curable. *L'Encéphale* 1912;**7**:18–29.

Contrepois, A. The clinician, germs and infectious diseases: the example of Charles Bouchard in Paris. *Medical History* 2002;**46**:197–220.

Cook, HJ. *Matters of Exchange: Commerce, Medicine and Science in the Dutch Golden Age.*

New Haven, CT, Yale University Press, 2007.

Cooke, J. *A Treatise on Nervous Diseases*. London, Longman, Hurst, Rees, Orme, and Brown, 1820.

Copeman, E. *A Collection of Cases of Apoplexy, with an Explanatory Introduction*. London, John Churchill, 1845.

Corday, E, SF Rothenberg, and TJ Putnam. Cerebral vascular insufficiency; an explanation of some types of localized cerebral encephalopathy. *Archives of Neurology and Psychiatry* 1953;**69**:551–70.

Cortnumm, J. *De morbo attonito*. Lipsiae, Heinricus Frommannus, 1677.

Crisp, E. Cases of cerebral disease, with observations. *The Lancet* 1840;**33**:863–72.

Crompton, MR. Retinal emboli in stenosis of the internal carotid artery. *The Lancet* 1963;**281**:886.

Crompton, MR. The pathogenesis of cerebral infarction following the rupture of cerebral berry aneurysms. *Brain* 1964;**87**:491–510.

Crompton, MR. Infarction following the rupture of cerebral berry aneurysms. *Brain* 1964;**87**:263–80.

Cruveilhier, J. *Anatomie pathologique du Corps humain, ou Descriptions, avec Figures lithographiées et coloriées des diverses Altérations morbides dont le Corps humain est susceptible*. Paris, J. B. Baillière, 1829–42.

Csiszar, A. *The Scientific Journal*. Chicago, IL, University of Chicago Press, 2018.

Cunningham, A. Peregrinatio medica. In Grell, OP, *et al.*, eds. *Centres of Medical Excellence? Medical Travel and Education in Europe, 1500–1789*. Farnham, Ashgate Publishing, 2009, 3–16.

Cunningham, A. *The Anatomist Anatomis'd: an Experimental Discipline in Enlightenment Europe*. Farnham, Ashgate Publishing, 2010.

Cushing, H. On routine determinations of arterial tension in operating room and clinic. *Boston Medical and Surgical Journal* 1903;**148**:250–6.

Czech, H. Vienna School of Medicine, 1939–1945. In Weindling, P, ed. *From Clinic to Concentration Camp: Reassessing Nazi Medical*

and Racial Research. London, Routledge, 2017, 138–62.

Da Carpi, B. *Isagogae breves et exactissimae in Anatomiam humani Corporis*. Argentoratum, Henricus Sybold, 1530.

Dandy, WE. Ventriculography following the injection of air into the cerebral ventricles. *Annals of Surgery* 1918;**68**:5–11.

Dandy, WE. Intracranial pressure without brain tumor: diagnosis and treatment. *Annals of Surgery* 1937;**106**:492–513.

Dandy, WE. Intracranial aneurysm of the internal carotid artery: cured by operation. *Annals of Surgery* 1938;**107**:654–9.

Dandy, WE. *Intracranial Arterial Aneurysms*. Ithaca, NY, Comstock Publishing Company, 1944.

Davidoff, LM. Pseudotumor cerebri: benign intracranial hypertension. *Neurology* 1956;**6**:605–15.

Davis, DB. Thrombosis of a superior cerebral vein. *Journal of Nervous and Mental Disease* 1933;**77**:22–6.

Davis, G. The most deadly disease of asylumdom: general paralysis of the insane and Scottish psychiatry, c.1840–1940. *Journal of the Royal College of Physicians of Edinburgh* 2012;**42**:266–73.

Dawber, TR, WB Kannel, PM McNamara, et al. An epidemiologic study of apoplexy ('strokes'). Observations in 5,209 adults in the Framingham study on association of various factors in the development of apoplexy. *Transactions of the American Neurological Association* 1965;**90**:237–40.

De Barahona Fernandes, HJ. Egas Moniz. In Kolle, K, ed. *Grosse Nervenärzte*. Stuttgart, Georg Thieme, 1956, 187–99.

De Graef, R. *De Succi pancreatici Natura et Usu*. Lugdunum Batavorum, Ex Officina Hackiana, 1664.

De Haen, A. *Ratio medendi in Nosocomio practico (pars quarta)*. Vindobonae, Johannae Thomae Trattner, 1759.

De Ridder-Symoens, H. The mobility of medical students. In Grell, OP, *et al.*, ed. *Centres of Medical Excellence? Medical Travel and Education in Europe, 1500–1789*. Farnham, Ashgate Publishing, 2009, 47–89.

De Visscher, C. Pathogénie et diagnostic de l'hémorrhagie et du ramollissement du cerveau. Thesis Bruxelles, Th. Lesigne, 1877.

Dechambre, A. Mémoire sur la curabilité du ramollissement cérébral. *Gazette Médicale de Paris* 1838;**II–6**:305–14.

Dei Liuzzi, M. *Anatomia*. Bologna, Monduzzi Editore, 1988 [1316].

Dei Poli, G and J Zucha. Beiträge zur Kenntnis der Anomalien und der Erkrankungen der Arteria carotis interna. *Zentralblatt für Neurochirurgie* 1940;**5**:209–38.

Dejerine, J and E Huet. Contribution à l'étude de l'aortite oblitérante. *Revue de Médecine* 1888;**8**:201–14.

Dejerine, J and G Roussy. Le syndrome thalamique. *Revue Neurologique* 1906;**14**:521–32.

Deniker, J. J. V. Laborde. *Nature* 1903;**69**:105–6.

Denman, FR, G Ehni, and WS Duty. Insidious thrombotic occlusion of cervical carotid arteries, treated by arterial graft: a case report. *Surgery* 1955;**38**:569–77.

Denny-Brown, D. The treatment of recurrent cerebrovascular symptoms and the question of 'vasospasm'. *Medical Clinics of North America* 1951;**35**:1457–74.

Denny-Brown, D. Recurrent cerebrovascular episodes. *Archives of Neurology* 1960;**2**:194–210.

Denny-Brown, D. Transient focal cerebral ischaemia. *British Medical Journal* 1963;**2**:930.

Descartes, R. *L'Homme et un Traitté de la Formation du Foetus*. Paris, Jacques Le Gras, 1664.

Deville, P. *Peste et Choléra*. Paris, Seuil, 2012.

Dewhurst, K. *Willis's Oxford Lectures*. Oxford, Sandford Publications, 1980.

Dijksterhuis, EJ. *The Mechanisation of the World Picture*. Oxford, Oxford University Press, 1961.

Diversus, PS. *De Febre pestilenti Tractatus et Curationes quorundam particularium Morborum, quorum Tractatio ab ordinariis Practicis non habetur*. Bononiae, Ioannes Rossius, 1584.

Dobson, J. Dr. Edwards Crisp: a forgotten medical scientist. *Journal of the History of Medicine and Allied Sciences* 1952;**7**:384–400.

Döhle, KG. Über Aortenerkrankung bei Syphilitischen und deren Beziehung zur Aneurysmabildung. *Deutsches Archiv für klinische Medicin* 1895;**55**:190–210.

Donatus, M. *De medica Historia mirabili Libri sex*. Mantuae, Franciscus Osana, 1586.

Dörfler, J. Ein Beitrag zur Frage der Lokalisation der Arteriosklerose der Gehirngefäße mit besonderer Berucksichtigung der Arteria carotis interna. *Archiv für Psychiatrie und Nervenkrankheiten* 1935;**103**:180–90.

Dos Santos, N. François-Nicolas Marquet. Sa vie, ses oeuvres et ses démêlés tardifs avec le Collège Royal de Médecine de Nancy. Thesis Nancy, 2008.

Dott, NM. Intracranial aneurysms: cerebral arterio-radiography: surgical treatment. *Edinburgh Medical Journal* 1933;**40**:T 219–34.

Dott, NM. Intracranial aneurysm formation. *Clinical Neurosurgery* 1969;**16** Suppl. 1:1–16.

Dow, DR. The incidence of arterio-sclerosis in the arteries of the body. *British Medical Journal* 1925;**2**:162–3.

Dowman, CE. Thrombosis of the Rolandic vein: report of a case. *Archives of Neurology and Psychiatry* 1926;**15**:110–12.

Drake, CG. Bleeding aneurysms of the basilar artery. Direct surgical management in four cases. *Journal of Neurosurgery* 1961;**18**:230–8.

Drake, CG. Further experience with surgical treatment of aneurysm of the basilar artery. *Journal of Neurosurgery* 1968;**29**:372–92.

Drake, CG. Ruptured intracranial aneurysms. *Proceedings of the Royal Society of Medicine* 1971;**64**:477–81.

Duchenne (de Boulogne). De l'ataxie locomotrice progressive; recherches sur une maladie caractérisée spécialement par des troubles généraux de la coordinations des mouvements. *Archives Générales de Médecine* 1858–9;**V–12–13**:641–52 (12), 36–62, 158–81, 417–51 (13).

Dupré, E and A Devaux. Foyers lacunaires de désintégration cérébrale (note sur le processus histogénique). *Revue Neurologique* 1901a;**71**:919–27.

Dupré, E and A Devaux. Rire et pleurer spasmodiques par ramollissement nucléocapsulaire antérieur: syndrome pseudo-bulbaire par désintégration lacunaire bilatérale des putamens. *Revue Neurologique* 1901b;**9**:919–26.

Durand, C. Des anévrysmes du cerveau. Thesis Paris, 1868.

Durand-Fardel, M. Mémoire sur une altération particulière de la substance cérébrale. *Gazette Médicale de Paris* 1842;**II–10**:23–6, 33–8.

Durand-Fardel, M. *Traité du Ramollissement du Cerveau*. Paris, J. B. Baillière and H. Baillière, 1843.

Durand-Fardel, M. *Traité clinique et pratique des maladies des Vieillards*. Paris, Germer Baillière, 1854.

Duretus, L. *Hippocratis Magni Coacae Praenotiones*. Parisiis, Batista Dupuys, 1588.

Dyken, ML, OJ Kolar, and FH Jones. Differences in the occurrence of carotid transient ischemic attacks associated with antiplatelet aggregation therapy. *Stroke* 1973;**4**:732–6.

Eadie, MJ. A pathology of the animal spirits – the clinical neurology of Thomas Willis (1621–1675). Part I – background, and disorders of intrinsically normal animal spirits. *Journal of Clinical Neuroscience* 2003;**10**:14–29.

Eastcott, HH, GW Pickering, and CG Rob. Reconstruction of internal carotid artery in a patient with intermittent attacks of hemiplegia. *The Lancet* 1954;**267**:994–6.

Ebbs, JH. Cerebral sinus thrombosis in children. *Archives of Diseases of Children* 1937;**12**:133–52.

Echlin, FA. Current concepts in the etiology and treatment of vasospasm. *Clinical Neurosurgery* 1968;**15**:133–60.

Ecker, A and PA Riemenschneider. Arteriographic demonstration of spasm of the intracranial arteries, with special reference to saccular arterial aneurysms. *Journal of Neurosurgery* 1951;**8**:660–7.

Ecker, AD. Linear fracture of the skull across the venous sinuses. *New York State Journal of Medicine* 1946;**46**:1120–1.

Editorial. Internal carotid stenosis. *British Medical Journal* 1974;**I**:258.

Ehlers, H and CB Courville. Thrombosis of internal cerebral veins in infancy and childhood: review of literature and report of five cases. *Journal of Pediatrics* 1936;**8**:600–23.

Ehrmann, JA. Des effets produits sur l'encéphale par l'oblitération des vaisseaux artériels qui s'y distribuent, avec une statistique des cas de ligature de l'artère carotide. Thesis Paris, J. B. Baillière, 1860.

Eichenberger, P. *Johann Jakob Wepfer als klinischer Praktiker*. Basel/Stuttgart, Schwabe & Co., 1969.

Eichler, G. Zur Pathogenese der Hirnhämorrhagie. *Deutsches Archiv für klinische Medizin* 1878;**22**:1–32.

Eliot, G. *Middlemarch*. London, Penguin Classics, 2011 [1872].

Ellis, AG. The pathogenesis of spontaneous cerebral hemorrhage. *Proceedings of the Pathological Society of Philadelphia* 1909;**12**:197–235.

Ellis, H. The story of peripheral vascular surgery. *Journal of Perioperative Practice* 2019;**29**:254–6.

Emch-Dériaz, A. Samuel-Auguste Tissot. In Bynum, WF and Bynum, H, eds. *Dictionary of Medical Biography*. Westport, CT, Greenwood Press, 2007, 1229.

Eppinger, H. *Pathogenesis, Histogenesis und Aetiologie der Aneurysmen, einschliesslich des Aneurysma equi verminosum*. Berlin, August Hirschwald, 1887.

Eppinger, H. Die miliare Hirnarterieaneurysmen (Charcot–Bouchard). *Archiv für pathologische Anatomie und Physiologie und für klinische Medicin* 1888;**III**:405–14.

Erb, W. Ein Fall von ausgedehnter Gehirnerweichung bei totaler Obliteration der Carotis communis sinistra. *Münchener Medizinische Wochenschrift* 1904;**51**:946–7.

Esmarch, F and W Jessen. Syphilis und Geistesstörung. *Allgemeine Zeitschrift für Psychiatrie* 1857;**14**:20–36.

Ettmüller, M. *Opera omnia theoretica et practica*. Lugduni [s.n.], 1685.

Eulenburg, A. Ueber den Einfluss von Herzhypertrophie und Erkrankungen der Hirnarterien auf das Zustandekommen von Haemorrhagia Cerebri. *Archiv für pathologische Anatomie und Physiologie und für klinische Medicin* 1862;**24**:329–62.

Eyerel, J. De vita et scriptis Maximiliani Stollii. In Stoll, M, ed. *Pars quarta Rationis medendi in Nosocomio practico Vindobonensi*. Ticini, Typographiae Monasterii S. Salvatoris et Balthassaris Comini Bibliopolae, 1790, 9–15.

Fabricius ab Aquapendente, H. *De Venarum Ostiolis*. Patavii, Laurentius Pasquatus, 1603.

Fabricius, G. *Observationum & Curationum chirurgicarum Centuriae*. Basiliae, Sumptibus Ludovici Regis, 1606.

Fabricius, G. *Observationum et Curationum chirurgicarum Centuria tertia*. In Nobili Oppenhemio, Johan-Theod. de Bry, 1614.

Fairburn, B. 'Twin' intracranial aneurysms causing subarachnoid haemorrhage in identical twins. *British Medical Journal* 1973;**1**:210–11.

Falconer, MA. The surgical treatment of bleeding intracranial aneurysms. *Journal of Neurology, Neurosurgery, and Psychiatry* 1951;**14**:153–86.

Falconer, MA. Surgery of intracranial aneurysms (correspondence). *British Medical Journal* 1959;**1**:743–4.

Falkhusius, MP. De Apoplexia Positiones. Thesis Basileae, 1641.

Fantini, B. Lancisi, Giovanni Maria. In Bynum, WF and Bynum, H, eds. *Dictionary of Medical Biography*. Westwood, CT, Greenwood Press, 2007, 766–8.

Fearnsides, EG. Intracranial aneurysms. *Brain* 1916;**39**:224–96.

Feigin, I and P Prose. Hypertensive fibrinoid arteritis of the brain and gross cerebral hemorrhage. *Archives of Neurology* 1959;**1**:98–110.

Feindel, W and R Leblanc. *The Wounded Brain Healed: The Golden Age of the Montreal Neurological Institute, 1934–1984*. Montreal, McGill-Queen's University Press, 2016.

Fernelius, J. *De abditis Rerum Causis*. Parisiis, Christianus Wechelus, 1548.

Fernelius, J. *Medicina*. Lutetiae, Andreas Wechelus, 1554.

Ferrand, J. Essai sur l'hémiplégie des vieillards: les lacunes de désintégration cérébrales. Thesis Paris, Jules Rousset, 1902.

Ferro, JM. Egas Moniz and internal carotid occlusion. *Archives of Neurology* 1988;**45**:563–4.

Fields, WS, ES Crawford, and ME Debakey. Surgical considerations in cerebral arterial insufficiency. *Neurology* 1958;**8**:801–8.

Fields, WS, V Maslenikov, JS Meyer, et al. Joint study of extracranial arterial occlusion. V. Progress report of prognosis following surgery or nonsurgical treatment for transient cerebral ischemic attacks and cervical carotid artery lesions. *JAMA* 1970;**211**:1993–2003.

Fischer-Wasels, B. Die funktionellen Störungen des peripheren Kreislaufs. *Frankfurter Zeitschrift für Pathologie* 1933;**45–1**:1–164.

Fisher, CM. Occlusion of the internal carotid artery. *Archives of Neurology and Psychiatry* 1951;**65**:346–77.

Fisher, CM. Transient monocular blindness associated with hemiplegia. *Archives of Ophthalmology* 1952;**47**:167–203.

Fisher, CM. Occlusion of the carotid arteries: further experiences. *Archives of Neurology and Psychiatry* 1954;**72**:187–204.

Fisher, CM. Cranial bruit associated with occlusion of the internal carotid artery. *Neurology* 1957a;**7**:299–306.

Fisher, CM. Cerebral thromboangiitis obliterans. *Medicine (Baltimore)* 1957b;**36**:169–209.

Fisher, CM. The use of anticoagulants in cerebral thrombosis. *Neurology* 1958;**8**:311–32.

Fisher, CM. Observations of the fundus oculi in transient monocular blindness. *Neurology* 1959;**9**:333–47.

Fisher, CM. Lacunes: small, deep cerebral infarcts. *Neurology* 1965a;**15**:774–84.

Fisher, CM. The vascular lesion in lacunae. *Transactions of the American Neurological Association* 1965b;**90**:243–5.

Fisher, CM. Pure sensory stroke involving face, arm, and leg. *Neurology* 1965c;**15**:76–80.

Fisher, CM. A lacunar stroke. The dysarthria–clumsy hand syndrome. *Neurology* 1967a;**17**:614–17.

Fisher, CM. Vertigo in cerebrovascular disease. *Archives of Otolaryngology* 1967b;**85**:529–34.

Fisher, CM. Some neuro-ophthalmological observations. *Journal of Neurology, Neurosurgery, and Psychiatry* 1967c;**30**:383–92.

Fisher, CM. The arterial lesions underlying lacunes. *Acta Neuropathologica* 1969;**12**:1–15.

Fisher, CM. Pathological findings in hypertensive cerebral haemorrhage. *Journal of Neuropathology and Experimental Neurology* 1971;**30**:536–50.

Fisher, CM. Cerebral miliary aneurysms in hypertension. *American Journal of Pathology* 1972;**66**:313–30.

Fisher, CM. Ataxic hemiparesis. A pathologic study. *Archives of Neurology* 1978;**35**:126–8.

Fisher, CM. 'Transient monocular blindness' versus 'amaurosis fugax'. *Neurology* 1989;**39**:1622–4.

Fisher, CM. Lacunar infarction: a personal view. In Donnan, GA, *et al.*, eds. *Lacunar and Other Subcortical Infarctions*. Oxford, Oxford University Press, 1995, 16–20.

Fisher, CM and DG Cameron. Concerning cerebral vasospasm. *Neurology* 1953;**3**:468–73.

Fisher, CM and LR Caplan. Basilar artery branch occlusion: a cause of pontine infarction. *Neurology* 1971;**21**:900–5.

Fisher, CM and M Cole. Homolateral ataxia and crural paresis: a vascular syndrome. *Journal of Neurology, Neurosurgery, and Psychiatry* 1965;**28**:48–55.

Fisher, CM and HB Curry. Pure motor hemiplegia of vascular origin. *Archives of Neurology* 1965;**13**:30–44.

Fisher, CM, I Gore, N Okabe, *et al.* Calcification of the carotid siphon. *Circulation* 1965;**32**:538–48.

Fleck, L. *Entstehung und Entwicklung einer wissenschaftliche Tatsache: Einführung in die Lehre vom Denkstil und Denkkollektiv*. Frankfurt am Main, Suhrkamp, 1980 [1935].

Fleming, JF and AM Park. Dissecting aneurysms of the carotid artery following arteriography. *Neurology* 1959;**9**:1–6.

Foderé, FE. *De Apoplexia: Disquisitio theoretico-practica*. Avenione/Parisiis, Seguin Fratres and Croullebois, 1808.

Foerster, O and L Guttman. Cerebrale Complicationen bei Thrombangiitis obliterans. *Archiv für Psychiatrie und Nervenkrankheiten* 1933;**100**:506–15.

Foerster, R. Amaurosis partialis fugax. *Klinische Monatsblätter für Augenheilkunde* 1869;**7**:422–30.

Foix, C, P Hillemand, and J Ley. Relativement au ramollissement cérébral, à sa fréquence et à son siège, et à l'importance relative des oblitérations artérielles complètes ou incomplètes dans sa pathogénie. *Bulletins et Mémoires de la Société Médicale des Hôpitaux de Paris* 1927;**III–51**:191–9.

Foix, C and M Lévy. Les ramollissements sylviens; syndromes des lésions en foyer du territoire de l'artère sylvienne et de ses branches. *Revue Neurologique* 1927;**35**:1–51.

Foix, C and J Ley. Contribution à l'étude du ramollissement cérébral envisagé en point de vue de sa fréquence, de son siège, et de l'état anatomique des artères du territoire nécrosé. *Journal de Neurologie et de Psychiatrie* 1927;**27**:658–84.

Foix, C and I Nicolescu. Contribution à l'étude des grands syndromes de désintégration sénile cérébro-mésencéphalique. *Presse Médicale* 1923;**31**:957–63.

Foley, J. Benign forms of intracranial hypertension: 'toxic' and 'otitic' hydrocephalus. *Brain* 1955;**78**:1–41.

Forestus, P. *Observationum en Curationum medicinalium ac chirurgicarum Opera omnia*, Tomus I. Rothomagi, J. and D. Berthelin, 1653 [1590].

Forsheim, A. Ein Beitrag zum Studium der spontanen Subarachnoidalblutung. *Deutsche Zeitschrft für Nervenheilkunde* 1913;**49**:123–32.

Foucault, M. *Naissance de la Clinique: une Archéologie du Regard médical*. Paris, Presses Universitaires de France, 1963.

France, JF. Examples of ptosis, with illustrative remarks. *Guy's Hospital Reports* 1846;**II–4**:37–63.

Frank-van Westrienen, A. *De groote Tour: Tekening van de Educatiereis der Nederlanders in de zeventiende Eeuw*. Amsterdam, Noord-Hollandsche Uitgeversmaatschappij, 1983.

Frederiks, JAM and PJ Koehler. The first lumbar puncture. *Journal of the History of the Neurosciences* 1997;**6**:147–53.

French, R. Harvey in Holland. In French, R and Wear, A, eds. *The Medical Revolution of the Seventeenth Century*. Cambridge, Cambridge University Press, 1989, 46–86.

French, R. *William Harvey's Natural Philosophy*. Cambridge, Cambridge University Press, 1994.

French, RK. Berengario. In Wear, A, *et al.*, eds. *The Medical Renaissance of the Sixteenth Century*. Cambridge, Cambridge University Press, 1985, 42–74.

Frenckner, P. Sinography: a method of radiography in the diagnosis of sinus thrombosis. *Journal of Laryngology and Otology* 1937;**52**:350–61.

Friedensburg, W. *Geschichte der Universität Wittenburg*. Halle a. S., Max Niemeyer, 1917.

Friedman, GD, WS Wilson, JM Mosier, *et al.* Transient ischemic attacks in a community. *JAMA* 1969;**210**:1428–34.

Fritsch, G and E Hitzig. Über die elektrische Erregbarkeit des Großhirns. *Archiv für Anatomie, Physiologie und Wissenschaftliche Medicin* 1870;**36**:300–32.

Frixione, E. Irritable glue. In Whitaker, H, *et al.*, eds. *Brain, Mind and Medicine: Essays in Eighteenth-Century Neuroscience*. New York, NY, Springer, 2007, 115–25.

Froin, G. Les hémorragies sous-arachnoidiennes et le méchanisme de l'hématolyse en général. Thesis Paris, G. Steinheil, 1904.

Frøvig, AG. Bilateral obliteration of the common carotid artery: thrombangiitis obliterans? *Acta Psychiatrica et Neurologica* 1946; Suppl. 39:3–78.

Fuchs, CH. *Beobachtungen und Bemerkungen über Gehirnerweichung*. Leipzig, Weygand'sche Verlag Buchhandlung (L. Gebhardt), 1838.

Fulton, J. *Harvey Cushing: A Biography*. Springfield, IL, Charles C. Thomas, 1946.

Galdston, M, SR Govons, SB Wortis, *et al.* Thrombosis of the common, internal and external carotid arteries. *Archives of Internal Medicine* 1941;**67**:1162–76.

Galenus. De Causis Pulsuum. In Brassavola, AM, ed. *Galeni Libri*. Venetiis, Apud Iuntas, 1625a [*c.*180], Classis 4.

Galenus. De Locis affectis. In Brassavola, AM, ed. Galeni Libri. Venetiis, Apud Iuntas, 1625b [*c.*180], Classis 4.

Galenus. De Usu Partium. In Brassavola, AM, ed. *Galeni Libri*. Venetiis, Apud Iuntas, 1625c [*c.*180], Classis 1.

Gallo, D. L'Età Medioevale. In Del Negro, P, ed. *L'Università di Padova: otto Secoli di Storia*. Padova, Signumpadova, 2001, 1–33.

Galvani, A. *De Viribus Electricitatis in Motu musculari Commentarius*. Bononiae, Ex Typographia Instituti Scientiarum, 1791.

Garcin, R and M Pestel. *Thrombo-phlébites cérébrales*. Paris, Masson, 1949.

Gass, HH, JF McGuire, and DR Simmons. Intracranial eradication of middle cerebral aneurysms. *Journal of Neurosurgery* 1958;**15**:223–32; discussion 232–3.

Gay, J-A. *Vues sur le Caractère et le Traitement de l'Apoplexie, dans lesquelles on réfute la Doctrine du Docteur Portal sur cette Maladie*. Paris, Didot Jeune, 1807.

Gay, J-A. *Traité contre la Saignée*. Paris, Frèrcs Manie, 1808.

Gay, J-A. *An Essay on the Nature and Treatment of Apoplexy*. London/Norwhich, John Churchill and Charles Muskett, 1843.

Geier, M. *Die Brüder Humboldt – eine Biographie*. Reinbek, Rowohlt, 2009.

Gély, A. Observation d'inflammation de la carotide interne, avec ramollissement du cerveau, suivie de réflections sur cette observation. *Archives Génerales de Médecine* 1837;**II–15**:331–46.

Gildemeester, JP and EF Hoyack. Syphilis secundaria, meningitis cerebralis circumscipta, obturatio art. fossae Sylvii dextrae, emollitio corp. striati dextri. *Nederlands Weekblad voor Geneeskunde* 1854;**4**:23–6.

Gillan, LA. Blood supply to brains of ungulates with and without a rete mirabile caroticum. *Journal of Comparative Neurology* 1974;**153**:275–90.

Gills, JP, Jr, JP Kapp, and GL Odom. Benign intracranial hypertension: pseudotumor cerebri from obstruction of dural sinuses. *Archives of Ophthalmology* 1967;**78**:592–5.

Giroud, F. *Une femme honorable: Marie Curie*. Paris, Arthème Fayard, 1991.

Glasser, O. *Wilhlelm Conrad Röntgen und die Geschichte der Röntgenstrahlen*, 2nd edn. Berlin, Springer Verlag, 1959.

Globus, JH and JA Epstein. Massive cerebral hemorrhage: spontaneous and experimentally induced. *Journal of Neuropathology and Experimental Neurology* 1953;**12**:107–31.

Globus, JH, JA Epstein, MA Green, *et al.* Focal cerebral hemorrhage experimentally induced. *Journal of Neuropathology and Experimental Neurology* 1949;**8**:113–16.

Globus, JH and I Strauss. Massive cerebral hemorrhage; its relation to preexisting cerebral softening. *Archives of Neurology and Psychiatry* 1927;**18**:215–39.

Gluge. Recherches microscopiques et expérimentales sur le ramollissement du cerveau. *Archives de Médecine Belge* 1840;**1**:180–98.

Goetz, CG. Pierre Marie: gifted intellect, poor timing and unchecked emotionality. *Journal of the History of the Neurosciences* 2003;**12**:154–66.

Goetz, CG, M Bonduelle, and T Gelfand. *Charcot: Constructing Neurology.* Oxford, Oxford University Press, 1995.

Goldflam, S. Beitrag zur Ätiologie und Symptomatalogie der spontanen subarachnoidalen Blutungen. *Deutsche Zeitschrft für Nervenheilkunde* 1923;**76**:158–82.

Goldner, J, JP Wisnant, and WF Taylor. Long-term prognosis of transient cerebral ischemic attacks. *Stroke* 1971;**2**:160–7.

Goldschmid, E. *Entwicklung und Bibliographie der pathologisch-anatomischen Abbildung.* Leipzig, Karl W. Hiersemann, 1925.

Gordon-Taylor, G and EW Walls. *Sir Charles Bell: His Life and Times.* Edinburgh, E. and S. Livingstone Ltd, 1958.

Goschler, C. *Rudolf Virchow: Mediziner, Anthropologe, Politiker.* Köln/Weimar/Wien, Böhlau Verlag, 2009.

Gouguenheim, A. Tumeurs anévrysmales des artères du cerveau. Thesis Paris, Adrien Delahaye, 1866.

Govons, SR and FC Grant. Angiographic visualisation of cerebrovascular lesions. *Archives of Neurology and Psychiatry* 1946;**55**:600–18.

Gowers, WR. *Manual and Atlas of Medical Ophthalmoscopy.* London, J. & A. Churchill, 1882.

Gowers, WR. *A Manual of Diseases of the Nervous System,* 2nd edn. London, J. & A. Churchill, 1893.

Graf, CJ. Prognosis for patients with nonsurgically-treated aneurysms. Analysis of the cooperative study of intracranial aneurysms and subarachnoid hemorrhage. *Journal of Neurosurgery* 1971;**35**:438–43.

Graf, CJ, JC Torner, GE Perret, *et al.* Long-term follow-up evaluation of randomised study. In

Sahs, AL, *et al.*, eds. *Aneurysmal Subarachnoid Hemorrhage.* Baltimore/Munich, Urban and Schwarzenberg, 1981, 203–48.

Grandjean de Fouchy, JP. Observation anatomique. In *Histoire de l'Académie royale des Sciences: année 1784.* Paris, Imprimerie Royale, 1787, 400.

Granier, JE. *Traité de l'Apoplexie, considerée en elle-même, d'après les Vues anciennes et modernes, et relativement aux Maladies qui la simulent, la précèdent, l'accompagnent ou lui succèdent.* Paris, Béchet Jeune, 1826.

Grasset, J. La cérébrosclérose lacunaire progressive d'origine artérielle. *Semaine Médicale* 1904;**24**:329–31.

Green, FHK. Miliary aneurysms in the brain. *Journal of Pathology and Bacteriology* 1930;**33**:71–7.

Greer, M. Benign intracranial hypertension. I. Mastoiditis and lateral sinus obstruction. *Neurology* 1962;**12**:472–6.

Gregory, F. *Natural Science in Western History.* Boston, MA, Houghton Mifflin Company, 2008.

Grenier, P-J. Du ramollissement sénile du cerveau. Thesis Paris, 1868.

Griesinger, W. Fortgesetzte Beobachtungen über Hirnkrankheiten. IV. Das Aneurisma der Basilararterie. *Archiv für Heilkunde* 1862;**3**:548–68.

Groch, SN, LJ Hurwitz, E McDevitt, *et al.* Problems of anticoagulant therapy in cerebrovascular disease. *Neurology* 1959;**9**:786–93.

Grzybowski, A and B Sobolewska. Carl Friedrich Richard Foerster (1825–1902): the inventor of perimeter and photometer. *Acta Ophthalmologica* 2015;**93**:586–90.

Guidetti, B, R Giuffre, and D Gambacorta. Follow-up study of 100 cases of pseudotumor cerebri. *Acta Neurochirurgica (Wien)* 1968;**18**:259–67.

Guillain, G and P Mathieu. *La Salpêtrière.* Paris, Masson et Cie, 1925.

Gulczynski, J, E Izycka-Swieszewska, and M Grzybiak. Short history of the autopsy. Part I. From prehistory to the middle of the 16th century. *Polish Journal of Pathology* 2009;**60**:109–14.

Gull, W. Thickening and dilatation of the arch of the aorta, with occlusion of the innominata and left carotid, atrophic softening of the brain. *Guy's Hospital Reports* 1855;**III–1**:12–18.

Gull, W. Cases of aneurisms of cerebral vessels. *Guy's Hospital Reports* 1859;**III–5**:283–304.

Gunewardene, HO. The stroke in high arterial pressure: a study of 150 cases. *British Medical Journal*, 1932;**1**:180–2.

Gurdjian, ES and LM Thomas. Cerebral vaso-spasm. *Surgery, Gynecology, and Obstetrics* 1969;**129**:931–48.

Guthrie, LG and S Mayou. Right hemiplegia and atrophy of left optic nerve. *Proceedings of the Royal Society of Medicine* 1908;**1**:180–4.

Hale-White, W. Intracranial aneurysm in young subjects unaffected with syphilis or malignant endocarditis. *British Medical Journal* 1894;**2**:869.

Hannaway, C. Cruveilhier, Jean. In Bynum, WF and Bynum, H, eds. *Dictionary of Medical Biography*. Westport, CT, Greenwood Press, 2007, 377–8.

Hannaway, C and A La Berge. Paris medicine: perspectives past and present. In Hannaway, C and La Berge, A, eds. *Constructing Paris Medicine*. Amsterdam/Atlanta, GA, Rodopi, 1998, 1–70.

Hanson, NR. *Patterns of Discovery: An Inquiry into the Conceptual Foundations of Science*. Cambridge, Cambridge University Press, 1958.

Harbridge, DF. Monocular visible spasm of the central artery of the retina. *Ophthalmology* 1906;**2**:647–53.

Hare, CJ. Case of complete paralysis of the motor oculi of the left side, dependent upon aneurysm of the left posterior communicating artery. *London Journal of Medicine* 1850;**2**:824–32.

Haroun, RI, D Rigamonti, and RJ Tamargo. Recurrent artery of Heubner: Otto Heubner's description of the artery and his influence on pediatrics in Germany. *Journal of Neurosurgery* 2000;**93**:1084–8.

Harris, CRS. *The Heart and the Vascular System in Ancient Greek Medicine: From Alcmaeon to Galen*. Oxford, Clarendon Press, 1973.

Harrison, MJG, J Marshall, JC Meadows, *et al.* Effect of aspirin in amaurosis fugax. *The Lancet* 1971;**2**:743–4.

Harveius, G. *Exercitatio anatomica de Motu Cordis et Sanguinis in Animalibus.* Francofurti, Guilelmus Fitzer, 1628.

Haslam, J. *Observations on Insanity, with Practical Remarks on the Disease, and an Account of the Morbid Appearances on Dissection.* London, F. and C. Rivington, 1798.

Hasse, KE. Ueber die Verschliessung der Hirnarterien als nächste Ursache einer Form von Hirnerweichung. *Zeitschrift für rationelle Medicin* 1846;**4**:91–111.

Hayem, G. Glio-sarcomes de la pie-mère – compression et oblitération des artères syl-viennes – ramollissement cérébrale consécutif – autopsie. *Archives de Physiologie Normale et Pathologique* 1869;**2**:126–31.

Heberden, G. *Commentarii de Morborum Historia et Curatione.* Londini, T. Payne, 1802.

Helm, J and K Stukenbrock. Hoffmann, Friedrich. In Bynum, WF and Bynum, H, eds. *Dictionary of Medical Biography*. Westport, CT, Greenwood Press, 2007, 657–8.

Helmholtz, H. *Beschreibung eines Augen-Spiegels.* Berlin, A. Förstnersche Verlagsbuchhandlung (P. Jeanrenaud), 1851.

Henderson, WG, JC Torner, and DW Nibbelink. Intracranial aneurysms and sub-arachnoid hemorrhage – report on a random-ized treatment study. IV-B. Regulated bed rest – statistical evaluation. *Stroke* 1977;**8**:579–89.

Henle, J. *Medizinische Wissenschaft und Empirie. Zeitschrift für rationelle Medicin* 1844;**1**:1–35.

Herpin, F. Discours sur la tombe de M. le doc-teur Louis Tonnellé. Tours, Imprimerie Ladevèze, 1860.

Heschl, R. Die Capillar-aneurysmen im Pons Varoli. *Wiener Medizinische Wochenschrift* 1865;**15**:1285–7, 1314–16.

Heubner, O. *Die luetische Erkrankung der Hirnarterien.* Leipzig, F. C. W. Vogel, 1874.

Hicks, SP and S Warren. Infarction of the brain without thrombosis: an analysis of one hun-dred cases with autopsy. *Archives of Pathology* 1951;**52**:403–12.

Hill, AB, J Marshall, and DA Shaw. A controlled clinical trial of long-term anticoagulant therapy in cerebrovascular disease. *Quarterly Journal of Medicine* 1960;**29**:597–609.

Hill, AB, J Marshall, and DA Shaw. Cerebrovascular disease: trial of long-term anticoagulant therapy. *British Medical Journal* 1962;**2**:1003–6.

Hiller, F. Zirkulationsstörungen im Gehirn: eine klinische und pathologisch-anatomische Studie. *Archiv für Psychiatrie und Nervenkrankheiten* 1935;**103**:1–52.

Hippocrates. On wounds in the head. In Withington, ET, ed. *Hippocrates, III (The Loeb Classical Library)*. London, William Heinemann, 1959a [*c.*400 BCE], 44–5.

Hippocrates. Aphorisms. In Jones, WHS, ed. *Hippocrates, IV (The Loeb Classical Library)*. London, William Heinemann, 1959b [*c.*400 BCE], 97–221.

Hippocrates. Epidemics 7. In Smith, WD, ed. *Hippocrates, VII (The Loeb Classical Library)*. Cambridge, MA, Harvard University Press, 1994 [*c.*400 BCE], 337–8.

Hirsch, A. *Biographisches Lexikon der hervorragenden Aertzte aller Zeiten und Völker*. Wien/Leipzig, Urban and Schwarzenberg, 1884–8.

Hirsch, C. Die Zirkulationsstörungen des Gehirns. In Curschmann, H, ed. *Lehrbuch der Nervenkrankheiten*. Berlin, Julius Springer, 1909, 586–617.

Hodgson, J. *A Treatise on the Diseases of Arteries and Veins, Containing the Pathology and Treatment of Aneurisms and Wounded Arteries*. London, Thomas Underwood, 1815.

Hoffmann, F. *Medicina rationalis systematica*. Halae Magdeburgicae, Renger, 1732.

Hofmann, C. *Institutionum medicarum Libri sex*. Lugdunum, Ioan. Antonius Huguetan, 1645.

Hollenhorst, RW. Significance of bright plaques in the retinal arterioles. *Transactions of the American Ophthalmological Society* 1961;**59**:252–73.

Holmes, G and P Sargent. Injuries of the superior longitudinal sinus. *British Medical Journal* 1915;**2**:493–8.

Horton, R. The moribund body of medical history. *The Lancet* 2014;**384**:292.

Howship, J. Observations on diseases of the brain, with cases and dissections. *Medical and Physical Journal* 1810;**14**:89–98.

Hughes, W, MCH Dodgson, and DC MacLennan. Chronic cerebral hypertensive disease. *The Lancet* 1954;**264**:770–4.

Huisman, F. The dialectics of understanding: on genres and the use of debate in medical history. *History and Philosophy of the Life Sciences* 2005;**27**:13–40.

Huizinga, J. *The Waning of the Middle Ages*. London, Penguin Books, 1922.

Hultquist, GT. *Über Thrombose und Embolie der Arteria carotis*. Jena, Gustav Fischer, 1942.

Hunt, JR. The role of the carotid arteries, in the causation of vascular lesions of the brain, with remarks on certain special features of the symptomatology. *American Journal of Medical Sciences* 1914;**147**:714–13.

Hunt, WE and RM Hess. Surgical risk as related to time of intervention in the repair of intracranial aneurysms. *Journal of Neurosurgery* 1968;**28**:14–20.

Hürlimann, B. Das Vermächtnis der Philipp Schwartz. *Neue Zürcher Zeitung* 2013;37.

Hurwitz, LJ, SN Groch, IS Wright, *et al.* Carotid artery occlusive syndrome. *Archives of Neurology* 1959;**1**:491–501.

Husemann, A. Konrad Heinrich Fuchs. In Traugott, RW, ed. *Allgemeine Deutsche Biographie*. Leipzig, Duncker & Humblot, 1878, 168–9.

Hutchinson, EC and PO Yates. The cervical portion of the vertebral artery: a clinico-pathological study. *Brain* 1956;**79**:319–31.

Hutchinson, EC and PO Yates. Caroticovertebral stenosis. *The Lancet* 1957;**272**:2–8.

Hutchinson, J. On a case of aneurysm of the internal carotid within the skull, diagnosed eleven years before the patient's death. Spontaneous cure. *Transactions of the Clinical Society of London* 1875;**8**:127–31.

Hutin, C. De la tempéture dans l'hémorrhagie cérébrale et le ramollissement. Thesis Paris, 1877.

Hyland, HH. Thrombosis of intracranial arteries; report of three cases involving, respectively, the anterior cerebral, basilar and internal carotid arteries. *Archives of Neurology and Psychiatry* 1933;**30**:342–56.

Imbert, M. Assoupissement extraordinaire. In *Histoire de l'Académie des Sciences, année 1713*.

Amsterdam, chez Pierre de Coup, 1717, 419–24.

Ingvar, S. Sur les hémorragies méningées. *Nouvelle Iconographie de la Salpêtrière* 1916;**28**:313–42.

Iragui, VJ. The Charcot–Bouchard controversy. *Archives of Neurology* 1986;**43**:290–5.

Irish, CW. Thrombosis of the superior cerebral vein. *Annals of Otology, Rhinology, and Laryngology* 1938;**47**:775–91.

JCR. Herbert Hylton Hyland. *Canadian Journal of Neurological Sciences* 1978;**5**:51.

JT. Robert Alexander Lundie. *Edinburgh Medical Journal* 1919;**22**:42–5.

Jaccoud, S. Bibliographie: clinical lectures on the principles and practice of medicine. *Gazette Hebdomadaire de Médecine et de Chirurgie* 1861;**8**:440–4.

Jackson, JH. A lecture on softening of the brain. *The Lancet* 1875;**106**:335–9.

Jaffé, R. Hypertonus und Apoplexie. *Zeitschrift für ärztliche Fortbildung* 1927;**24**:477–81.

James, TGI. Thrombosis of the internal carotid artery. *British Medical Journal* 1949;**2**:1264–7.

Jelliffe, SE and WA White. *Diseases of the Nervous System: A Textbook of Neurology and Psychiatry*, 4th edn. London, H. K. Lewis & Co., 1923.

Jennings, EA. Case of aneurism of the basilar artery. *Transactions of the Provincial Medical and Surgical Society* 1836;**1**:270–4.

Joffroy, A. Rhumatisme articulaire aigu, affection cardiacque, embolie cérébrale, hémiplégie gauche, embolie dans les artères des membres inférieurs, gangrène de la jambe gauche, autopsie, coagulations anciennes dans l'auricule gauche, retablissement du circulation cérébrale par organisation et retraction du caillot embolique. *Comptes Rendus des Séances et Mémoires de la Société de Biologie* 1869;**V–I**:230–4.

Johnson, HC and AE Walker. The angiographic diagnosis of spontaneous thrombosis of the internal and common carotid arteries. *Journal of Neurosurgery* 1951;**8**:631–59.

Johnson, J. Case of meningeal apoplexy, with some remarkable phenomena, and the appearances of dissection. *The London Medical and Physical Journal* 1824;**51**:364–9.

Johnson, RV, SR Kaplan, and ZR Blailock. Cerebral venous thrombosis in paroxysmal nocturnal hemoglobinuria. Marchiafava-Micheli syndrome. *Neurology* 1970;**20**:681–6.

Johnston, I and A Paterson. Benign intracranial hypertension. I. Diagnosis and prognosis. *Brain* 1974;**97**:289–300.

Jones, EWP. The life and works of Guilhelmus Fabricius Hildanus (1560–1634): part I. *Medical History* 1960;**4**:112–34.

Jones, PM. Reading medicine. In Nutton, V and Porter, R, eds. *The History of Medical Education in Britain*. Amsterdam/Atlanta, GA, Rodopi, 1995, 153–83.

Kalbag, RM and AL Woolf. *Cerebral Venous Thrombosis*. Oxford, Oxford University Press, 1967.

Kannel, WB. Role of blood pressure in cardiovascular disease: the Framingham study. *Angiology* 1975;**26**:1–14.

Kannel, WB, TR Dawber, A Kagan, *et al.* Factors of risk in the development of coronary heart disease: six year follow-up experience. The Framingham Study. *Annals of Internal Medicine* 1961;**55**:33–50.

Karenberg, A and I Hort. Medieval descriptions and doctrines of stroke: preliminary analysis of select sources. Part I: The struggle for terms and theories – late antiquity and early Middle Ages. *Journal of the History of the Neurosciences* 1998a;**7**:162–73.

Karenberg, A and I Hort. Medieval descriptions and doctrines of stroke: preliminary analysis of select sources. Part II: between Galenism and Aristotelism – Islamic theories of apoplexy (800–1200). *Journal of the History of the Neurosciences* 1998b;**7**:174–85.

Karenberg, A and I Hort. Medieval descriptions and doctrines of stroke: preliminary analysis of select sources. Part III: multiplying speculation – the high and late Middle Ages (1000–1450). *Journal of the History of the Neurosciences* 1998c;**7**:186–200.

Karp, HR, A Heyman, S Heyden, *et al.* Transient cerebral ischemia. Prevalence and prognosis in a biracial rural community. *JAMA* 1973;**225**:125–8.

Kass, AM and EH Kass. *Perfecting the World: The Life and Times of Dr. Thomas Hodgkin*

1798–1866. New York, NY, Harcourt Brace Jovanovich, 1988.

Kaufman, MH. Bell, Charles. In Bynum, WF and Bynum, H, eds. *Dictionary of Medical Biography*. Westport, CT, Greenwood Press, 2007, 183–5.

Keele, CA. Pathological changes in the carotid sinus and their relation to hypertension. *Quarterly Journal of Medicine* 1933;**II–2**:213–20.

Kelly, C. Thrombosis of the middle cerebral artery: white softening of the brain. *The Lancet* 1870;**95**:409.

Kendell, RE and J Marshall. Role of hypotension in the genesis of transient focal cerebral ischaemic attacks. *British Medical Journal* 1963;**2**:344–8.

Key, A and G Retzius. Studien in der Anatomie des Nervensystems. *Archiv für mikroskopische Anatomie* 1873;**9**:308–86.

Key, A and G Retzius. *Studien in der Anatomie des Nervensystems und des Bindegewebes*. Stockholm, Samson and Wallin, 1875–6.

Kinal, ME. Traumatic thrombosis of dural venous sinuses in closed head injuries. *Journal of Neurosurgery* 1967;**27**:142–5.

King, AB and OR Langworthy. Neurologic symptoms after extensive occlusion of the common or internal carotid artery. *Archives of Neurology and Psychiatry* 1941;**46**:835–42.

King, LS and MC Meehan. A history of the autopsy: a review. *American Journal of Pathology* 1973;**73**:514–44.

King, T. Remarks on aneurysms of the cerebral arteries. *The Medical Quarterly Review* 1835;**3**:434–8.

Kirkes, WS. On some of the principal effects resulting from the detachment of fibrinous deposits from the interior of the heart, and their mixture with the circulating blood. *Medico-Chirurgical Transactions* 1852;**II–17**:281–324.

Kirkes, WS. On apoplexy in relation to chronic renal disease. *The Times and Medical Gazette* 1855;**II**:515–17.

Kirkland, T. A. *Commentary on Apoplectic and Paralytic Affections and on Diseases Connected with the Subject*. London, William Dawson, 1792.

Kluyskens, C. Des maladies inflammatoires survenant pendant les suites de couches. Thesis Louvain, 1876.

Knapp, H. Ueber Verstopfung der Blutgefässe des Auges. *Archiv für Ophthalmologie* 1868;**14**:207–56.

Knoeff, R, ed. *Histories of Healthy Ageing*. Groningen, Bakhuis and University Museum Groningen, 2017.

Koch, GP. De apoplexiae ex praecordiorum origine. In Ackermann, JGC, ed. *Philippi Georgii Schroeder Opuscula omnia*. Norimbergiae, Ioh. Georg. Lochner, 1779 [1767], 338–84.

Koppe, FAH. Dr. med. Heinrich Wichern. *Berichte des Naturwissenschaftlichen Verein für Bielefeld und Umgegend* 1950;**II**:12–13.

Korotkoff, NS. Concerning the problem of the methods of blood pressure measurement. *Proceedings of the Emperor's Military Medical Academy St Petersburg* 1905;**II**:365–7. [in Russian; reprinted and translated in *Journal of Hypertension* 2005;23:5]

Krayenbühl, H. Zur Diagnostik und chirurgische Therapie der zerebralen Erscheinungen bei der Endangiitis obliterans v. Winiwarter-Buerger. *Schweizerische Medizinische Wochenschrift* 1945;**75**:1025–9.

Krayenbühl, H. Cerebral venous thrombosis. The diagnostic value of cerebral angiography. *Schweizer Archiv für Neurologie und Psychiatrie* 1954;**74**:261–87.

Krayenbühl, H and G Weber. Die Thrombose der Arteria carotis interna und ihre Beziehung zur Endangiitis obliterans v. Winiwarter-Buerger. *Helvetica Medica Acta* 1944;**II**:289–333.

Kubik, CS and RD Adams. Occlusion of the basilar artery: a clinical and pathological study. *Brain* 1946;**69**:73–121.

Kühn, CG, ed. *Claudii Galeni Opera omnia*. Lipsiae, Karl Cnobloch, 1821–33.

Kussmaul, A. Zwei Fälle von spontaner allmähliger Verschliessung grosser Halsarterienstämme. *Deutsche Klinik* 1872;461–5, 473–4.

Laborde, J-V. *Le Ramollissement et la Congestion du Cerveau, principalement considérés chez le Vieillard*. Paris, Adrien Delahaye, 1866.

Lallemand, F. *Recherches anatomopathologiques sur l'Encéphale et ses Dépendances*. Paris, Baudoin Frères, 1820–34.

Lancereaux, É. De la thrombose et de l'embolie cérébrales, considérées principalement dans leur rapports avec le ramollissement du cerveau. Thesis Paris, 1862.

Lancisius, JM. *De Mortibus subitaneis.* Luca, Peregrinus Fredianus, 1707.

Lazerme, J. *Tractatus de Morbis internis Capitis.* Amstelodami, Sumptibus societatis, 1748.

Le Roy Ladurie, E. *Le siècle des Platter (1499–1628). Tome 1: le Mendiant et le Professeur.* Paris, Fayard, 1995.

Lebert, H. Ueber Aneurysmen der Hirnarterien. *Berliner klinische Wochenschrift* 1866;**3**:209–12, 229–31, 249–51, 281–5, 336–8, 345–7, 386–90, 402–5.

Leriche, R. Experimental and clinical basis for arterectomy in the treatment of localized arterial obstructions. *American Journal of Surgery* 1931;**14**:55–67.

Leriche, R, R Fontaine, and SM Dupertuis. Arterectomy: with follow-up studies on 78 operations. *Surgery, Gynaecology, and Obstetrics* 1937;**64**:149–55.

Leune, JCF. *De Apoplexia.* Lipsiae, Apud Joan. Ambros. Barthium, 1817.

Lhermitte, F, JC Gautier, and C Derouesne. Nature of occlusions of the middle cerebral artery. *Neurology* 1970;**20**:82–8.

Lieutaud, J. *Essais anatomiques, contenant l'Histoire exacte de tous les Parties qui composent le Corps de l'Homme, avec la Manière de dissequer.* Paris, P. M. Huart, 1742.

Lieutaud, J. *Historia anatomico-medica, sistens numerosissima Cadaverum humanorum Extispicia, quibus in apricum venit genuina Morborum Sedes; horumque referantur Causae, vel patent Effectus.* Parisiis, Vincent, 1767.

Limb, M. Michael Harrison: clinical neurologist and stroke researcher. *British Medical Journal* 2019;**336**:l5502.

Lin, PM, H Javid, and EJ Doyle. Partial internal carotid artery occlusion treated by primary resection and vein graft: report of a case. *Journal of Neurosurgery* 1956;**13**:650–5.

Lindeboom, GA. *Dutch medical Biography: A biographical Dictionary of Dutch Physicians and Surgeons 1475–1975.* Amsterdam, Rodopi, 1984a.

Lindeboom, GA. *Herman Boerhaave: The Man and His Work.* London, Methuen & Co. Ltd, 1984b.

Lindemann, H. Die Hirngefässe in apoplektischen Blutungen. *Virchow's Archiv für pathologische Anatomie und Physiologie und für klinische Medizin* 1924;**253**:27–44.

Lindenberg, R and H Spatz. Über die Thromboendarteriitis der Hirngefäße (cerebrale Form der v. Winiwarter-Buergerschen Krankheit). *Virchow's Archiv für pathologische Anatomie und Physiologie und für klinische Medizin* 1939;**305**:531–56.

Litten, M. Apoplexie des Gehirns und der Retina bedingt durch miliare Aneurysmen. *Berliner klinische Wochenschrift* 1881;**18**:25–7.

Locksley, HB, AL Sahs, and L Knowler. Report on the cooperative study of intracranial aneurysms and subarachnoid hemorrhage. Section II. General survey of cases in the central registry and characteristics of the sample population. *Journal of Neurosurgery* 1966;**24**:922–32.

Loeper, M. Bouchard. In Dumesnil, R and Bonnet-Roy, F, eds. *Die berühmten Ärzte.* Genf, Lucien Mazenod, 1947, 248–9.

Logue, V. Surgery in spontaneous subarachnoid haemorrhage: operative treatment of aneurysms on the anterior cerebral and anterior communicating artery. *British Medical Journal* 1956a;**1**:473–9.

Logue, V. Surgery of intracranial aneurysms. *British Medical Journal* 1956b;**1**:986.

Loman, J and A Myerson. Visualisation of cerebral vessels by direct intracarotid injection of thorium dioxide (thorotrast). *American Journal of Roentgenology and Radium Therapy* 1936;**35**:188–93.

Lorry, A-C. *De Melancholia et Morbis Melancholicis.* Paris, Guillelmus Cavelier, 1765.

Löwenfeld, L. *Studien über Aetiologie und Pathogenese der spontanen Hirnblutungen.* Wiesbaden, J. F. Bergmann, 1886.

Lucretius. *De Rerum Natura* (Bailey, C, ed.). Oxford, Oxford University Press, 1947 [*c.*59 BCE].

Lundie, RA. Transient blindness due to spasm of the retinal artery. *The Ophthalmic Review* 1906;**25**:129–40.

Lycosthenes, C. *Prodigiorum ac Ostentorum Chronicon*. Basileae, Henricus Petri, 1557.

Lyons, C and G Galbraith. Surgical treatment of atherosclerotic occlusion of the internal carotid artery. *Annals of Surgery* 1957;**146**:487–96; discussion 496–8.

Lysak, WR and HJ Svien. Long-term follow-up on patients with diagnosis of pseudotumor cerebri. *Journal of Neurosurgery* 1966;**25**:284–7.

Macewen, JAC. Purulent mastoiditis: sinus thrombosis, threatened cerebral abscess, recovery after operation. *Annals of Surgery* 1904;**40**:348–9.

Maclean, I. *Logic, Signs and Nature in the Renaissance: The Case of Medicine*. Cambridge, Cambridge University Press, 2002.

Macmillan, M. Localization and William Macewen's early brain surgery – part II: the cases. *Journal of the History of the Neurosciences* 2005;**14**:24–56.

Maire, I, ed. *Recentiorum Disceptationes de Motu Cordis, Sanguinis et Chili in Animalibus*. Lugduni Batavorum, Ioannes Maire, 1647.

Malpigius, M. De pulmonibus epistola II. In Malpigius, M. *Exercitationes de Structura Viscerum*. Francofurti, Augustus Boetius, 1683 [1661], 241–52.

Mangetus, JJ. *Theophili Boneti Medicinae Doctoris Sepulchretum, sive Anatomia practica ex Cadaveribus Morbo denatis*. Genevae, Cramer and Perachon, 1700.

Manschot, WA. The fundus oculi in subarachnoid haemorrhage. *Acta Ophthalmologica* 1944;**22**:281–91.

Manschot, WA. Subarachnoid hemorrhage: intraocular symptoms and their pathogenesis. *American Journal of Ophthalmology* 1954;**38**:501–5.

Marais, S, G Thwaites, JF Schoeman, *et al.* Tuberculous meningitis: a uniform case definition for use in clinical research. *The Lancet Infectious Diseases* 2010;**10**:803–12.

Marey, ÉJ. *Recherches sur le pouls au moyen d'un nouvel appareil enregistreur: le sphygmographe*. Paris, E. Thunot & Co., 1860.

Marie, P. Des foyers lacunaires de désintégration et de différents autres états cavitaires du cerveau. *Revue de Médecine* 1901;**21**:281–98.

Marie, P and G Guillain. Existe-t-il en clinique des localisations dans la capsule interne? *Semaine Medicale* 1902;**22**:209–13.

Marinesco, G and A Kreindler. Oblitération progressive et complète des deux carotides primitives: accès épileptiques, considérations sur le rôle des sinus carotidiens dans la pathogénie de l'accès épileptique. *Presse Médicale* 1936;**44**:833–6.

Markham, WO. Case of disease of the aorta: aneurysms at the aortic sinuses, clots in the arteria innominata and middle cerebral arteries. *British Medical Journal* 1857;**1**:187–8.

Marquet, M. *Traité de l'Apopléxie, Paralysie*. Paris, J. P. Costard, 1770.

Marshall, J. The natural history of transient ischaemic cerebro-vascular attacks. *Quarterly Journal of Medicine* 1964;**33**:309–24.

Marshall, J and EH Reynolds. Withdrawal of anticoagulants from patients with transient ischaemic cerebrovascular attacks. *The Lancet* 1965;**285**:5–6.

Martial, R. L'étiologie de la paralysie générale. *Revue de Médecine* 1905;**25**:728–38.

Martin, JP and HL Sheehan. Primary thrombosis of cerebral veins (following childbirth). *British Medical Journal* 1941;**1**:349–53.

Martin, MJ, JP Whisnant, and GP Sayre. Occlusive vascular disease in the extracranial cerebral circulation. *Archives of Neurology* 1960;**3**:530–8.

Massaria, A. *Practica medica, seu Praelectiones academicae, continentes Methodum ac Rationem cognoscendi et curandi*. Francoforti, Melchior Hartmann, 1601.

Mattern, SP. *The Prince of Medicine: Galen in the Roman Empire*. Oxford, Oxford University Press, 2013.

Matthews, B. The investigation of cerebrovascular disease. *Proceedings of the Royal Society of Medicine* 1972;**65**:75–8.

Matthews, JR. *Quantification and the Quest for Medical Certainty*. Princeton, NJ, Princeton University Press, 1995.

McAllen, PM and J Marshall. Cardiac dysrhythmia and transient cerebral ischaemic attacks. *The Lancet* 1973;**301**:1212–14.

McBrien, DJ, RD Bradley, and N Ashton. The nature of retinal emboli in stenosis of the internal carotid artery. *The Lancet* 1963;**281**:697–9.

McCarthy, LR. Dandy, Walter Edward. In Bynum, WF and Bynum, H, eds. *Dictionary of Medical Biography*. Westport, CT, Greenwood Press, 2007, 397–9.

McKissock, W and KWE Paine. Subarachnoid haemorrhage. *Brain* 1959;**82**:356–66.

McKissock, W, KWE Paine, and LS Walsh. The value of hypothermia in the surgical treatment of ruptured intracranial aneurysms. *Journal of Neurosurgery* 1960a;**17**:700–7.

McKissock, W, KWE Paine, and LS Walsh. An analysis of the results of treatment of intracranial aneurysms: report of 772 consecutive cases. *Journal of Neurosurgery* 1960b;**17**:761–76.

McKissock, W, A Richardson, and L Walsh. 'Posterior-communicating' aneurysms: a controlled trial of the conservative and surgical treatment of ruptured aneurysms of the internal carotid artery at or near the point of origin of the posterior communicating artery. *The Lancet* 1960c;**275**:1203–6.

McKissock, W, A Richardson, and L Walsh. Middle-cerebral aneurysms: further results in the controlled trial of conservative and surgical treatment of ruptured intracranial aneurysms. *The Lancet* 1962;**280**:417–21.

McKissock, W, A Richardson, and L Walsh. Anterior communicating aneurysms: a trial of conservative and surgical treatment. *The Lancet* 1965;**285**:874–6.

Medical Research Council. Streptomycin treatment of pulmonary tuberculosis. *British Medical Journal* 1948;**2**:769–82.

Mehnert, E. Ueber die topographische Verbreitung der Angiosclerose, nebst Beiträgen zur Kenntnis des normalen Baues der Aeste des Aortenbogens und einiger Venenstämme. Thesis Dorpat, 1888.

Melicher, LJ. Tractatus de Apoplexia. Thesis Vindobonae, 1840.

Mendel, E. Ueber die apoplexia cerebri sanguinea. *Berliner medizinische Wochenschrift* 1891;**28**:577–82 and 594–5 (discussion).

Mercurialis. H. Responsio. In Varolio, C, ed. *De Nervis opticis, nonnullisque aliis praeter communem Opinionem in humano Capite observatis ad Hieronimum Mercurialem*. Patavii: Paulus and Antonius Meiettus, 1573, 20v–5r.

Meyer, A and R Hierons. A note on Thomas Willis' views on the corpus striatum and the internal capsule. *Journal of the Neurological Sciences* 1964;**1**:547–54.

Meynert, T. Ueber Gefässentartungen in den Varolsbrücke und den Gehirnschenkeln. *Allgemeine Wiener medizinische Zeitung* 1864;**9**:220–1.

Middlemore, R. *Treatise on Diseases of the Eye and Its Appendages*. London, Longman, Rees, Orme, Brown, Green, and Longman, and James Drake, Birmingham, 1835.

Millikan, CH. Ccrebral vasospasm and ruptured intracranial aneurysm. *Archives of Neurology* 1975;**32**:433–49.

Millikan, CH, RG Siekert, and JP Whisnant. Intermittent carotid and vertebral-basilar insufficiency associated with polycythemia. *Neurology* 1960;**10**:188–96.

Minkenhof, JE. De behandeling van bacteriële meningitides. *Nederlands Tijdschrift voor Geneeskunde* 1953;**97**:2857–64.

Mistichelli, D. *Trattato dell' Apoplessia, in cui con nove Osservazioni anatomiche, e Riflessioni fisiche si richercano tutte le Cagioni, e Spezie di quel Male, e vi se palesa frà gli altri un nuovo, & efficace Rimedio*. Roma, Antonio de' Rossi, 1709.

Mistichelli, D. *Aggiunta al Trattato dell' Apoplessia*. Padova, Giovanni Manfrè, 1715.

Moll, IG. De Apoplexia biliosa. Thesis Academia Georgia Augusta, Gottingae, 1780.

Mommsen, TE. Petrarch's conception of the Dark Ages. *Speculum Artium* 1942;**17**:226–42.

Moniz, E. L'encéphalographie artérielle, son importance dans la localisation des tumeurs cérébrales. *Revue Neurologique* 1927;**48**:72–90.

Moniz, E. *L'angiographie cérébrale*. Paris, Masson et Cie, 1934.

Moniz, E, A Lima, and R de Lacerda. Hémiplégies par thrombose de la carotide interne. *Presse Médicale* 1937;**45**:977–80.

Monneret, JAÉ, A Bouchardat, E-N Vigla, *et al*. Discours prononcés le samedi 6 octobre 1866 aux obsèques de M. Rostan. Paris, Imprimerie Félix Malteste et Cie, 1866.

Monro, A. *Observations on the Structure and Function of the Nervous System*. Edinburgh/London, William Creech and Joseph Johnson, 1783.

Montain, JFF and GAC Montain. *Traité de l'Apoplexie, contenant l'Énumeration des Causes de cette Maladie, la Description de ses différentes Espèces, son Traitement, et les Moyens de la prévenir*. Paris, Brunot-Labbé, 1811.

Moore, MT. Perivascular encephalolysis: histology and pathogenesis. *Archives of Neurology and Psychiatry* 1954;**71**:344–57.

Moore, W. *The Knife Man: The Extraordinary Life and Times of John Hunter, Father of Modern Surgery*. New York, NY, Broadway Books, 2005.

Moore, WS and AD Hall. Importance of emboli from carotid bifurcation in pathogenesis of cerebral ischemic attacks. *Archives of Surgery* 1970;**101**:708–16.

Morgagni, JB. *Adversaria anatomica VI*. Patavii, Josephus Cominus, 1719.

Morgagni, JB. *De Sedibus et Causis Morborum per Anatomen indagatis*. Venetiis, Ex Typographia Remondiana, 1761.

Moulin, É. *Traité de l'Apoplexie ou Hémorrhagie cérébrale: Considérations sur les Hydrocéphales, Description d'une Hydropisie cérébrale particulière aux Vielliards récemment observée*. Paris, J. B. Baillière, 1819.

Moxon, A. A contribution to the history of visceral syphilis. *Guy's Hospital Reports* 1868;**13**:329–407.

Mushet, WB. *A Practical Treatise on Apoplexy (Cerebral Haemorrhage): Its Pathology, Diagnosis, Therapeutics, and Prophylactics*. London, John Churchill and Sons, 1866.

Nebel, DGH. *Dissertatio inauguralis medica exhibens observationem aneurysmatum duorum rariorum, quorum alterum ex arcu aortae, alterum ex arteria corporis callosi ortum est*. Thesis Heidelbergae, 1834.

Neubürger, K. Zur Frage der funktionellen Gefässstörungen unter besonderer Berücksichtigung des Zentralnervensystems. *Klinische Wochenschrift* 1926;**5**:1689–92.

Neuburger, M. *Die historische Entwicklung der experimentellen Gehirn-und Rückenmarksphysiologie vor Flourens*. Stuttgart, Ferdinand Enke, 1897.

New, PFJ and WR Scott. *Computed Tomography of the Brain and Orbit (EMI Scanning)*. Baltimore, MD, Williams & Wilkins, 1975.

Nibbelink, DW and LA Knowler. Cooperative study of intracranial aneurysms and subarachnoid hemorrhage. Report on a randomized treatment study. II. Objectives and design of randomized aneurysm study. *Stroke* 1974;**5**:552–6.

Nibbelink, DW, JC Torner, and WG Henderson. Intracranial aneurysms and subarachnoid hemorrhage: report on a randomized treatment study. IV-A. Regulated bed rest. *Stroke* 1977;**8**:202–18.

Nicolson, M. Baillie, Matthew. In Bynum, WF and Bynum, H, eds. *Dictionary of Medical Biography*. Westport, CT, Greenwood Press, 2007, 147–8.

Nitrini, R. The history of tabes dorsalis and the impact of observational studies in neurology. *Archives of Neurology* 2000;**57**:605–6.

Noguchi, H and JW Moore. A demonstration of *Treponema pallidum* in the brain in cases of general paralysis. *Journal of Experimental Medicine* 1913;**17**:232–8.

Nonne, M. Uber Fälle vom Symptomenkomplex 'Tumor cerebri' mit Ausgang in Heilung (Pseudotumor cerebri). Über letal verlaufene Fälle von 'Pseudotumor cerebri' mit Sektions-befund. *Deutsche Zeitschrift für Nervenheilkunde* 1904;**27**:169–216.

Nonne, M. Der heutige Standpunkt der Lues-Paralysefrage. *Deutsche Zeitschrift für Nervenheilkunde* 1913;**49**:384–446.

Nordmann, M. Referat über die Spontanblutungen im menschlichen Gehirn. *Verhandlungen der Deutschen Pathologischen Gesellschaft* 1937;**29**:11–54.

Norlén, G and H Olivecrona. The treatment of aneurysms of the circle of Willis. *Journal of Neurosurgery* 1953;**10**:404–15.

Northcroft, GB and AD Morgan. A fatal case of traumatic thrombosis of the internal carotid artery. *British Journal of Surgery* 1944;**32**:105–7.

Nutton, V. Books, printing and medicine in the Renaissance. *Medicina nei Secoli – Arte e Scienza* 2005;**17**:421–42.

Nutton, V. *Galen: A Thinking Doctor in Imperial Rome.* New York, NY, Routledge, 2020.

Nymmanus, G. *Tractatus de Apoplexia.* Wittebergae, J. W. Fincelius, 1629.

Odom, GL. Cerebral vasospasm. *Clinical Neurosurgery* 1975;**22**:29–58.

Oliveira, V. History of carotid occlusions: the contribution of Egas Moniz. *Journal of Stroke and Cerebrovascular Diseases* 2018;**27**: 3626–9.

O'Malley, CD. *Michael Servetus.* Philadelphia, PA, American Philosophical Society, 1953.

O'Malley, CD. *Andreas Vesalius of Brussels 1514–1564.* Berkeley, CA, University of California Press, 1965.

Ongaro, G. Mercuriale, Girolamo. In Bynum, WF and Bynum, H, eds. *Dictionary of Medical Biography.* Westport, CT, Greenwood Press, 2007a, 871–3.

Ongaro, G. Morgagni, Giovanni Battista. In Bynum, WF and Bynum, H, eds. *Dictionary of Medical Biography.* Westport, CT, Greenwood Press, 2007b, 897–900.

Ooneda, G, Y Yoshida, K Suzuki, *et al.* Morphogenesis of plasmatic arterionecrosis as the cause of hypertensive intracerebral hemorrhage. *Virchows Archiv, Abt. A Pathologie und Pathologische Anatomie* 1973;**361**:31–8.

Oppenheim, H. *Lehrbuch der Nervenkrankheiten, für Ärzte und Studierende,* 6th edn. Berlin, S. Karger, 1913.

Osler, W. *The Principles and Practice of Medicine.* New York, NY, D. Appleton and Company, 1892.

Osler, W. Transient attacks of aphasia and paralyses in states of high blood pressure and arterio-sclerosis. *Canadian Medical Association Journal* 1911;**1**:919–26.

Otis, L. *Müller's Lab.* Oxford, Oxford University Press, 2007.

Ott, JM. Dissertatio inauguralis medico-anatomica, historiam renis sinistri maxime tumidi atque corrupti, in cadavere humano reperti, pandens et explicans. Thesis Basileae, 1719.

Ott, JM. Historia renis sinistri maxime tumidi. In *Acta Helvetica Physico-Mathematico-Botanico-Medica.* Basileae, Joh. Rudolphus Imhof, 1751, 30–48.

Pagel, J. *Lexicon hervorragender Ärzte des neunzehnten Jahrhunderts.* Berlin/Wien, Urban and Schwarzenberg, 1901.

Pagel, W. *Harvey's Biological Ideas: Selected Aspects and Historical Background.* Basel/New York, NY, S. Karger, 1967.

Pagel, W. *Joan Baptista van Helmont: Reformer of Science and Medicine.* Cambridge, Cambridge University Press, 1982.

Paget, J. Fatty degeneration of the small blood vessels of the brain, and its relation to apoplexy. *The London Medical Gazette* 1850;**II–X**:229–35.

Parish, LC. Hutchinson, Jonathan. In Bynum, WF and Bynum, H, eds. *Dictionary of Medical Biography.* Westport, CT, Greenwood Press, 2007, 680–1.

Paterson, R, N Depasquale, and S Mann. Pseudotumor cerebri. *Medicine (Baltimore)* 1961;**40**:85–99.

Payne, FJ. Dictionary of National Biography, 1885–1900/Carswell, Robert. https://en .wikisource.org/wiki/Carswell,_Robert_ (DNB00). [Accessed 6 September 2021]

Peacock, TB. Intracranial aneurisms. *Saint Thomas's Hospital Reports* 1876;**7**:119–74, 317–23.

Pearce, JMS. A brief history of the clinical thermometer. *Quarterly Journal of Medicine* 2002;**95**:251–2.

Pearce, JMS. Brain disease leading to mental illness: a concept initiated by the discovery of general paralysis of the insane. *European Neurology* 2012;**67**:272–8.

Pearce, JMS, SS Gubbay, and JN Walton. Long-term anticoagulant therapy in transient cerebral ischaemic attacks. *The Lancet* 1965;**285**:6–9.

Peitzman, SJ. Bright, Richard. In Bynum, WF and Bynum, H, eds. *Dictionary of Medical Biography.* Westport, CT, Greenwood Press, 2007, 259–61.

Penzoldt, F. Ueber Thrombose (autochthone oder embolische) der Carotis. *Deutsches Archiv für klinische Medicin* 1881;**28**:80–93.

Pestronk, A. The first neurology book. 'De Cerebri Morbis' (1549) by Jason Pratensis. *Archives of Neurology* 1988;**45**:341–4.

Pick, L. Ueber die sogenannten miliare Aneurysmen der Hirngefässe. *Berliner klinische Wochenschrift* 1910;**47**:325–9, 382–6.

Pickering, A. Against putting the phenomena first: the discovery of the weak neutral current. *Studies in History and Philosophy of Science* 1984;**15**:85–117.

Pickering, GW. Transient cerebral paralysis in hypertension and in cerebral embolism with special reference to the pathogenesis of chronic hypertensive encephalopathy. *Journal of the American Medical Association* 1948;**137**:423–30.

Pickering, GW. *High Blood Pressure*. London, J. & A. Churchill, 1955.

Pinel, S. *Traité du Pathologie cérébrale ou des Maladies du Cerveau*. Paris, Just Rouvier, 1844.

Pioch. Observation relative à un cas de gangrène partielle du pied attribuée à un caillot détaché du coeur. *Gazette Médicale de Paris* 1847;**III–2**:671–2.

Piso, C. *De praetervisis hactenus Morbis Affectibusque praeter Naturam, ab Aqua seu serosa Colluvie & Diluvie ortis*. Ponte ad Monticulum, Carolus Mercator, 1618.

Pitt, GN. On cerebral embolism and aneurysm. *British Medical Journal.* 1890;**I**:827–32.

Platerus, F. *Praxeos, seu de cognoscendis, praedicendis, praecavendis curandisque Affectibus Homini incommodantibus: Tractatus de Functionum Laesionibus*. Basileae, Conradus Waldkirchius, 1602.

Platerus, F. *Observationum in Hominis Affectibus plerisque, Corpori & Animo, Functionum Laesione, Dolore, aliave Molestia & Vitio accomodantibus, Libri tres*. Basileae, Ludovicus König, 1614.

Poirier, J. Claude François Lallemand (1790–1854). *Journal of Neurology* 2010;**257**:681–2.

Poirier, J. Le docteur Jean-Baptiste Vincent Laborde (1830–1903), neurologue et neurophysiologiste oublié. *Gériatrie et Psychologie Neuropsychiatrie du Vieillissement* 2015;**13**:73–82.

Poirier, J-P. *Lavoisier*. Paris, Éditions Pygmalion, 1993.

Pomata, G. Observation rising. In Daston, L and Lunbeck, E, eds. *Histories of Scientific Observation*. Chicago, IL, University of Chicago Press, 2011, 45–80.

Pomme, P. *Traité des affections vaporeuses des deux sexes*. Lyon, Benoit Duplain, 1765.

Pomme, P. *Traité des Affections vaporeuses des deux Sexes*. Paris, Imprimerie Royale, 1782.

Ponfick, E. Ueber embolische Aneurysmen, nebst Bemerkungen über das akute Herzaneurysma (Herzgeschwür). *Archiv für pathologische Anatomie und Physiologie und für klinische Medicin* 1873;**58**:528–71.

Ponsart, GB. *Traité de l'Apoplexie et de ses differentes Espèces*. Liège, L. J. Demany, 1775.

Portal, A. Observations sur l'apoplexie. *Mémoires de l'Académie Royale des Sciences* 1781;623–30.

Portal, A. *Mémoires sur la Nature et le Traitement de plusieurs Maladies*. Paris, Bertrand et Moutardier, 1800.

Portal, A. *Observations sur la Nature et le Traitement de l'Apoplexie, et sur les Moyens de la prévenir*. Paris, Crochard, 1811.

Posey, WC. Transient monocular blindness. *Journal of the American Medical Association* 1902;**38**:1418–21.

Postel, M and J Postel. La découverte de l'étiologie syphilitique de la paralysie générale et ses incidences idéologiques sur la prévention des maladies mentales. *Histoire des Sciences Médicales* 1982;**17**:83–7.

Pratensis, I. *De Cerebri Morbis*. Basileae, Henrichus Petri, 1549.

Prévost, J-L. De la déviation conjuguée des yeux et de la rotation de la tête dans certains cas d'hémiplégie. Thesis Paris, 1868.

Prévost, J-L and J Cotard. *Études physiologiques et pathologiques sur le Ramollissement cérébral*. Paris, Adrien Delahaye, 1866.

Primirosius, J. Antidotum adversus Henrici Regii Utrajectensis Medicinae Professoris venenatam Spongiam, sive Vindiciae Animadversationum. In *Recentiorum Disceptationes de Motu Cordis, Sanguinis et Chili in Animalibus*. Lugduni Batavorum, Ioannes Maire, 1644.

Proust, A. Des différentes formes de ramollissement du cerveau. Thesis Paris, 1866.

Quincke, H. Die Lumbalpunktion des Hydrocephalus. *Berliner klinische Wochenschrift* 1891;**28**:929–33, 965–8.

Quincke, H. Über Meningitis serosa. In *Sammlung klinischer Vorträge, innere Medizin no. 23*. Leipzig, Breitkopf und Härtel, 1893, 655–94.

Raige-Delorme. Notice nécrologique sur le Dr. Rochoux. *Archives Générales de Médecine* 1852;**28**:503–8.

Ramsey, M. Portal, Antoine. In Bynum, WF and Bynum, H, eds. *Dictionary of Medical Biography*. Westport, CT, Greenwood Press, 2007, 1029–30.

Ray, BS and HS Dunbar. Thrombosis of the dural venous sinuses as a cause of pseudotumor cerebri. *Annals of Surgery* 1951;**134**:376–86.

Ray, BS, HS Dunbar, and CT Dotter. Dural sinus venography. *Radiology* 1951;**57**:477–86.

Reading, PV and PH Schurr. Thrombosis of the sigmoid sinus: past and present. *The Lancet* 1956;**271**:473–6.

Reed, RL, RG Siekert, and J Merideth. Rarity of transient focal cerebral ischemia in cardiac dysrhythmia. *Journal of the American Medical Association* 1973;**223**:893–5.

Regli, F. Die flüchtigen ischämischen zerebralen Attacken. Naturlicher Verlauf und Pathogenese. *Deutsche Medizinische Wochenschrift* 1971;**96**:525–30.

Reynolds, EH and JV Kinnier Wilson. Stroke in Babylonia. *Archives of Neurology* 2004;**61**:597–601.

Reynolds, JR and HC Bastian. Softening of the brain. In Reynolds, JR, ed. *System of Medicine*. London/Philadelphia, PA, Macmillan and Co., Lippincott and Co., 1868, 434–77.

Ribes, F. Exposé succinct des recherches faites sur la phlébite. *Revue Médicale Française et Étrangére et Journal de Clinique de l'Hôtel Dieu et de la Charité de Paris* 1825;**3**:5–41.

Richardson, JC and HH Hyland. A clinical and pathological study of subarachnoid and intracerebral haemorrhage caused by berry aneurysms. *Medicine* 1941;**20**:1–84.

Richelmi, P. *Essai sur l'Apoplexie, ou Pathologie, Séméiotique, Hygiène et Thérapeutique de cette Maladie, considérée dans ses différentes Espèces*. Marseille, Joseph-François Achard, 1811.

Richerand, A. *Nosographie chirurgicale*. Paris, Crapard, Caille, et Ravier, 1806.

Ricord, P. *Traité pratique des Maladies vénériennes*. Paris, Just Rouvier et E. Le Bouvier, 1838.

Ridley, H. *The Anatomy of the Brain, Containing its Mechanism and Physiology, Together with Some New Discoveries and Corrections of Ancient and Modern Authors on That Subject, to which Is Annexed a Particular Account of Animal Functions and Muscular Motion*. London, Sam. Smith and Benj. Walford, 1695.

Ridley, H. Experimentum anatomicum ad veram durae matris motus causam detegendam institutum. *Philosophical Transactions of the Royal Society of London* 1703;**23**:1480–4.

Riechert, T. Die Arteriographie der Hirngefässe bei einseitingem Verschluß der Carotis interna. *Der Nervenarzt* 1938;**11**:290–7.

Riobé, M. Observations propres à résoudre cette question: l'apoplexie dans laquelle il se fait un épanchement de sang dans le cerveau, est-elle susceptible de guérison? Thesis Paris, 1814.

Riolan, J. *Encheiridium anatomicum et pathologicum*. Lugduni Batavorum, Ex Officina Adriani Wyngaerden, 1649a.

Riolan, J. *Opuscula anatomica nova*. Londini, Milo Flesher, 1649b.

Riva-Rocci, S. Un nuovo sfigmomanometro. *Gazzetta medico di Torino 1896–1897*; **47–8**:981–96, 1001–17, 161–72, 181–91.

Rob, C and EB Wheeler. Thrombosis of internal carotid artery treated by arterial surgery. *British Medical Journal* 1957;**2**:264–6.

Robin, C. Recherches sur quelques particularités de la structure des capillaires de l'encéphale. *Journal de la Physiologie de l'Homme et des Animaux* 1859;**2**:537–48.

Robinson, RG. Ruptured aneurysms of the middle cerebral artery. *Journal of Neurosurgery* 1971;**35**:25–33.

Rocca, J. *Galen on the Brain: Anatomical Knowledge and Physiological Speculation in the Second Century AD*. Leiden and Boston, MA, Brill, 2003.

Rochoux, J-A. *Recherches sur l'apoplexie*. Paris, Méquignon-Marvis, 1814.

Rochoux, J-A. *Recherches sur l'Apoplexie, et sur plusieurs autres Maladies de l'Appareil nerveux cérébro-spinal*. Paris, Béchet Jeune, 1833.

Rochoux, J-A. Sur l'hypertrophie du coeur considérée comme cause de l'apoplexie et sur le système de Gall. *Archives Générales de Médecine* 1836;II–**11**:167–88.

Rochoux, J-A. Du ramollissement du cerveau et de sa curabilité. *Archives Générales de Médecine* 1844;**IV–6**:265–82, 401–30.

Rokitansky, C. *Handbuch der speciellen pathologischen Anatomie*. Wien, Braumüller and Seidel, 1844.

Romberg, M. Ueber den Schlagfluss in pathologisch-anatomischer Hinsicht: aus der neueren Untersuchungen der Herren Dr. Dr. Cheyne, Rochoux, Riobé und Bricheteau. *Horn's Archiv für Medizinische Erfahrung im Gebiete der praktischen Medizin, Chirurgie, Geburtshülfe und Staatsarzneikunde* 1819;**36**:533–70.

Romberg, M. Ueber den Schlagfluss in pathologisch-anatomischer Hinsicht aus den neueren Untersuchungen englischer und französischer Aertzte. *Horn's Archiv für Medizinische Erfahrung im Gebiete der praktischen Medizin, Chirurgie, Geburtshülfe und Staatsarzneikunde* 1820;**38**:1–112.

Romberg, M. Kritische Prüfung von J. Abercrombie's Abhandlung über die Krankheiten de Gehirns und des Rückenmarks (zweiter Teil). *Horn's Archiv für Medizinische Erfahrung im Gebiete der praktischen Medizin, Chirurgie, Geburtshülfe und Staatsarzneikunde* 1822;**41**:458–87.

Romberg, M. Ergebnisse einiger Leichenöffnungen; zweite Klasse der Hirn- und Rückenmarkskrankheiten: Hämorrhagieen. *Horn's Archiv für Medizinische Erfahrung im Gebiete der praktischen Medizin, Chirurgie, Geburtshülfe und Staatsarzneikunde* 1823;**43**:405–47.

Romberg, M. *Lehrbuch der Nervenkrankheiten des Menschen*. Berlin, Alexander Duncker, 1840–1846.

Romberg, MH. Commentationes quaedam de Cerebri Haemorrhagia. Thesis Berolini, 1830.

Röntgen, WC. Ueber eine neue Art von Strahlen. *Sitzungsberichte der Würzburger physikalisch-medicinische Gesellschaft* 1895;**137**:132–41.

Rosenberg, CE. Introduction. In *Framing Disease: Illness, Society and History*. New Brunswick, NJ, Rutgers University Press, 1992.

Rosenblath, W. Über die Entstehung der Hirnblutung bei dem Schlaganfall. *Deutsche Zeitschrift für Nervenheilkunde* 1918;**61**:10–143.

Ross Russell, RW. Observations on the retinal blood-vessels in monocular blindness. *The Lancet* 1961;**280**:1422–8.

Ross Russell, RW. Observations on intracerebral aneurysms. *Brain* 1963;**86**:425–42.

Ross Russell, RW. From the retired. Changing ideas on the pathogenesis of stroke. *Practical Neurology* 2003;**3**:240–5.

Ross, S. 'Scientist': the story of a word. *Annals of Science* 1962;**18**:65–85.

Rostan, L. *Recherches sur une Maladie encore peu connue, qui a reçu le Nom de Ramollissement du Cerveau*. Paris, Béchet et Crevot, 1820.

Rostan, L. *Recherches sur le Ramollissement du Cerveau*. Paris, Béchet, Gabon, et Crevot, 1823.

Rostan, L. *Untersuchungen über die Erweichung des Gehirns, zugleich eine Unterscheidung der verschiedenen Krankheiten dieses Organs durch characteristische Zeichen beabsichtigend*. Leipzig, Leopold Boß, 1824.

Roth, M. Ueber Gehirnapoplexie. *Correspondenzblatt für Schweizer Aerzte* 1874;**4**:145–52.

Rothenberg, SF and E Corday. Etiology of the transient cerebral stroke. *Journal of the American Medical Association* 1957;**164**:2005–8.

Rühl, A. Atheroskerotische Gefässruptur oder Spasmus als Ursache der apoplektischen Gehirnblutung? *Beiträge zur pathologischen Anatomie und zur allgemeinen Pathologie* 1927;**78–2**:160–86.

Rush, C and JF Shaw. *With Sharp Compassion: Norman Dott, Freeman Surgeon of Edinburgh*. Aberdeen, Aberdeen University Press, 1990.

Russell, DS. The pathology of spontaneous intracranial haemorrhage. *Proceedings of the Royal Society of Medicine* 1954;**47**:689–93.

Russell, W. A postgraduate lecture on intermittent closing of the cerebral arteries: its relation to temporary and permanent paralysis. *British Medical Journal* 1909;**2**:1109–10.

Ruysch, F. Responsio ad Goelicke. In *Frederici Ruyschii Opera omnia Anatomico-Medica-Chirurgica*, vol. 2. Amstelodami, Apud Janssonio-Waesbergios, 1743 [1697], 1–11.

Sahs, AL. Cooperative study of intracranial aneurysms and subarachnoid hemorrhage.

Report on a randomized treatment study. I. Introduction. *Stroke* 1974;**5**:550–1.

Sahs, AL, GE Perret, HB Locksley, *et al.*, eds. *Intracranial Aneurysms and Subarachnoid Hemorrhage*. Philadelphia, PA, J. B. Lippincott Company, 1969.

Samuel, KC. Atherosclerosis and occlusion of the internal carotid artery. *Journal of Pathology and Bacteriology* 1956;**71**:391–401.

Sanders, TE. Intermittent occlusion of the central retinal artery. *American Journal of Ophthalmology* 1939;**22**:861–9.

Savory, WS. Case of a young woman in whom the main arteries of both upper extremities and of the left side of the neck were throughout completely obliterated. *Medico-Chirurgical Transactions* 1856;**39**:205–19.

Sawday, J. *The Body Emblazoned*. London, Routledge, 1995.

Saxonia, H. *Prognoseon Practicarum, Libri duo*. Francofurti, Zacharia Palthenius, 1610.

Saxonia, H. *Opera practica*. Patavinum, Franciscus Bolzetta, 1639.

Scardona, JF. *Aphorismi de cognoscendis et curandis Morbis*. Patavii, Joannis Manfrè, 1746.

Schaudinn, F and E Hoffmann. Vorläufiger Bericht über das vorkommen von Spirochaeten in syphilitischen Krankheitsprodukten und bei Papillomen. *Arbeiten aus dem Kaiserlichen Gesundheitsamte* 1905;**22**:527–34.

Scheinker, IM. Changes in cerebral veins in hypertensive brain disease and their relation to cerebral hemorrhage: clinical pathologic study. *Archives of Neurology and Psychiatry* 1945;**53**:395–408.

Schenck von Grafenberg, J. *Paratereseon, sive Observationum medicarum, rararum, novarum, admirabilium & monstrosarum Volumen, Tomis septem*. Francofurti, Nicolaus Hoffmann, 1609.

Schiffter, R. Moritz Heinrich Romberg (1795–1873). *Journal of Neurology* 2010;**257**:1409–10.

Schmahmann, JD, RM Nitsch, and DN Pandya. The mysterious relocation of the bundle of Turck. *Brain* 1992;**115**:1911–24.

Schneider, CV. *Liber de Osse cribriformi, & Sensu ac Organo odoratus, & Morbis ad utraque spectantibus*. Wittebergae, Tobias Mevius and Elardus Schumacher, 1655.

Schneider, CV. *Liber primus de Catarrhis, quo agitur de Species Catarrhorum, & de Osse Cuneiformi, per quod Catarrhi decurrere finguntur*. Wittebergae, Tobias Mevius and Elardus Schumacher, 1660.

Scholz, W and D Nieto. Studien zur Pathologie der Hirngefässe; I. Fibrose und Hyalinose. *Zeitschrift für die gesamte Neurologie und Psychiatrie* 1938;**162**:675–93.

Schutta, HS and HM Howe. Seventeenth century concepts of 'apoplexy' as reflected in Bonet's 'Sepulchretum'. *Journal of the History of the Neurosciences* 2006;**15**:250–68.

Schützenberger, C. *De l'Oblitération subite des Artères par des Corps solides ou des Concrétions fibrineuses détachées du Coeur ou des gros Vaisseaux à Sang rouge*. Strasbourg, G. Silbermann, 1857.

Schwartz, CJ and JRA Mitchell. Atheroma of the carotid and vertebral arterial systems. *British Medical Journal* 1961;**2**:1057–63.

Schwartz, D, R Flamant, and J Lellouch. *L'essai thérapeutique chez l'homme*. Paris, Flammarion-Médecine, 1970.

Schwartz, P. *Die Arten der Schlaganfälle des Gehirns und ihre Entstehung*. Berlin, Julius Springer, 1930a.

Schwartz, P. Apoplektische Schädigungen bei der essentiellen Hypertonie. *Der Nervenarzt* 1930b;**3**:450–62.

Schwartz, P. *Cerebral Apoplexy: Types, Causes and Pathogenesis*. Springfield, IL, Charles C. Thomas, 1961.

Schwencke, T. *Rari Casus Explicatio anatomico-medica*. Hagae-Comitum, Petrus de Hondt, 1733.

Scott, A, M Eadie, and A Lees. *William Richard Gowers 1845–1915: Exploring the Victorian Brain*. Oxford, Oxford University Press, 2012.

Scougal, EF. Hemiplegia occurring nine days after parturition: death; partial post mortem examination. *Transactions of the Obstetrical Society of London* 1888;**30**:214–17.

Sédillot, CE. Blessure de l'artère carotide externe droite; hémorragies successives; tentatives infructueuses de ligature de la carotide primitive, le cinquième jour; continuation des hémorragies; ligature immédiate du tronc carotidien le treizième jour; hémiplégie complète du côté gauche; paralysie de la face et de les sens du côté droit; résorption purulente; mort le vingt-troisième jour de l'accident et le dixième de l'opération. *Gazette Médicale de Paris* 1842;**II–10**:367–71.

Sée, M. Discussion sur l'artérite. *Gazette Hebdomadaire de Médecine et de Chirurgie* 1857;**4**:601–4.

Seldinger, SI. Catheter replacement of the needle in percutaneous arteriography: a new technique. *Acta Radiologica* 1953;**39**:368–76.

Serbinenko, FA. Balloon catheterization and occlusion of major cerebral vessels. *Journal of Neurosurgery* 1974;**41**:125–45.

Serres, A. Nouvelle division des apoplexies. *Annuaire Médico-chirurgical des Hôpitaux et Hospices Civiles de Paris.* 1819;**1**:246–363.

Serres, A. Observations sur la rupture des anévrysmes des artères du cerveau. *Archives Générales de Médecine* 1926;**10**:419–31.

Shapin, S. *The Social History of Truth.* Chicago, IL, University of Chicago Press, 1994.

Shapin, S. *The Scientific Revolution.* Chicago, IL, University of Chicago Press, 1996.

Shennan, T. Miliary aneurysms, in relation to cerebral haemorrhage. *Edinburgh Medical Journal* 1915;**15**:245–52.

Sherrington, CS. *The Endeavour of Jean Fernel.* Cambridge, Cambridge University Press, 1946.

Shimidzu, K. Beiträge zur Arteriographie des Gehirns – einfache percutane Methode. *Archiv für klinische Chirurgie* 1937;**188**:295–316.

Shlyakhto, E and A Conrady. Korotkoff sounds: what do we know about its discovery? *Journal of Hypertension* 2005;**23**:3–5.

Shorvon, S and A Compston. *Queen Square: A History of the National Hospital and Its Institute of Neurology.* Cambridge, Cambridge University Press, 2019.

Sicard, J-A. Chromodiagnostic du liquide céphalorachidien dans les hémorragies du névraxe. Valeur de la teinte jeunatre. *Comptes Rendus des Séances et Mémoires de la Société de Biologie* 1901;**23**:1050–2.

Sicard, J-A and J Forestier. Méthode radiographique d'exploration de la cavité épidurale par le Lipiodol. *Revue Neurologique* 1921;**37**:1264–6.

Sie-Boen-Lian. Spasm of macular arteries. *Archives of Ophthalmology* 1948;**39**:267–72.

Siegert, P. Die ursächliche Bedeutung einer Verkalkung oder Thrombose der Carotis interna für Funktionsstörungen des Auges. *Archiv für Ophthalmologie* 1938;**138**:798–844.

Siekert, RG. Cardiac dysrhythmia and transient cerebral ischaemic attacks. *The Lancet* 1973;**302**:444–5.

Siekert, RG, CH Millikan, and JP Whisnant. Anticoagulant therapy in intermittent cerebrovascular insufficiency. Follow-up data. *JAMA* 1961;**176**:19–22.

Sigerist, HE. *The Great Doctors: A Biographical History of Medicine.* New York, NY, W. W. Norton, 1933.

Silversides, JL. Basilar artery stenosis and thrombosis. *Proceedings of the Royal Society of Medicine* 1954;**47**:290–3.

Siraisi, NG. The Canon of Avicenna. In Wear, A, *et al.*, eds. *The Medical Renaissance of the Sixteenth Century.* Cambridge, Cambridge University Press, 1985, 16–41.

Siraisi, NG. *The Clock and the Mirror: Girolamo Cardano and Renaissance Medicine.* Princeton, NJ, Princeton University Press, 1997.

Smith, CUM. Brain and mind in the 'long' eighteenth century. In Whitaker, H, *et al.*, eds. *Brain, Mind and Medicine: Essays in Eighteenth-Century Neuroscience.* New York, NY, Springer, 2007, 15–28.

Sömmerring, ST. *Das Organ der Seele.* Königsberg, Friedrich Nicolovius, 1796.

Sorgo, W. Über den Art. carotis interna-Verschluss bei jüngeren personen. *Zeitschrift für die gesamte Neurologie und Psychiatrie.* 1939;**167**:581–5.

Sorgo, W. Über den durch Gefässprozesse bedingten Verschluss der Art. carotis interna. *Zentralblatt für Neurochirurgie* 1939;**4**:161–79.

Soulier, H. Étude critique sur le ramollissement cérébral. Thesis Lyon, 1867.

Sponer, E. Beitrag zu dem durch Gefäßveränderungen bedingten Verschluß der Arteria carotis interna. *Bruns' Beiträge zur klinischen Chirurgie* 1941;**172**:481–95.

Sprengel, K. *Versuch einer pragmatischen Geschichte der Arzneykunde*, 3rd edn. Halle, Gebauersche Buchhandlung, 1821–1828.

Spurgin, T. Case of aneurysm of the anterior cerebral artery. *The London Medical Repository* 1825;**3**:443–5.

Staemmler. Zur Lehre von der Entstehung des Schlaganfalles. *Klinische Wochenschrift* 1936;**15**:1300–6.

Stein, L. Beitrag zur Ätiologie der Gehirnblutungen. *Deutsche Zeitschrift für Nervenheilkunde* 1895;**7**:314–29.

Steinke, H. Haller, Albrecht von. In Bynum, WF and Bynum, H, eds. *Dictionary of Medical Biography*. Westport, CT, Greenwood Press, 2007, 603–5.

Stevens, DL and WB Matthews. Cryptogenic drop attacks: an affliction of women. *British Medical Journal* 1973;**1**:439–42.

Stoll, M. *Pars prima Rationis medendi in Nosocomio practico Vindobonensi*. Lugduni Batavorum, Apud Haak, Socios, A., and J. Honkoop, 1786.

Sträuli, P. Die Ärztefamilie Brunner aus Diessenhofen. In Nägeli, E and Speich, HM, eds. *Thurgauer Jahrbuch 1980*. Frauenfeld, Huber, 1979, 69–78.

Strümpell, A and C Seyfarth. *Lehrbuch der speziellen Pathologie und Therapie der inneren Krankheiten, für Studierende und Ärzte*, 25th edn. Leipzig, F. C. W. Vogel, 1926.

Stumpff, AAA. De aneurysmatibus arteriarum cerebri. Thesis Berolini, 1836.

Sudhoff, K, ed. *Theophrast von Hohenheim gen. Paracelsus, Sämtliche Werke*. München/Berlin, K. Oldenbourg, 1931.

Sugar, HS, JE Webster, and ES Gurdjian. Ophthalmologic findings in spontaneous thrombosis of the carotid arteries. *Archives of Ophthalmology* 1950;**44**:823–32.

Sundt, TM, Jr. Management of ischemic complications after subarachnoid hemorrhage. *Journal of Neurosurgery* 1975;**43**:418–25.

Suy, R. The varying morphology and aetiology of the arterial aneurysm: a historical study. *Acta Chirurgica Belgica* 2006;**106**:354–60.

Sydenham, T. *Observationes medicae circa Morborum acutorum Historiam et Curationem*, 4th edn. Londini, Gualtherus Kettelby, 1676.

Sydenham, T. *De Podagra et Hydrope*. Lugduni Batavorum, Adrianus Marston, 1684.

Sydenham, T. *Dissertatio epistolaris ad spectatissimum doctissimumque Virum Guilelmum Cole de*

Observationibus nuperis circa Curationem Variolarum confluentium, nec non de Affectione hysterica. Genevae, Samuel de Tournes, 1684.

Symonds, C. Otitic hydrocephalus. *Neurology* 1956;**6**:681–5.

Symonds, C. Autobiographical introduction. In Symonds, C, ed. *Studies in Neurology*. Oxford, Oxford University Press, 1970, 1–23.

Symonds, CP. Spontaneous subarachnoid haemorrhage. *Quarterly Journal of Medicine* 1924;**18**:93–122.

Symonds, CP. Otitic hydrocephalus. *Brain* 1931;**54**:55–71.

Symonds, CP and H Cushing. Contributions to the clinical study of cerebral aneurysms. *Guy's Hospital Reports* 1923;**73**:139–58.

Szekely, P. Systemic embolism and anticoagulant prophylaxis in rheumatic heart disease. *British Medical Journal* 1964;**1**:1209–12.

Tachenius, O. *Hippocrates Chymicus*. Venetiis, Combi & La Nou, 1666.

Teasdale, G and B Jennett. Assessment of coma and impaired consciousness. A practical scale. *The Lancet* 1974;**304**:81–4.

Teitelbaum, GP, DW Larsen, V Zelman, et al. A tribute to Dr. Fedor A. Serbinenko, founder of endovascular neurosurgery. *Neurosurgery* 2000;**46**:462–9; discussion 469–70.

Teive, H, MG Ferreira, CHF Camargo, et al. The duels of Pierre Marie and Jules Dejerine. *European Neurology* 2020;**83**:345–50.

Témoin, S. *La maternité de Paris, pendant l'an 1859*. Paris, Adrien Delahaye, 1860.

Terson, A. De l'hémorrhagie dans le corps vitré au cours de l'hémorrhagie cerebrale. *La Clinique Ophthalmologique* 1900;**6**:309–12.

Thuillier, J. *Monsieur Charcot de la Salpêtrière*. Paris, Robert Laffond, 1993.

Tissot, SAD. *Nobilissimo et illustrissimo Alb. v. Hallero de Variolis, Apoplexia, et Hydrope*. Lausannae, Ex Typographia Antonii Chapuis, 1761.

Tissot, SAD. *Avis au Peuple, sur sa Santé*, 3rd edn. Lyon, Jean-Marie Bruyset et Benoit Duplain le jeune, 1764.

Todd, NV, JE Howie, and JD Miller. Norman Dott's contribution to aneurysm surgery. *Journal of Neurology, Neurosurgery, and Psychiatry* 1990;**53**:455–8.

Todd, RB. Account of a case of a dissecting aneurism of the aorta, innominata, and right carotid arteries, giving rise to suppression of urine and white softening of the brain. *Medico-Chirurgical Transactions* 1844;**27**:301–24.

Todd, RB. *Clinical Lectures on Paralysis, Certain Diseases of the Brain, and Other Affections of the Nervous System.* London, John Churchill, 1856.

Tonnellé, L. *Mémoire sur les Maladies des Sinus veineux de la Dure-mère.* Paris, Académie Royale de Médecine, 1829.

Towbin, A. The syndrome of latent cerebral venous thrombosis: its frequency and relation to age and congestive heart failure. *Stroke* 1973;**4**:419–30.

Troupp, H and G af Björkesten. Results of a controlled trial of late surgical versus conservative treatment of intracranial arterial aneurysms. *Journal of Neurosurgery* 1971;**35**:20–4.

Trousseau, A. *Clinique médicale de l'Hôtel-Dieu de Paris.* Paris, J. B. Baillière, 1882.

Tubbs, RS, M Loukas, MM Shoja, *et al.* Costanzo Varolio (Constantius Varolius 1543–1575) and the Pons Varolli. *Neurosurgery* 2008;**62**:734–7.

Tulpius, N. *Observationum medicarum Libri tres; cum aeneis Figuris.* Amstelredami, Apud Ludovicum Elzevirum, 1641.

Türck, L. Über die Beziehung gewisser Krankheitsherde des grossen Gehirnes zur Anästhesie. *Sitzungsberichte der kaiserlichen Akademie der Wissenschaften, mathematischnaturwissenschaftlichte Klasse* 1859;**36**:191–9.

Turnbull, HM. Alterations in arterial structure, and their relation to syphilis. *Quarterly Journal of Medicine* 1915;**8**:201–54.

Turner, AL. Patient operated upon for sigmoid sinus thrombosis. *Proceedings of the Royal Society of Medicine* 1908;**1**:137.

Turner, FC. Arteries of the brain from cases of cerebral haemorrhage. *Transactions of the Pathological Society of London* 1882;**33**:96–101.

Turner, WA and TG Stuart. *A Textbook of Nervous Diseases.* London, J. & A. Churchill, 1910.

Ullersperger, JB. *Der Hirnnervenschlag (Apoplexia nervosa).* Neuwied und Leipzig, J. H. Heuser, 1864.

Unger, W. Beiträge zur Lehre von den Aneurysmen. *Beiträge zur pathologischen Anatomie und zur allgemeinen Pathologie* 1911;**51**:137–77.

Vallisneri, A. *Dell'Uso e dell'Abuso di Bevande e Bagnature calde o freddo.* Napoli, Felice Mosca, 1727.

Van den Berg, JH. *Het menselijk Lichaam.* Nijkerk, G. F. Callenbach, 1965.

Van der Korst, JK. *Een Dokter van Formaat: Gerard van Swieten, Lijfarts van Keizerin Maria Theresia.* Houten/Bohn, Stafleu and van Loghum, 2003.

Van Gehuchten, A. *Les maladies nerveuses.* Louvain, Librairie Universitaire, 1920.

Van Gijn, J. A patient with word blindness in the seventeenth century. *Journal of the History of the Neurosciences* 2015;**24**:352–60.

Van Gijn, J and B Bonke. Interpretation of plantar reflexes: biasing effect of other signs and symptoms. *Journal of Neurology, Neurosurgery, and Psychiatry* 1977;**40**:787–9.

Van Helmont, JB. *Ortus Medicinae, id est, Initia Physicae inaudita. Progressus Medicinae novus, in Morborum Ultionem, ad Vitam longam.* Amsterodami, Apud Ludovicum Elzevirum, 1648.

Van Swieten, GLB. *Commentaria in Hermanni Boerhaave Aphorismos de cognoscendis et curandis Morbis.* Lugduni Batavorum, Johannes et Hermannus Verbeek, 1755–72.

Varolio, C. *De Nervis opticis, nonnullisque aliis praeter communem Opinionem in humano Capite observatis ad Hieronimum Mercurialem.* Patavii, Paulus and Antonius Meiettus, 1573.

Vesalius, A. *Tabulae anatomicae sex.* Venetiis, D. Bernardini, 1538.

Vesalius, A. *De humani Corporis Fabrica Libri septem.* Basileae, Ioannis Oporinus, 1543.

Vesalius, A. *De humani Corporis Fabrica Libri septem,* 2nd edn. Basileae, Ioannis Oporinus, 1555.

Vesling, J. *Syntagma Anatomicum, Locis plurimis auctum, emendatum, novisque Iconibus diligenter exornatum,* 2nd edn. Patavii, Typis Pauli Frambotti Bibliopolae, 1647.

Vesselle, B and G Vesselle. Sur les traces du docteur François Ribes, chirurgien de la 1ère division d'ambulance dite du champ de bataille. *Histoire des Sciences Médicales* 2014;**48**:405–16.

Vessier, M. *La Pitié-Salpêtrière: quatre siècles d'histoire et d'histoires.* Paris, Assistance Publique et Hôpitaux de Paris, 1999.

Viets, HR. Heinrich Erb. In Haymaker, W and Schiller, F, eds. *The Founders of Neurology.* Springfield, IL, Charles C. Thomas, 1970, 435–8.

Vincent, JP. Tying the common carotid artery – death. *The Lancet* 1829;**12**:570–2.

Virchow, R. Faserstoff; form der Gerinnung. *Neue Notizen aus dem Gebiete der Natur- und Heilkunde* 1845;**35**:323–30.

Virchow, R. Ueber die chemischen Eigenschaften des Faserstoffs. *Zeitschrift für rationelle Medicin* 1846a;**4**:262–92.

Virchow, R. Ueber die physikalische Eigenschaften und das Zerfallen des Faserstoffs. *Zeitschrift für rationelle Medicin* 1846b;**5**:213–42.

Virchow, R. Die Verstopfung der Lungenarterie und ihre Folgen. *Beiträge zur experimentellen Pathologie und Physiologie* 1846c;1–90.

Virchow, R. Ueber die akute Entzündung der Arterien. *Archiv für pathologische Anatomie und Physiologie und für klinische Medicin* 1847a;**1**:272–378.

Virchow, R. Zur pathologischen Physiologie des Bluts. *Archiv für pathologische Anatomie und Physiologie und für klinische Medicin* 1847b;**1**:547–83.

Virchow, R. Ueber die Erweiterung kleinerer Gefässe. *Archiv für pathologische Anatomie und Physiologie und für klinische Medicin* 1851;**3**:427–62.

Virchow, R. Ueber die Natur der constitutionell-syphilitischen Affectionen. *Archiv für pathologische Anatomie und Physiologie und für klinische Medicin* 1858;**15**:217–336.

Virchow, R. Verstopfung der Gekrösarterie. In Kölliker, A, *et al.*, eds. *Verhandlungen der physicalisch-medicinischen Gesellschaft in Würzburg.* Würzburg, Stahel, 1854, 341–9.

Virchow, R. *Gesammelte Abhandlungen zur wissenschaftlichen Medicin.* Frankfurt a.M., Meidinger, 1856a.

Virchow, R. Verstopfung der Lungenarterie. In Virchow, R, ed. *Gesammelte Abhandlungen zur wissenschaftlichen Medicin.* Frankfurt a.M., Meidinger, 1856b, 227–94.

Virchow, R. Ursprung des Faserstoffs. In Virchow, R, ed. *Gesammelte Abhandlungen zur Wissenschaftlichen Medicin.* Frankfurt a.M., Meidinger, 1856c, 104–46.

Vogt, C and O Vogt. Zur Lehre der Erkrankungen des striären Systems. *Journal für Psychologie und Neurologie* 1920;**25**:631–846.

Von Bergmann, G. Das spasmogene Ulcus pepticum. *Münchener medizinische Wochenschrift* 1913;**60**:169–74.

Von Bonin, G. Walter Campbell. In Haymaker, W and Schiller, F, eds. *The Founders of Neurology.* Springfield, IL, Charles C. Thomas, 1970, 102–4.

Von Haller, A. *Primae Lineae physiologiae, in Usum Praelectionum academicarum. ad secundam Editionem Gottingensem* [1st edn 1747]. Prostant Lovanii, Apud L. J. van Rossum, 1758.

Von Hofmann, E. Ueber Aneurysmen der Basilararterien und deren Ruptur als Ursache des plötzlichen Todes. *Wiener Medizinische Wochenschrift* 1894;**7**:823–6, 848–50, 867–8, 886–8.

Von Monakow, C. *Gehirnpathologie.* Wien, Alfred Hölder, 1897.

Von Staden, H. The discovery of the body: human dissection and its cultural contexts in ancient Greece. *Yale Journal of Biology and Medicine* 1992;**65**:223–41.

Von Weismayr, A. Ein Fall der Stenose der Carotis und Subclavia. *Wiener klinische Wochenschrift* 1894;**7**:906–8, 925–7.

Von Zenker, FA. Spontane Hirnhämorrhagien. In Winter, A, ed. *Tageblatt der 45. Versammlung Deutscher Naturforscher und Aerzte.* Leipzig, C. Wilfferodt, 1872, 159–60.

Vulpian, A. Note sur l'état des nerfs sensitifs, des ganglions spinaux et du grand sympathique dans les cas de sclerose des faisceaux postérieurs de la moelle épinière avec atrophie des racines postérieurs. *Archives de Physiologie Normale et Pathologique* 1868;**1**:128–56.

Waga, S, K Otsubo, and H Handa. Warning signs in intracranial aneurysms. *Surgical Neurology* 1975;**3**:15–20.

Waggoner, RW. Thrombosis of a superior cerebral vein: clinical and pathological study of a case. *Archives of Neurology and Psychiatry* 1928;**20**:580–4.

Walker, AE. Egas Moniz. In Haymaker, W and Schiller, F, eds. *The Founders of Neurology*. Springfield, IL, Charles C. Thomas, 1970, 489–92.

Walker, E. Ueber Verstopfung der Hirnarterien. Thesis Zürich, 1872.

Walsh, FB. *Clinical Neuro-ophthalmology*. Baltimore, MD, Williams & Wilkins Company, 1947.

Walter, PF, SD Reid, Jr, and NK Wenger. Transient cerebral ischemia due to arrhythmia. *Annals of Internal Medicine* 1970;**72**:471–4.

Walton, JN. *Subarachnoid Haemorrhage*. Edinburgh, E. & S. Livingstone Ltd, 1956a.

Walton, JN. Surgery of intracranial aneurysms. *British Medical Journal* 1956b;**1**:859–60.

Walusinski, O. Jean-Martin Charcot's house officers at La Salpêtrière Hospital. *Frontiers of Neurology and Neuroscience* 2011;**29**:9–35.

Walusinski, O. Jean-André Rochoux (1787–1852), a physician philosopher at the dawn of vascular neurology. *Revue neurologique* 2017a;**173**:532–41.

Walusinski, O. Jean-Martin Charcot (1825–1893): a treatment approach gone astray? *European Neurology* 2017b;**78**:296–306.

Ward, J. Case of hemiplegia, with softening of the brain. *London Medical Repository* 1824;**1**:46–7.

Wassermann, A, A Neisser, and C Bruck. Eine serodiagnostische Reaktion bei Syphilis. *Deutsche medizinische Wochenschrift* 1906;**32**:745–6.

Watkins, R. *The Miraculous Deliverance of Anne Greene*. Oxford, Leonard Lichfield and H. Hall, for Thomas Robinson, 1651.

Wear, A. Early modern Europe. In Conrad, LI, et al., eds. *The Western Medical Tradition 800 BC to AD 1800*. Cambridge, Cambridge University Press, 1995, 215–361.

Wear, A, RK French, and IM Lonie, eds. *The Medical Renaissance of the Sixteenth Century*. Cambridge, Cambridge University Press, 1985.

Webster, JE, S Dolgoff, and ES Gurdjian. Spontaneous thrombosis of the carotid arteries in the neck: report of four cases. *Archives of Neurology and Psychiatry* 1950;**63**:942–53.

Weisberg, LA. Benign intracranial hypertension. *Medicine (Baltimore)* 1975;**54**:197–207.

Weiss, A. Zur Pathogenese der Gehirnhämorrhagie. Thesis Erlangen, 1869.

Weiss, KE. Amaurosis fugax durch Krampf der Retinalgefässe. *Bericht über die Versammlung der opthalmologische Gesellschaft Heidelberg* 1912;**38**:205–13.

Welch, FJ. Aortic aneurism in the army, and the conditions associated with it. *The Lancet* 1875;**106**:769–71.

Wendeler, P. Zur Histologie der syphilitischen Erkrankung der Hirnarterien. *Deutsches Archiv für klinische Medicin* 1895;**55**:161–72.

Wepfer, JJ. *Observationes anatomicae ex Cadaveribus eorum, quos sustulit Apoplexia, cum Exercitatione de eius Loco affecto*. Schaffhusii, Caspar Suter, 1658.

Wepfer, JJ. *Observationes anatomicae, ex Cadaveribus eorum, quos sustulit Apoplexia, cum Exercitatione de eius Loco affecto; novae Editioni accessit Auctuarium Historiarum & Observationum similium, cum Scholiis*. Schaffhusii, Onophrii A Waldkirch, 1675.

Wepfer, JJ. *Historiae Apoplecticorum, Observationibus & Scholiis anatomicis & medicis quamplurimis elaboratae & illustratae*. Amstelaedami, Janssonius van Waesberge, 1724.

Wepfer, JJ. *Observationes medico-practicae de Affectibus Capitis internis & externis*. Scaphusii, Typis and Impensis Joh. Adami Ziegleri, 1727.

Westphal, K. Über die Entstehung des Schlaganfalles. II. Klinische Untersuchungen zum Problem der Entstehung des Schlaganfalles. *Deutsches Archiv für klinische Medicin* 1926a;**151**:31–95.

Westphal, K. Über die Entstehung des Schlaganfalles. III. Experimentelle Untersuchungen zum Apoplexieproblem. *Deutsches Archiv für klinische Medicin* 1926b;**151**:96–109.

Westphal, K. Über die Entstehung und Behandlung der Apoplexia sanguinea. *Deutsche Medizinische Wochenschrift* 1932;**58**:685–90.

Westphal, K. Über die Spontanblutungen des Gehirns. *Verhandlungen der Deutschen Pathologischen Gesellschaft* 1937;**29**:55–73.

Westphal, K and R Bär. Über die Entstehung des Schlaganfalles. I. Pathologisch-anatomische Untersuchungen zur Frage der Entstehung des Schlaganfalles. *Deutsches Archiv für klinische Medicin* 1926;**151**:1–30.

Whitaker, H, CUM Smith, and S Finger. Introduction. In Whitaker, H, et al., eds. *Brain, Mind and Medicine: Essays in Eighteenth-Century Neuroscience.* New York, NY, Springer, 2007, 3–4.

Wichern, H. Klinische Beiträge zur Kenntnis der Hirnaneurysmen. *Deutsche Zeitschrift für Nervenheilkunde* 1912;**44**:220–63.

Widal, F. Le diagnostic de l'hémorragie meningée. *Presse Médicale* 1903;**11**:413–15.

Wiener, LM, RG Berry, and J Kundin. Intracranial circulation in carotid occlusion. *Archives of Neurology* 1964;**11**:554–61.

Wiesendanger, M. Constantin von Monakow (1853–1930): a pioneer in interdisciplinary brain research and a humanist. *Comptes Rendus Biologies* 2006;**329**:406–18.

Wilks, S. Sanguineous meningeal effusion (apoplexy): spontaneous and from injury. *Guy's Hospital Reports* 1859;**III–5**:119–27.

Wilks, S. On the syphilitic affections of internal organs. *Guy's Hospital Reports* 1863;**III–9**:1–64.

Wilks, S. *Lectures on Diseases of the Nervous System, Delivered at Guy's Hospital.* London, J. & A. Churchill, 1878.

Williams, D and TG Wilson. The diagnosis of the major and minor syndromes of basilar insufficiency. *Brain* 1962;**85**:741–74.

Williams, DJ. Central vertigo. *Proceedings of the Royal Society of Medicine* 1967;**60**:961–4.

Willis, T. *Cerebri Anatome, cui accessit Nervorum Descriptio et Usus.* Londini, Typis Ja. Flesher, Impensis Jo. Martyn, and Ja. Allestry, 1664.

Willis, T. *De Anima Brutorum, quae Hominis vitalis ac sensitiva est, Exercitationes duae.* Londini, Ric. Davis, 1672.

Wilson, DH and WJ Gardner. Benign intracranial hypertension with particular reference to its occurrence in fat young women. *Canadian Medical Association Journal* 1966;**95**:102–5.

Wilson, PJ and IP Cast. 'Twin' intracranial aneurysms. *British Medical Journal* 1973;**1**:484.

Wilson, SAK and AN Bruce. *Neurology.* London, Edward Arnold & Co., 1940.

Wolfe, HRI. Unexplained thrombosis of the left internal carotid artery. *The Lancet* 1948;**252**:567–9.

Wolff, K. Grundlagen zu dem Problem der spontanen apoplektischen Hirnblutungen; Teil I. *Beiträge zur pathologischen Anatomie und zur allgemeinen Pathologie* 1932a;**89**:249–310.

Wolff, K. Grundlagen zu dem Problem der spontanen apoplektischen Hirnblutungen; Teil II. *Beiträge zur pathologischen Anatomie und zur algemeinen Pathologie* 1932b;**89**:487–512.

Wolff, K. Untersuchungen und Bemerkungen zur Lehre von der hypertonischen apoplektischen Hirnblutung. *Virchow's Archiv für pathologische Anatomie und Physiologie und für klinische Medizin* 1937;**299**:573–628.

Wright, JR and L McIntyre. Misread and mistaken: Étienne Lancereaux's enduring legacy in the classification of diabetes mellitus. *Journal of Medical Biography* 2022;**30**:15–20.

Wright, T. *Circulation: William Harvey's Revolutionary Idea.* London, Chatto and Windus, 2012.

Wüllenweber, G. Fortdauer des Lebens bei doppelseitigem vollständigen Verschluß der Aa. Carotides internae. *Deutsche Zeitschrift der Nervenkrankheiten* 1928;**105**:283–8.

Yasargil, MG and JL Fox. The microsurgical approach to intracranial aneurysms. *Surgical Neurology* 1975;**3**:7–14.

Yates, PO. Cerebral pathology following carotid spasm. *Proceedings of the Royal Society of Medicine* 1954;**47**:606–7; discussion, 607–8.

Yates, PO and EC Hutchinson. *Cerebral Infarction: The Role of Stenosis of the Extracranial Cerebral Arteries.* London, Her Majesty's Stationary Office, 1961.

Yelloly, J. Case of preternatural growth in the lining membrane covering the trunks of the vessels proceeding from the arch of the aorta. *Medico-Chirurgical Transactions* 1823;**12**:565–9.

Zago, S and MV Meraviglia. Costanzo Varolio (1543–1575). *Journal of Neurology* 2009;**256**:1195–6.

Zanchetti, A and G Mancia. The centenary of blood pressure measurement: a tribute to Scipione Riva-Rocci. *Journal of Hypertension* 1996;**14**:1–12.

Zarranz, JJ. Bourneville: a neurologist in action. *Neurosciences and History* 2015;**3**:107–15.

Zeidman, LA, MG Ziller, and M Shevell. Ilya Mark Scheinker: controversial neuroscientist and refugee from National Socialist Europe. *Canadian Journal of Neurological Sciences* 2016;**43**:334–44.

Zentmayer, W, J Rowan, and AK. William Campbell Posey (1866-1934). *Archives of Ophthalmology* 1934;**12**:931–8.

Ziegler, DK and RS Hassanein. Prognosis in patients with transient ischemic attacks. *Stroke* 1973;**4**:666–73.

Zulian, F. *Ueber den Schlagfluss, vorzüglich der Nerven (in freien Uebersetzung von Wilhelm Friederich Domeier)*. Hannover, Helwigschen Hofbuchhandlung, 1791.

Zulianius, F. *De Apoplexia, praesertim nervea, Commentarius*. Brixiae, Fratres Pasini, 1789.

Zylberszac, S. Gottlieb Gluge. Biographie Nationale de l'Académie Royale des Sciences, des Lettres et des Beaux Arts de Belgique. www.academieroyale.be/academie/documents/FichierPDFBiographieNationaleTome2098.pdf#page=182. [Accessed 1 May 2022]

INDEX

Printed in the United States
by Baker & Taylor Publisher Services